Critical Approaches to Car

What does 'care' mean in contemporary society? How are caring relationships practised in different contexts? What resources do individuals and collectives draw upon in order to care for, care with and care about themselves and others? How do such relationships and practices relate to broader social processes?

Care shapes people's everyday lives and relationships, and caring relations and practices influence the economies of different societies. This interdisciplinary book takes a nuanced and context-sensitive approach to exploring caring relationships, identities and practices within and across a variety of cultural, familial, geographical and institutional arenas. Grounded in rich empirical research and discussing key theoretical, policy and practice debates, it provides important, yet often neglected, international and cross-cultural perspectives. It is divided into four parts covering: caring within educational institutions; caring amongst communities and networks; caring for and about families; and caring across the life course.

Contributing to broader theoretical, philosophical and moral debates associated with the ethics of care, citizenship, justice, relationality and entanglements of power, *Critical Approaches to Care* is an important work for students and academics studying caring and care work in the fields of health and social care, sociology, social policy, anthropology, education, human geography and politics.

Chrissie Rogers is a Reader in Education and Director of the Childhood and Youth Research Institute at Anglia Ruskin University, UK.

Susie Weller is a Senior Research Fellow in the Families & Social Capital Research Group at London South Bank University, UK.

Relationships & resources
Series Editors: Janet Holland and Rosalind Edwards

A key contemporary political and intellectual issue is the link between the relationships that people have and the resources to which they have access. When people share a sense of identity, hold similar values, trust each other and reciprocally do things for each other, this has an impact on the social, political and economic cohesion of the society in which they live. So, are changes in contemporary society leading to deterioration in the link between relationships and resources, or new and innovative forms of linking, or merely the reproduction of enduring inequalities? Consideration of relationships and resources raises key theoretical and empirical issues around change and continuity over time as well as time use, the consequences of globalisation and individualisation for intimate and broader social relations, and location and space in terms of communities and neighbourhoods. The books in this series are concerned with elaborating these issues and will form a body of work that will contribute to academic and political debate.

Available titles include:

Marginalised Mothers: Exploring Working-Class Experiences of Parenting
Val Gillies

Sibling Identity and Relationships: Sisters and Brothers
Rosalind Edwards, Lucy Hadfield, Helen Lucey and Melanie Mauthner

Teenagers' Citizenship: Experiences and Education
Susie Weller

Researching Families and Communities: Social and Generational Change
Edited by Rosalind Edwards

Interdependency and Care over the Lifecourse
Sophia Bowlby, Linda McKie, Susan Gregory and Isobel MacPherson

Transnational Families: Ethnicities, Identities and Social Capital
Harry Goulbourne, Tracey Reynolds, John Solomos and Elisabetta Zontini

International Perspectives on Racial and Ethnic Mixedness and Mixing
Edited by Rosalind Edwards, Suki Ali, Chamion Caballero and Miri Song

Critical Approaches to Care: Understanding Caring Relations, Identities and Cultures
Edited by Chrissie Rogers and Susie Weller

Forthcoming titles include:

Moving On: The Changing Lives of Young People after Parental Divorce
Bren Neale and Jennifer Flowerdew

Critical Approaches to Care

Understanding caring relations,
identities and cultures

Edited by
Chrissie Rogers and Susie Weller

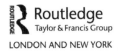
Routledge
Taylor & Francis Group

LONDON AND NEW YORK

First published 2013
by Routledge
2 Park Square, Milton Park, Abingdon, Oxon, OX14 4RN

Simultaneously published in the USA and Canada
by Routledge
711 Third Avenue, New York, NY 10017

Routledge is an imprint of the Taylor & Francis Group, an informa
business

First issued in paperback 2014

British Library Cataloguing in Publication Data
A catalogue record for this book is available from the British Library

Library of Congress Cataloging in Publication Data
Critical approaches to care : understanding caring relations, identities and
cultures / edited by Chrissie Rogers and Susie Weller.
p. cm. -- (Relationships & resources)
1. Caregivers. 2. Interpersonal relations. 3. Helping behavior. 4.
Responsibility. 5. Families. 6. Women--Family relationships. 7. Social
networks. 8. Social service. I. Rogers, Chrissie. II. Weller, Susie.
HM1146.C75 2012
362′.0425--dc23
2011052349

ISBN: 978-0-415-61329-3 (hbk)
ISBN: 978-1-138-78178-8 (pbk)

Typeset in Times
by Saxon Graphics Ltd, Derby

Contents

Notes on contributors   *viii*
Endorsements   *xii*

1   **Understanding care and thinking with care**   1
    GEORGIA PHILIP, CHRISSIE ROGERS AND SUSIE WELLER

PART I
Caring within educational institutions   13

Part I Summary: caring within educational institutions   15
PAULETTE LUFF, UTHEL LAURENT, VAL GILLIES,
YVONNE ROBINSON AND MABELLE VICTORIA

2   **Reclaiming care in early childhood education and care**   18
    PAULETTE LUFF

3   **Revisiting care in schools: exploring the caring experiences
    of disengaged young people**   30
    UTHEL LAURENT

4   **At risk pupils and the 'caring' curriculum**   42
    VAL GILLIES AND YVONNE ROBINSON

5   **A discourse analytic study of power as caring relations in
    Philippine university classrooms**   54
    MABELLE VICTORIA

PART II
Caring amongst communities and networks   67

Part II Summary: caring amongst communities and networks   69
MAXINE BIRCH, NINA NISSEN, TRACEY REYNOLDS, ANDREA DOUCET,
NATASHA MAUTHNER AND LINDA BELL

6 **A different way of caring? An exploration of alternative
   health care relationships**   72
   MAXINE BIRCH AND NINA NISSEN

7 **'Men's business'? Black men's caring within black-led
   community organisations**   82
   TRACEY REYNOLDS

8 **Tea and Tupperware: mommy blogging as care, work,
   and consumption**   92
   ANDREA DOUCET AND NATASHA MAUTHNER

9 **Researching 'care', family and neighbourhood in Tehran, Iran**   105
   LINDA BELL

PART III
Caring for and about families   117

Part III Summary: caring for and about families   119
LINDA NUTT, CHRISSIE ROGERS AND GEORGIA PHILIP

10 **Foster care in ambiguous contexts: competing understandings
    of care**   122
    LINDA NUTT

11 **Intellectual disability and mothering: an engagement with
    ethics of care and emotional work**   132
    CHRISSIE ROGERS

12 **Working at post-divorce family life: the feminist ethics of care as
    a framework for exploring fathering after divorce or separation**   144
    GEORGIA PHILIP

PART IV
Caring across the life course   155

Part IV Summary: caring across the life course   157
SUSIE WELLER, ELISABETTA ZONTINI AND JANE RIBBENS McCARTHY

13 **Who cares? Exploring the shifting nature of care and caring**
    practices in sibling relationships   160
    SUSIE WELLER

14 **Care arrangements of transnational migrant elders:**
    between family, community and the state   171
    ELISABETTA ZONTINI

15 **Caring after death: issues of embodiment and relationality**   183
    JANE RIBBENS McCARTHY

    References   *195*
    Index   *221*

Contributors

Linda Bell is Principal Lecturer in the School of Health and Social Sciences, Middlesex University. She is an anthropologist whose publications relate to mothering and aspects of health and social care, and is a long-standing member of the *Women's workshop*. Her PhD, entitled 'My child, your child; mothering in a Hertfordshire town in the 1980s' was completed in 1994. She teaches research methods and works extensively with research students. Recent research focuses around professional identity, including gender issues, parenting, and ethics. She has also researched inter-professionalism and social work education, care worker training and women's experiences of a therapy centre concerned with male violence, when based at King's College, London. She is co-reviews editor for the *International Journal of Social Research Methodology*.

Maxine Birch is a Senior Lecturer in the Faculty of Health and Social Welfare at the Open University. Maxine's teaching and research interests centre on experiences of health and well-being, qualitative research methods, especially ethnography and narrative studies. Maxine's interest in ethics and feminist research developed in the first edition of *Ethics and Qualitative Research* (2002, co-edited with Melanie Mauthner, Julie Jessop and Tina Miller).

Andrea Doucet is the Canada Research Chair in Gender, Work and Care and Professor of Sociology and Gender Studies at Brock University. Her research and writing focuses on gender and care work, mothering and fathering, parental leave policies, embodiment, reflexive sociology, and knowledge construction processes. Her book *Do Men Mother?* (2006) was awarded the John Porter Tradition of Excellence Book Award from the Canadian Sociology Association. She is currently working on two book projects, one on breadwinning mothers and caregiving fathers and a co-authored book, *Narrative Analysis: The Listening Guide Approach* (with Natasha Mauthner). She is editor of the international journal *Fathering*.

Val Gillies is a Professor of Social Research and a co-director of the Families and Social Capital Research Group at London South Bank University. She has researched and published in the area of family, social class and marginalised children and young people, producing a wide range of journal articles and book chapters on parenting, young people at risk of school exclusion, home–school relations as well as qualitative research methods. Her book: *Marginalised Mothers: Exploring Working Class Parenting* (Routledge) was published in 2007.

Uthel Laurent began her teaching career in 1990, where she taught various subjects across the age and ability level at different secondary schools and lectured at a Further Education College in the Caribbean. She came to Britain in 2004 to complete a PGCE in Social Science at Keele University. She then taught for two years at a secondary school in the Midlands, UK, before accepting a 1 + 3 funded studentship to pursue studies leading to a PhD (Education) at the Open University in 2007. Her wider research interests include: Disengagement across settings, times and cultures; Youth Studies and Caribbean Pedagogies.

Paulette Luff (MA, PhD) is a Senior Lecturer in Early Childhood Studies at Anglia Ruskin University, where she has worked since 2003. Her main teaching, writing and research interest is in early years pedagogy, with a current focus on ways of documenting young children's learning as a means of supporting thoughtful, responsive care and education. Her doctoral research explored early years practitioners' uses of child observation. Paulette has enjoyed working in the field of early childhood for nearly thirty years, as a teacher, foster carer, school–home liaison worker and as a lecturer in Further and Higher Education.

Natasha Mauthner is a Reader at the University of Aberdeen Business School. Her research interests lie in the areas of health and well-being; gender, work and family; and knowledge-making in the academy (including interpretive, collaborative, and data sharing practices). Her current research on the digital data sharing movement is funded by a grant from the Society for Research into Higher Education. She is author of *The Darkest Days of my Life* (2002), and is writing a book with Andrea Doucet on *Narrative Analysis: The Listening Guide Approach*.

Nina Nissen is an anthropologist currently based at the University of Southern Denmark, where she is researching EU citizens' attitudes and needs concerning complementary and alternative medicine. For her PhD she examined the multiple change processes associated with women's contemporary practice and use of western herbal medicine, an alternative health modality she also practised and taught for more than 20 years in the UK and the Caribbean. Her research interests include feminist practice and scholarship, health social movements, and the interplay between healthcare practices, gender, and personal and social change processes.

Linda Nutt is an independent researcher. Her doctorate was a qualitative research project on the perspectives of foster carers. Whilst there had been considerable research on the fostered children there has been little on the carers. Her book *The Lives of Foster Carers: Private Sacrifices, Public Restrictions* (2006) therefore makes an original contribution to the theorising of foster care. She is currently totally absorbed in reading French history together with some of its literature (very slowly in the original), learning the language and assimilating the mores and customs of its society.

Georgia Philip completed her MA in Sociology at the University of Essex in 2000. She has spent many years lecturing in Sociology at West Suffolk College; a regional satellite of University Campus Suffolk. During this time she completed a PGCE and began her PhD part-time with the Open University. In 2006 she was awarded funding to complete her PhD and was awarded her doctorate in July 2010. Since November 2011 Georgia has been an Economic and Social Research Council (ESRC) funded postdoctoral fellow at the University of East Anglia, developing her work on fathers with Professor Margaret O'Brien. Her research interests include post-divorce parenting, fathers, gender, care and feminist moral philosophy.

Tracey Reynolds is a Reader in the Families and Social Capital ESRC Research Group, which is situated within the Weeks Centre for Social and Policy Research at London South Bank University. Tracey's research interests focus on transnational families and kinship networks; constructions of motherhood, parenting and childrearing. She has conducted extensive empirical research in the UK across a range of social issues including black and minority families living in disadvantaged communities. She has also extended her research interests to include developments in the Caribbean and North America. Her current research examines Caribbean youths and transnational identities and, more recently, care planning among black, Asian and minority ethnic (BAME) older people in London (with Age Concern Lewisham and Southwark, funded by the Big Lottery). Previous publications include 'Exploring the absent/present dilemma: Black fathers, family relationships and social capital in Britain', *Annals of the American Academy of Political and Social Science* (2009). She is also the author of *Caribbean Mothers: Identity and Experience in the UK* (2005); *Transnational Families: Ethnicities, Identities and Social Capital,* with Harry Goulbourne, John Solomos and Elisabetta Zontini (Routledge, 2010) and editor of the Special Issue 'Young People, Ethnicity and Social Capital' in the *Journal of Ethnic and Racial Studies* (May 2010).

Jane Ribbens McCarthy is Reader in Family Studies at the Open University. She has researched and published widely in the areas of family relationships, and relationships at the end of life. Recent and forthcoming publications include: *Family Troubles: Exploring Changes and Challenges in the Family Lives of Children and Young People* (2012, edited with Carol-Ann Hooper and Val Gillies); *Understanding Family Meanings* (2012, with Megan Doolittle and Shelley Day Sclater), *Key Concepts in Family Studies* (2010, with Rosalind Edwards), and *Young People's Experiences of Loss and Bereavement: Towards an Interdisciplinary Approach* (2006).

Yvonne Robinson is a Senior Research Fellow in the Families and Social Capital Research Group at London South Bank University. Her background is in Human Geography and her research interests include children and young people, education, race, ethnicity and the arts. Yvonne has successfully undertaken research and evaluation for the ESRC and a number of UK government departments, producing articles and reports on excluded and vulnerable groups as well as arts based research methodologies as a means to understanding marginalised group experiences. Yvonne is currently working on an ESRC follow-on study with students marginalised from education.

Chrissie Rogers is a Reader in Education and Director of the Childhood and Youth Research Institute at Anglia Ruskin University, UK. Her main interests are related to intellectual disability, 'inclusive' education, mothering and intimacy. Chrissie began her research journey due to her own mothering experiences with an intellectually disabled daughter. She completed her Sociology PhD (ESRC) at the University of Essex, UK, and her postdoctoral fellowship (ESRC) at Cambridge University, UK. She has held lectureships at Keele University and Brunel University and is author of *Parenting and Inclusive Education* and various journal articles. Chrissie also has a forthcoming book *Intellectual Disability and Social Theory: Philosophical and Sociological Debates on Being Human* with Routledge.

Mabelle Victoria is a PhD student at the Open University. She has an MRes in Education from the same university and an MA in TEFL from the University of Birmingham. Her projects have been shaped by her fascination with language, culture and communication. Her current research focuses on exploring how individuals from different cultural and linguistic backgrounds use English as a common language to build social relations, negotiate meaning, and construct identities. She is interested in applying insights from linguistic ethnography, discourse analysis and pragmatics to the analysis of spoken interaction.

Susie Weller is a Senior Research Fellow in the Families and Social Capital Research Group at London South Bank University. Her background is in Human Geography and she is particularly interested in citizenship and participation, friendships and social networks, family relationships and the development of youth-centred research methods. She has published widely on these subjects, notably *Teenagers' Citizenship: Experiences and Education* (2007, Routledge). Since 2000 she has been working on a number of projects that hold central the voices and experiences of children and teenagers. Most recently she has been researching the changing nature of young people's sibling relationships and friendships as part of the ESRC Timescapes programme, the first major qualitative longitudinal study to be funded in the UK.

Elisabetta Zontini is a Lecturer in Sociology in the School of Sociology and Social Policy at the University of Nottingham. Previously, she was a Visiting Fellow at the International Gender Studies Centre at Oxford University and Research Fellow in the Families and Social Capital ESRC Research Group at London South Bank University. She has published extensively in the areas of gender and migration and transnational families. She is the author of *Transnational Families, Migration and Gender: Moroccan and Filipino Women in Bologna and Barcelona* (2010) and of *Transnational Families: Ethnicities, Identities and Social Capital* (with Harry Goulbourne, Tracey Reynolds and John Solomos) (2010, Routledge).

Endorsements

'*Critical Approaches to Care* is a rich and engaging work, both theoretically and empirically. Its richness is enhanced through its cross-disciplinary and cross-cultural focus. Through a series of case studies, it explores the moral dilemmas, power relations, ethical considerations, and even unwelcome demands of care from a range of perspectives and across different political contexts. It is a feminist-inspired work that is both inclusionary and respectful of diversity. It examines the many equality and gender justice dilemmas posed by care work, be it through caring for intellectually disabled children, fostering, transnational caring, fathering or mothering. At a theoretical level, it addresses the tensions between an ethics of care and an ethic of justice. The book challenges us to consider how an ethic of care can reinvent understanding of what is socially just in a deeply uncaring and unequal world. It should be read not only by academics and students but by all of those with a public policy remit.'
Kathleen Lynch, Professor of Equality Studies in the School of Social Justice, UCD, Ireland.

'Care is both deeply unfashionable in contemporary social policy, and an enduring focus for understanding everyday lives and social practices. This collection is a major contribution to the re-emergence of applied research and scholarship recognizing the centrality of care in diverse personal and professional relationships, and as a political value.'
Marian Barnes, Professor of Social Policy, University of Brighton.

1 Understanding care and thinking with care

Georgia Philip, Chrissie Rogers and Susie Weller

Care in context

> People do not spring up from the soil like mushrooms. People produce people. People need to be cared for and nurtured throughout their lives by other people, at some times more urgently and more completely than at other times.
>
> (Kittay 2005: 1)

What does 'care' mean in contemporary society? How are caring relationships practised in different contexts? How do conceptions and experiences of care continue to both inform and become shaped by wider societal, political and theoretical ideas and institutions? What resources do individuals and collectives draw upon in order to care *for*, care *with* and care *about* themselves and others?

Addressing such questions, this book takes a nuanced and context-sensitive approach to exploring caring relationships, identities and practices *within* and *across* a variety of cultural, familial, geographical and institutional arenas. It aims to explore care as both an analytical and theoretical resource, and to continue the debate over the value of expanding and deepening understandings of care in order to inform and reform policy contexts and political thinking (Bowlby *et al.* 2010; Lynch *et al.* 2009; Nussbaum 2006; Robinson 2011). Globally, care is high on current policy agendas, but only in a service or professionalised context or in response to demographic changes, such as an ageing population. Even then this is not sufficient. Care as an ethical position, applicable to much broader and deeper questions of how lives might be lived in contemporary societies, remains absent from the political agenda. Critically there ought to be good public arrangements for all care-givers, as it is they who often are poorly paid, marginalised and socially restricted.

This collection represents attempts to develop thinking about and with 'care' in this more moral philosophical direction; to apply, test or explore the concepts of care and caring in a range of research settings, and to offer suggestions about the potential of 'care' for responding to pertinent current issues such as social justice, exclusion and connection. Ultimately being deprived of care or being unable to develop a supportive caring environment is 'a serious human deprivation for most people' (Lynch *et al.* 2009: 1).

Key contributions and concerns

The principal aim of this volume is to energise and contribute to key theoretical, policy and practice debates concerning *'who cares, how, why and when?'* Through a critical and reflexive approach, the book examines theoretical constructions of care and caring relations, providing empirically embedded ways of thinking about and understanding care in contemporary society. In different ways, many of the chapters engage imaginatively and critically with the feminist ethics of care in particular, as an important source of moral philosophical thinking about 'care'. Some of the chapters adopt care perspectives to provide new substantive insights, whilst others use the focus of their research to challenge and reframe conceptualisations of care. Various chapters present alternative perspectives regarding flows of care and power within families and communities, whilst some challenge assumptions about the contexts in which caring practices take place, thus advancing discussions surrounding care beyond private and/or commercial domains.

In addition to the particular contributions of each chapter, the book also aims to highlight a number of common concerns and propose some broader arguments arising from the collection as a whole. First, the book draws attention to the importance of defining and understanding care and caring, arguing for the cross-cultural significance, if not universality, of human vulnerability, interdependence and the need for care, as ongoing, not just at the beginning and end of life. Equally, the book highlights the importance of cultural context and cultural differences, in relation to both conceptions of care and to lived caring relationships and practices. This recognition of both the more generalised and the particular aspects of care are important for its development as a broader ethical resource or position. In theoretical terms, the argument is also that care can do important conceptual work and contribute not only to theories of relationality or moral reasoning on a personal level, but also to theories of citizenship, justice and equality (Lynch *et al.* 2009; Nussbaum 2006; Sayer 2011).

Third, at the level of specific societal analysis, this book highlights a number of constraints and tensions which are revealed through studying how care is operationalised in particular institutions. This examination of how policy ideals, organisational objectives, political rhetoric and professional practice intersect when care is institutionalised or commodified is highly relevant, and offers suggestions and directions beyond the particular settings illustrated here. Similarly, whilst each of the chapters points to policy implications in relation to their specific topics, including for example inclusion in education, holistic health care, foster carers and parenting after divorce or separation, there is also an overarching position taken by the book as a whole. This is to highlight and advocate the significance and potential of care to policy debates at the broadest level; around social justice, exclusion, social cohesion, ethical or sustainable living (including production and consumption) and well-being.

A further common concern across this book is with the ongoing significance of gender in relation to the experience, social organisation and political understanding of care. All the authors represented here share a critical interest in feminist theoretical and methodological perspectives, expressed in this book through the exploration of care. Continuing the trajectory of feminist work, this collection makes the general arguments that all human societies require the provision of love and care, that interdependency is the 'condition' of human beings, and that love and care cannot be understood without recognition of the 'gendered order of caring' (Lynch *et al.* 2009: 219). In this way, the chapters in this book also highlight the need to expand understandings and recognition of care beyond the 'private', 'domestic' or personal arenas and insist on the 'salience of care and love as goods of public significance' (Lynch *et al.* 2009: 2). One final articulation of this common interest in feminist approaches to ethics and to care is through the methodological insights offered by a number of the chapters. Another important contribution made by this book is the exploration and application of feminist ethics to the process of research. There are reflexive discussions of caring relations, practices and dilemmas within research relationships that readers with a particular interest in qualitative or feminist research will find useful. The book therefore encourages questions of how to think and write about care, with care, and how to be attentive and responsive to research participants; to be competent and responsible as a researcher (Tronto and Fisher 1990).

As outlined above, this book includes important, and yet often neglected, international and cross-cultural perspectives. Research within the book has been undertaken in Canada, Iran, the Philippines and the UK. The chapters cover a wide range of multicultural settings, thereby encompassing the perspectives and experiences of those from different cultural, ethnic and racial backgrounds. For example, chapters include work on: Filipino students (Chapter 5), family and neighbourhoods in Tehran, Iran (Chapter 9), sibling relationships of young people from different backgrounds (Chapter 13) and an analysis of care amongst transnational families (Chapter 14). Grounded in rich empirical work and illustrated with in-depth examples, the book presents the perspectives of a wide range of people including but not limited to: children, parents and grandparents; students and teachers; healthcare professionals and patients; consumers; and communities.

In doing so, we aim to contribute to the growth of interest in care and the way that people care *for, with* and *about* others. This is of importance not only because care shapes people's everyday lives and relationships, but also because caring relations and practices influence the economies and welfare systems of different societies. The collection also considers ways in which feminist conceptions of care can challenge persisting assumptions about human relationships, decision making and the allocation of resources; including time, emotions, love and labour, in personal, social and institutional contexts. This is important in order to avoid limiting care as either a taken-for-granted idea or as a professionalised term to describe a commercial service. All the explorations of care, caring practices and relationships offered here, in different ways, use care as a lens to reveal insights about practical, moral, emotional and ethical aspects of human relationships and to consider the centrality and complexity of our vital connections with others. Alongside other contemporary authors in this field, we aim to argue that, '[T]he notion of care is a valuable political concept and that how we think about care is deeply implicated in existing structures of power and inequality' (Robinson 2011: 3).

Thinking about and with care

Whilst each of the chapters engages extensively with literature covering many aspects of care, the book contributes particularly to debates surrounding a feminist ethics of care. Chapters either explicitly use work by key authors in this field to frame their empirical research, or nod towards them whilst using subject-specific authors who directly engage with different critical literature and research. Given this focus we would like to map out the feminist ethics of care in more detail.

Feminist ethics of care

The body of literature that defines and defends a feminist ethics of care contributes important critiques of established ways of thinking about ethics, morality, citizenship and care. It also provides alternatives to them; operating at an epistemological and theoretical level but also at the level of practical application (Sevenhuijsen 2003). Spanning the last thirty years, this literature can loosely be divided into two waves, with Gilligan and Noddings as central figures in the early 1980s, and Tronto and Sevenhuijsen forming the core of a second wave from the early 1990s onwards (Williams 2004). In Northern Europe and the UK particularly, there has been a consistent empirical, sociological and feminist engagement with care and caring, with writers such as Ve (1989), Waerness (1989), Graham (1983) and Finch and Mason (1993) being important early examples. This engagement has continued to develop across a number of disciplines, including Sociology, Geography, Psychosocial Studies and Social Policy and there has been particular interest from those studying family lives and relationships (Duncan and Edwards 1999; Smart and Neale 1999; Thomson and Holland 2002; Ribbens McCarthy *et al.* 2003; Doucet 2006a). Here a focus has been on revealing the moral and ethical aspects of family lives and extending the range of contexts in which caring relations and responsibilities are seen to exist and be struggled with. More recently still, the debate on care has been reinvigorated by those such as Barnes (2006), Bowlby *et al.* (2010), Lynch *et al.* (2009) and Robinson (2011) who argue the relevance of care for political and policy responses to social and economic inequalities and opportunities.

Originally, many of the key thinkers, including Noddings (2003), Ruddick (1995) and Tronto (1987, 1993) included accounts of the particular relationship between women and the ethic of care. This often involved a consideration of the mother–child relationship as a specific and significant example of where ethics and everyday life are intertwined. Whilst the embodied aspects of motherhood are fully recognised, it is the gendering of the social roles of women, and indeed of morality, that is emphasised, producing accounts of moral reasoning which are grounded in, but not limited to, women's experiences of care. From this care is understood and presented as a practice and as a way of thinking. The development of a feminist ethics of care then, sought to define care in more grounded terms, but also at a philosophical level it has aimed to reposition and argue the value of care as a basis for moral and political theory and also for social policy.

Noddings (2003) is significant in the conceptualisation of care and caring as a starting point for an alternative moral theory, and offers a detailed definition of care as a central, crucial and *human* practice. She presents care, as do others (for example Ruddick 1995), as a practice and therefore as learnt and, importantly, as improvable, but also argues that experiences of being cared for are definitively human, or 'universally accessible' (Noddings 2003: 5). This point illustrates a significant theme in feminist ethics, which is to highlight the commonality of human vulnerability, not just at the beginning and end of life, but as a constant and fundamental condition. This conception forms the basis for the recognition and valuing of care and caring relations, and provides an important platform for the concepts of interdependence and a relational self (Ruddick 1995; Tronto 1993; Sevenhuijsen 1998).

Noddings presents a central relation between the 'one-caring' and the 'cared-for'; arguing that while this relationship involves both parties, it is neither symmetrical nor equal. Understanding the relationship between those caring and those cared-for is seen to have important implications for developing a feminist moral theory which does not relegate or romanticise women's experiences of care, and which does not reduce caring to a selfless or self-sacrificial act. Related to this, Noddings distinguishes between 'natural caring', which she sees as spontaneous and most evident within the mother–child relationship, and caring as an 'ethical ideal', which refers to the process by which we struggle to reason, act and relate to others in an ethical way. Noddings also makes a distinction between 'caring for', which she sees as involving caring activities and responsibilities experienced directly, and 'caring about', which involves a more indirect concern and potential for caring activity with those at greater distance.

Tronto and Fisher (1990: 40), also key authors in this field, offer a slightly different, broader definition of caring:

> A species activity that includes everything that we do to maintain, continue and repair our 'world', so that we can live in it as well as possible. That world includes our bodies, ourselves, and our environment, all of which we seek to interweave in a complex, life-sustaining web.

Tronto and Fisher (1990) set out what they describe as four aspects of care: caring about, taking care of, care-giving and care-receiving. Alongside these are corresponding ethical values: attentiveness, responsibility, competence and responsiveness, each of which also acts as evaluative criteria, producing both the possibility to consider good enough caring, and to define moral or ethical failings such as 'inattentiveness' or 'privileged irresponsibility' (Tronto 2004). Tronto, and Tronto and Fisher, also define these ethical values from the premise of a connected, relational and socially situated self, and of care as a practice, with both cognitive and affective elements, rather than by constructing or drawing on notions of abstract and formal moral principles. This concern with developing a moral theory grounded in context and practice, and emphasising the process of moral deliberation and decision making, rather than detached conformity to absolute moral rules, is, again, a central preoccupation of writers in this field. A number of recurring debates have emerged from the process of seeking to reposition and enrich understandings of care. Three of these – the value of care for moral and political theory, the relationship between care and gender, and between justice and care – are directly relevant to this book and will now be briefly outlined.

An ongoing central argument from feminist moral philosophy has been for the potential and value of care for moral and political theory. Sevenhuijsen (1998: 6) is a highly significant figure here, and shares with Tronto an interest in 'a search for an appropriate vocabulary for making care into a political issue from a feminist perspective'. The focus of Sevenhuijsen's work, more specifically, has been to explore and argue the value of care in relation to citizenship; again seeking to critique traditional models of both the citizen and the nature of citizenship. For her, ethics and morality are intimately linked to citizenship as: 'judging is a principle task of citizenship and thus of collective action in a democratic context' (1998: 15). Sevenhuijsen also asserts the way in which a feminist ethics of care can offer not only new ways of thinking about citizenship as an aspect of ethical life, but also about morality itself and the process of 'judging'. Sevenhuijsen continued to develop this relationship between an ethic of care and a political theory of citizenship in her later work, and, like Tronto (2004), valued care as a political concept, arguing for it to be fully transferred to the public sphere.

The second key area of debate is that of the relationship between care and gender. Whilst Gilligan (1982) claimed not to be presenting an essentialist account of the 'different voice', she remains a focal point for the question of whether the different voice is definitively female. The development of a feminist ethics of care has provided opportunities for fruitful discussions of gender difference and, alongside this, a critical consideration of the risks and implications of attempting to theorise difference in feminist terms. Significant contributions here come from Ruddick (1995) and Tronto (1993) who explicitly state that they use women's caring experiences as mothers in order both to make visible their deeply ethical, deliberative and relational qualities and to demonstrate the value of such experiences as a model for ethical reasoning in other contexts. Alongside the re-valuing of women's experiences of caring, there is also the aim of critiquing the gendered, unequal distribution of caring labour and seeking to establish care as a central social and political issue. In this way, then, the literature on a feminist ethics of care provides another example of a much wider and long-standing feminist concern with pursuing equality without equating this with sameness (Sevenhuijsen 2000: 28).

The third area of debate relevant to the contributions in this collection, concerns the relationship between care and justice. Since Gilligan's initial proposal of an *alternative* ethic of care, these two core ideas, of care and justice, have been contrasted:

> An ethic of justice focuses on questions of fairness, equality, individual rights, abstract principles, and the consistent application of them. An ethic of

care focuses on attentiveness, trust, responsiveness to need, narrative nuance and cultivating caring relations.

(Held 2006: 3–4)

Much attention has been paid to questions over the nature and extent of differences between justice and care, and the implications of such differences in terms of the epistemological, cultural and practical value of each. If justice and care are seen as oppositional, then the ethic of care must either be convincingly presented as a preferable or superior alternative, or risk being relegated as secondary.

For writers such as Tronto, this risk is associated particularly with what she sees as 'feminine' accounts of an ethics of care: 'As long as women's morality is viewed as different and more particular than mainstream moral thought, it inevitably will be treated as a secondary form of moral thinking' (Tronto 1987, in Larrabee 1993: 246). If an ethic of care is seen as a replacement for an ethic of justice, then this could be detrimental to the pursuit of equality; a conception and language of 'rights' has long been a resource for those challenging prejudice and discrimination. An alternative strategy is to see justice and care as, in some ways, and to some extent, compatible or integrated, and that both may be necessary for a systematic theory of morality and ethics. However, there are a number of significant issues involved in attempting to reconcile or combine care and justice such as the conception and evaluation of needs.

Part of exploring the extent to which care and justice perspectives may share common concerns or contain elements of one another, has been to consider the kinds of moral questions they ask, or the moral problems they raise. One such question, as identified by Tronto (1993) is how best to understand human 'needs' and how competing needs may be evaluated and met. She offers a critical consideration of the conception of need, to argue that a care perspective may offer a more appropriate means of understanding, and judging between, complex human needs. For example, she argues that a traditional model of justice among rights-bearing individuals tends to reduce or alienate those deemed 'needy', presenting a skewed and inaccurate picture of the characteristics of both people and needs themselves. Because the ethic of care foregrounds human vulnerability and the need for care, where care is seen as relating to material, emotional and psychological well-being, Tronto (1993) argues that it not only incorporates justice questions, but is equally, if not better, placed to respond to them. This concern with asserting the relevance of care to issues of justice and equality is one that has continued in feminist care ethics, political philosophy and sociology over the past two decades. It has been articulated in terms of 'affective inequality' (Lynch *et al.* 2009), 'interdependency and caringscapes' (Bowlby *et al.* 2010), 'species membership' (Nussbaum 2006) and most recently 'human survival and security' (Robinson 2011).

About the book

This book brings together authors from a broad range of disciplines, theoretical perspectives and at different stages in their careers. Intended to highlight the complexity of care giving/receiving over time and in different spaces, it is divided into four themed parts: caring – 'within educational institutions', 'amongst communities and networks', 'for and about families' and 'across the life course', and each part seeks to explore *'who cares, how, why and when'*. In doing so, the parts examine the ways in which care and caring practices are conceived, articulated and manifest in different contexts. In line with our collective approach each themed part has a summary, written by the collective in that part, that synthesises key themes emerging from the chapters with the aim of providing a critical edge to contemporary conceptual, as well as policy-oriented, debates on care.

In more detail then, the first part focuses on 'caring within educational institutions'. Drawing on examples from the Philippines and the UK, the four chapters relocate discourses on care from dominant discussions surrounding the home to educational institutions thereby considering the, often neglected, caring practices and relations amongst students, and between students and teachers. The chapters examine formal and informal dimensions of 'care' from the standpoint of both teachers and students with respect to: the place of care in early childhood education and care (Chapter 2 by Paulette Luff); how adolescent students think about and experience 'care' in their lives at the intersection of home and school (Chapter 3 by Uthel Laurent); how individualised notions of care problematically infuse school curriculums and shape student–teacher relationships (Chapter 4 by Val Gillies and Yvonne Robinson); and how university professors show care in lessons (Chapter 5 by Mabelle Victoria).

The second part then considers 'caring amongst communities and networks' and turns to care in a range of different 'community-based' contexts within the UK, Canada and Iran. Recognising the complexity of 'community' the four chapters focus particularly on the significance of culture, ethnicity/race, gender and religion in shaping perceptions and experiences of care. The contributions seek to challenge engrained assumptions about caring relationships, practices and resources in different geographical and cultural contexts, as well as conceptualisations of consumption and care including: alternative care relationships and the ways in which care can become a networked activity (Chapter 6 by Maxine Birch and Nina Nissen); Black men's involvement in community care work and the ways in which intersections between race and gender produce particular forms of care experiences and provision for Black men and women (Chapter 7 by Tracey Reynolds); the explicit consumption discourses and practices on marketing parenthood (Chapter 8 by Andrea Doucet and Natasha Mauthner); and women's responsibilities and attitudes towards child care, family, neighbourhoods and the state, within the highly gendered Islamic society of Iran (Chapter 9 by Linda Bell).

The third part builds on the collective's long-standing interest in 'families' and family relationships to emphasise caring relationships and practices within often neglected areas of family life, not least those where a range of problematic assumptions surrounding mothering, fathering and parenting more generally exist in particular in policy and practice debates. Drawing on UK-based empirical studies the three chapters examine: the experiences of foster carers (Chapter 10 by

Linda Nutt); caring and emotional work for mothers with intellectually disabled children (Chapter 11 by Chrissie Rogers); and the perceptions and lived experiences of fathers trying to adjust to and sustain relationships with children and mothers beyond the ending of a marriage or partnership (Chapter 12 by Georgia Philip).

Finally the fourth part explores examples of the dynamic nature of care in different life-course contexts. The three chapters focus on the perspectives of children, elders and bereaved families. In doing so, the part seeks to challenge preconceptions about flows of care *within* and *across* generations. Rather than replicate well-rehearsed discussions about hierarchical flows of care and power and more conventional caring relationships, the chapters examine shifts in caring practice and relations over different dimensions of time including a focus on: caring practices within lateral sibling relationships (Chapter 13 by Susie Weller); inter-generational and transnational care dilemmas and the experiences of ageing Italian migrants (Chapter 14 by Elisabetta Zontini); and relationality with respect to bereaved families and the continuation of care after death (Chapter 15 by Jane Ribbens McCarthy).

Collectively thinking and writing with care

Before we move into the substantive part of the book, we would like to talk a little about how we have worked in a collective way, and how we have developed this volume, outlining the origins and ethos of the research network to which we belong and the writing process itself. Established in 1987 the 'Women's Workshop on Qualitative Family and Household Research' (hereafter the group) originated as a small informal support group for five PhD students who met and discovered their shared interest in qualitative research on families and households at a British Sociological Association summer school (Ribbens and Edwards 1995, 1998). By the mid-1990s the group had grown to almost 20 members, principally by word of mouth. Although not originally intended to be so, over time the group developed into a valued women-only forum, united by an interest in feminist epistemologies and methods, and a concern for the peripheral position of women's experiences in academia (Ribbens and Edwards 1998; Mauthner *et al.* 2002; Gillies and Lucey 2007).

Whilst the structure of the group was formalised through the appointment of a coordinator, to this day, it endeavours to retain an informal, supportive and collaborative ethos that enables members to experiment with new ideas, discuss tentative thoughts, ask challenging questions, share current and ongoing research, and provide constructive criticism on work-in-progress (Ribbens and Edwards 1995, 1998; Mauthner *et al.* 2002). The group currently comprises 43 members from doctoral students to research professors from over 20 institutions, primarily although not exclusively based in the UK. Members also reside in Canada, Denmark, France and Switzerland.

Reflecting the multidisciplinary nature of the group this volume contains chapters from those with backgrounds in Anthropology, Education, Geography,

Psychology, Health and Social Care, Sociology and Social Policy. We meet on a bi-monthly basis to discuss individual's work-in-progress (e.g. journal articles, book chapters, funding applications) and also to develop joint ventures. The group has a strong track record of collective work and authorship within the areas of family, intimacy and research methods producing a Special Issue of the *Women's Studies International Forum* (Ribbens and Edwards 1995), and edited collections on *Feminist Dilemmas in Qualitative Research: Public Knowledge and Private Lives* (Ribbens and Edwards 1998), *Ethics in Qualitative Research* (Mauthner, Birch, Jessop and Miller 2002) and *Power, Knowledge and the Academy: The Institutional Is Political* (Gillies and Lucey 2007) along with many single and co-authored papers and books enhanced by the groups' discussions.

The emphasis on collaboration is set within an environment imbued with competition (Gillies and Lucey 2007). As Jane Ribbens and Rosalind Edwards (1998: 6) note, 'Members have been drawn to the group by the need for a setting which recognises the significance of privately based everyday knowledge and ways of knowing instead of simply prioritising the drive towards institutional, public, academic output and credentials.' When reflecting on earlier manifestations of the group they suggest that members often research areas of great personal interest and, therefore, there is a sense in which they *care* deeply about their subject and participants. Care is also apparent in the ethos of the group; members care *for* and *about* the group and its members, often sharing in both personal and professional elations and sadness. Published 25 years after the establishment of the Women's Workshop, we feel this book is highly apt in its emphasis on re-visiting feminist ethics of care with respect to contemporary caring relations and practices across a wide variety of contexts.

The original concept for the book emerged, as many writing projects do, from a relatively casual conversation about how 'care' across a wide variety of contexts and manifestations traversed the interests of many group members. The idea followed a number of meetings in which individuals shared and sought feedback on papers relating to the subject. Fundamentally, these discussions instigated others to think about their work through a similar lens and in particular to consider areas where caring relations and practices had been overlooked. Members' interests proved to be multifarious with some having a long-term interest in care as an explicit part of their research within the context of, for example, mothering and fathering, transnational networks and a feminist ethics of care. For others the subject formed an implicit or emerging part of their work, that was, as yet, under-explored. A number of members suggested that, as a collective, we would have a great deal to say about care in different contexts and, more specifically, that our work could re-energise debates surrounding the feminist ethics of care.

Collaboration forms a key part of the group's ethos and, as in the case of previous writing projects, discussion soon turned to the most appropriate and effective way of working together; a task Val Gillies and Helen Lucey (2007) suggest is challenging, particularly given the differing statuses and experience of members. We do not wish to paint a harmonious picture of group decision making, nor would we want or have expected it to be so. Rather, decision making was constantly negotiated, generally lively and constructive, and based on majority consensus. The selection of editors, for instance, was not always without controversy. This volume has been no different in that way.

Whilst the ideal might be to write the entire book collectively the experience of established members suggested that nominated editors would be necessary to organise and drive forward the project ensuring it retained momentum and coherence. Members nominated themselves or others, with the decision-making process based on the advice of established members with experience of putting together previous collections. It was suggested that the editors ought to constitute slightly more established members familiar with group dynamics, those able to attend all meetings, and those who had contributed to previous writing projects and were familiar with the group's working practices.

Chrissie and Susie were nominated, having 'served their apprenticeship' by contributing co-authored chapters to the previous book, and they had attended the majority of meetings for over seven years. This 'unwritten' aspect of the apprenticeship has proved to be caring and supportive, as members join the group and see how status and commitment to the group is played out. Chrissie, for example, said that when she first arrived as a PhD student she saw and participated in working together in a safe, but nonetheless critical, environment. The space to critically engage with ideas and writing, away from the conference circuit and research seminar scene can be crucial in academic development. This apprenticeship meant that both Chrissie and Susie began by contributing verbally, then writing with other more senior group members, before moving to editorial roles. Via two books their experience and confidence grew, as they became 'more senior' group members. Neither had edited a book before but had edited working papers and journal Special Issues. For Chrissie and Susie, the passing of the mantle of co-editorship felt like a significant responsibility and almost a rite of passage. Not only did they feel accountable for the successful completion of the book, but also for the future longevity and well-being of the group and its growing reputation for collaborative authorship.

On the basis of group discussion and brainstorming sessions in 2008/09 we developed a basic rationale and structure for the volume and then requested abstracts from which we developed a book proposal. This was then circulated to the group for revisions. The selection of potential publishers was also subject to collective decision making on the basis of a number of criteria including the willingness to publish in paperback and the likely international reach of the publication. Based on such criteria the Resources and Relationships book series published by Routledge proved most popular. Established member Rosalind Edwards is co-editor of the series, and several members had published books as part of the collection. After a lengthy wait we were delighted to receive a contract with only a few revisions to the original proposal requested. These amendments included the addition of further contributions on social care, to which we responded by inviting colleagues Paulette Luff and Linda Nutt to join the process and share their expertise. We also asked Georgia Philip to join us in writing this introduction. Georgia, a newer member to the group, has significant expertise in the area of feminist ethics and had recently finished her PhD, and has now moved on to her ESRC postdoctoral fellowship, and we wanted to work with her on the introduction in a mutually advantageous relationship.

In previous edited collections developed by the group the emphasis has been on the co-authorship of chapters to foster collaboration (Mauthner *et al.* 2002). This volume takes a slightly different approach, comprising both single and co-authored chapters. Rather, the collaborative process centres on the detailed discussion of each chapter during meetings enabling members to fully engage with the other chapters in the volume. Authors and other group members also worked in small teams to develop of summaries of the themed parts in order to elucidate the critical stance of the book, extrapolate key theoretical and substantive messages, and highlight methodological, policy and practice insights. We coordinated this process in order to foster coherence and 'cross-fertilisation'. As already mentioned, on average the group has met on a bi-monthly basis, with each session attended by 12–15 members. Those unable to participate have offered their feedback electronically. Those not writing chapters have also provided design and editorial ideas, along with constructive criticism. Digital recordings of each discussion have been uploaded onto a shared, but private, electronic folder accessible by all members. Whilst we had some reservations about doing so, such as concerns about deterring members from divulging particular issues or talking without fear of repercussions, the process has enabled more remote members, not least those living overseas, to feel part of the discussions. The recording also provides a useful documentation allowing authors to make any necessary revisions. Chapters were submitted for group discussions in varying levels of completeness; some as outlines, others as polished drafts. Members then resubmitted their chapters for review by the editors.

Whilst we have been keen to maintain a collective ethos, over time it has felt as though our role as editors guiding and shaping the process had increased. Susie, as coordinator of the meetings, was particularly concerned as she had to instigate a lot of organisation and decision making processes. A significant proportion of the way through the process Susie announced she was expecting a baby three months before the submission of the manuscript, which meant that we were even more keen for deadlines to be met and, to some degree, had to balance being, at times, a little authoritarian with maintaining a caring ethos understanding the immense pressures of work and personal lives. Susie went on to have a baby boy, and two other group members had babies during the course of developing the book. Whilst Susie was on maternity leave Chrissie took the reins in the final stages of the group meetings and chapter editing, but then Susie, with it seems a very helpful baby, was able to complete the final edit with Chrissie. All in all, three babies and a book.

Part I
Caring within educational institutions

Caring within educational institutions

Part I Summary

Caring within educational institutions

Paulette Luff, Uthel Laurent, Val Gillies,
Yvonne Robinson and Mabelle Victoria

The following four chapters piece together many aspects of relational care and engage with care discourses in educational settings within the UK and the Philippines. Care practices are usually construed as duties practised within the home domain in relation to significant others, which implies that in other relations with generalised others in the public sphere care should take on alternative forms. Within educational settings, such care is viewed in terms of the dual relation involving the care-giver and those cared-for. This part examines care from the standpoint of both parties at three educational levels, namely the early years and primary schooling, compulsory secondary level and the higher education phase. While three of the chapters focus on how the carers (childcare practitioners, behaviour support staff and professors) think about and show care in their practice, the other chapter explores how the cared-for (students) experience care in their lives at the intersection of home and school. At pre-adult developmental level, government policies play a huge part in the way that care is expressed, interpreted and experienced at school. Over the years, increasing government preoccupation with care has resulted in a shift from general concerns of the well-being of all learners to specialised concerns about the specific care needs of vulnerable groups of learners within an educational setting, e.g. toddlers in a nursery and disruptive pupils attending Behaviour Support Units. This is seen in Chapter 2 by Paulette, where centralised regulation of early childhood education and care and the assessment demands of a national curriculum run counter to the traditional values of caring for young children upheld by practitioners; and Val and Yvonne's chapter (4), where a policy focus on the emotional well-being of challenging pupils interweaves with discourses of professional caring and carelessness to produce complex and sometimes contradictory expressions of teacher–pupil care. Within the secondary school setting this practice precludes the majority of teachers from demonstrating care. Moreover, schools are preoccupied with meeting educational objectives in keeping with governmental policies, which is at odds with how students expect care to be demonstrated.

A common thread running through the chapters is the way in which formal professional requirements and responsibilities translate into informal relational care. Val and Yvonne's and Paulette's chapters (4 and 2) focus on how care is interpreted and practised by practitioners; Uthel's chapter (3) explores care from the learner's point of view; Mabelle (in Chapter 5) explores how professors discursively demonstrate care through the downplaying of institutional power.

The establishment and management of formal caring practices within educational institutions have been driven by government policies as well as guidelines and policies that operate in schools. The aim is to ensure that caring practices are properly discharged. Val and Yvonne's chapter (4) shows that formal caring is a professional responsibility where the focus is on 'professional competence, neutrality, and detachment'. They focus on how care, which is geared at meeting the psychological needs of challenging students, is controlled and monitored within specific boundaries that regulate staff–pupil relationships and limit expressive relational caring. Their chapter argues for the need to go beyond the boundaried exercise of care, a position made visible when care is seen from students' perspectives as emphasised in Uthel's chapter. In Chapter 3 she shows that students' engagement at school was linked to their experiences of care received and depended to a great extent on whether needs and interests, including their 'lives out of school' were taken into consideration.

There are informal caring practices and moments of caring that occur within professional settings. However, where such informal relational caring is realised, it is often overshadowed by the statutory frameworks that structure and regulate the way that proper care should be expressed and experienced. This is the point explicitly raised by Paulette in Chapter 2, which highlights the prevalence of informal care shown by early years practitioners in the nurseries in which she observed. For these toddlers, informal care was based on meeting their need for protection, physical and intellectual growth, as well as social acceptance. However, within early childhood settings emphasis is placed on the curriculum and learner achievement. Caring practices are often in tension with, and obscured by, a preoccupation with documenting and monitoring progress, meeting educational objectives, the need to adhere to rigid procedures, and assessment of care based on official frameworks. This diminishes the priority placed on informal care which is, nevertheless, a main concern of early years practitioners and an important aspect of their professional identity.

All the chapter authors argue for the need to focus more on informal caring practices as demonstrated by the impulse to care on the part of the care-giver. Such informal care would also centre on concerns for the 'total' well-being of students, including the home and school lives of individual students. This is especially important for those precluded from fully participating in mainstream education. Yet, within a teaching/learning context this informal caring is often separated from the teaching act. Besides, where caring is shown within mainstream or ordinary schooling it is often partial because focus on the committed concerns shown to the academically able students is often done at the expense of the less able students. However, where students experience a neglect of care, they show their dissatisfaction in various ways including through forms of disengaged, difficult or disruptive behaviour. Yet, Chapter 5 by Mabelle shows that caring can be embedded within pedagogical practices where caring is given priority. She highlights this capacity to demonstrate care for learners as 'persons' and as 'students', illustrated by the way Filipino professors use linguistic devices to downplay their institutional authority, thus reducing the asymmetry between students and academics. Each chapter uses a different lens to add to our multifaceted view of what it means to care from the perspective of the carer and the cared-for. The point that perhaps does not need emphasising is the fact that caring practices in institutions reflect the complex interplay between schools, government policies, educators and those at the receiving end of care.

2 Reclaiming care in early childhood education and care

Paulette Luff, Anglia Ruskin University

If our actions make the world then we can act to change the very conditions under which we love, laugh, trust, work. We can bring a caring and trusting world into being through acts of caring and trusting.

(Koehn 1998: 9)

In this chapter I present some findings from ethnographic research carried out in two day nurseries and an infant school and use these as the basis for an argument for reconsidering the place of care in Early Childhood Education and Care (ECEC). The chapter begins with an account of the current context for ECEC in England, and highlights the challenge of integrating education and care effectively at a time when increasing emphasis is placed upon the achievement of formal educational outcomes by 5 years of age. This is followed by a short description of the original research project and key insights from the study, in relation to early years practitioners' 'ways of knowing' (Belenky *et al.* 1997) and ways of seeing the young children with whom they work. The main discussion then draws upon notions of maternal thinking (Ruddick 1989), analysing caring work with children in relation to key themes of protection, nurturance and social training. In the final part of the chapter some of the implications of these understandings for ECEC are considered.

Child care and early education in an English context

Early childhood education and care developed throughout the twentieth century, initially to improve the health and physical well-being of children living in poverty in industrial areas. This is exemplified in the campaigning work of Margaret McMillan (1919) and her sister, Rachel, who set up an open-air nursery school in Deptford, London. Child care then expanded during a period of increased maternal employment through the years of the Second World War (1939–45). The twin aims of increasing children's welfare and allowing parents to work continue to drive ECEC policy today (OECD 2006; Penn 2008; Pugh 2010).

In the latter part of the twentieth century, provision for the care and education of children under 5 grew unevenly with local authority day care provided for families in need and, from the 1960s, the expansion of preschool playgroups run by parents and voluntary agencies. Some extension of state nursery schools and nursery classes occurred following the publication of the Plowden Report[1] (HMSO 1967). In addition to this, private sector day-care centres expanded, particularly during the 1990s, to cater for children of working parents who required full-time care for their children (a service also provided by registered childminders and by private nannies). Access and affordability varied, according to local priorities, and these services differed in their aims and purposes, with a divide existing between child care and early years education (Anning *et al.* 2004; Penn 2008; Pugh 2010).

From 1997, the UK Labour Government showed commitment to young children and families; investing significant sums of money in the expansion of early childhood services, as a strategy for reducing child poverty and increasing children's well-being and educational achievement. A National Childcare Strategy (DfEE 1998) led to the expansion of care and education provision and the establishment of local Sure Start[2] programmes; and was followed by the UK government's ten-year childcare strategy 'Choice for Parents, the Best Start for Children' (DfES 2004a). This led to the creation of integrated children's services, a new Office for Standards in Education[3] (Ofsted) inspection regime (see below) and workforce reform. Influenced by the UN Convention on the Rights of the Child (United Nations 1989), and first published alongside the report of the inquiry into the death of Victoria Climbié[4] (Laming 2003), the Every Child Matters (ECM) programme of reform (DfES 2003; DfES 2004b; HM Government 2004) summed up positive aspirations for children in its five principles: being healthy; staying safe; enjoying and achieving; making a positive contribution; and achieving economic well-being.

Increased government funding for early years education was accompanied by the introduction of a national curriculum for this age group. The Curriculum Guidance for the Foundation Stage (CGFS) (QCA 2000) contained stepping stones and early learning goals for six areas of learning, to be met through child-centred, playful learning, for 3 to 5 year olds. 'Birth to Three Matters' (DfES 2002) was subsequently introduced, as a framework to promote and support effective practice for those caring for babies and very young children. These two documents, together with national standards for the registration and inspection of child care, are now combined within the Early Years Foundation Stage (EYFS) curriculum guidance for the care and education of children from birth to age 5 (DCSF 2008; National Strategies 2009).

It is mandatory for all registered early years settings in England to implement the statutory elements of the EYFS (DCSF 2008), which are legally binding and enforced by Ofsted. Quality and standards in early years care and education have been monitored by Ofsted since 2001, when the registration and inspection of childcare settings moved from local authority control to a centralised government system. Under the current regime, Ofsted inspectors visit in order to assess and grade provision, according to the extent to which each setting is perceived to be providing for the welfare of children, and promoting their learning and progress in relation to the ECM outcomes (Ofsted 2009).

Within the field of ECEC in England there has been enthusiasm for the increased recognition of the importance of the sector and acknowledgement of the progress made in developing a play-based curriculum and extending provision. Nevertheless, there is also disappointment with the lack of a clear long-term vision for the early years and the proliferation of existing types of early years care and education, rather than the implementation of a new comprehensive strategy at national, regional and local level (Penn 2008; Fawcett 2009), and there is some discomfort with the external regulation of standards and emphasis upon children's formal academic attainment (Papatheodorou 2008; Ellyatt 2009).

Pugh (2010) notes that the dual aims of increasing daycare provision, as part of a strategy to support parental employment and alleviate child poverty, and of ensuring high quality learning environments, in order to promote positive educational outcomes, are sometimes at variance. There is a potential conflict of interest between accepting the 'child as being', part of a caring community whose human worth is rooted in belonging and mutual interdependence, and a focus upon the individual 'child as becoming' whose progress is objectively mapped and measured (Papatheodorou 2008: 9). Elfer (2007) uses the psychodynamic concept of 'primary task', to describe such confusion within the work of early years settings, and draws attention to the uncertainties that staff may experience when there is personal or institutional conflict between the tasks of caring for and educating young children.

Osgood (2006), writing from a post-structuralist feminist perspective, represents these same tensions slightly differently. She describes a culture of conscientious caring, which characterises the emotional labour of early years practitioners, as 'hyper-feminine and therefore unmanageable, unquantifiable and impossible for the state to regulate' (9). In her view, the demands for measurement of professional competence, quality of provision and outcomes for children focus upon regulation of standards and thus undermine understandings of professionalism based upon emotion, nurturance and care.

Researching care in ECEC

Against this background of policy and debate, the research took the form of a collective case study[5] (Stake 1995). This focused upon ten newly qualified early years practitioners, all of whom had recently acquired a level three qualification[6] in early years education and care (either a National Vocational Qualification or a Council for Awards in Care, Health and Education Diploma). The main aim of the research was to investigate these participants' understandings and uses of child observation during their first year in the workplace. The topic of observation was chosen as learning to observe children plays an important part in the training of early years practitioners. It is also a key tool for assessing young children and planning their care and education. The EYFS requires practitioners to make systematic observations of each child's achievements and interests and to use these as a basis for designing relevant learning experiences and for assessing their progress (DCSF 2008).

The participants were all female, which reflects the gender bias within a profession where only 2 per cent of workers are men (Kahn 2011). They were, however, a heterogenous group ranging in age from 18 to 40, coming from different cultural and ethnic backgrounds, and having followed different routes into childcare work. Their workplaces varied, reflecting the diverse provision for young children discussed above. The first was a small (36 places) not-for-profit day nursery in London, serving the staff and students of a college and the surrounding community. The second was also a day nursery in a rural location, which was privately owned and run. It was larger (103 places) and catered for children of working parents. The third was a large infant school in a town, and the participants worked in a reception class with 4–5-year-old children. In all these early years settings the same EYFS curriculum, described above, applied.

Taking an ethnographic approach, the year-long project used participant observation in the three settings, combined with semi-structured interviews with each of the ten practitioners and their mentors (at the beginning, mid-point and end of the study), to collect evidence of child observation in practice. Thematic content analysis of data focused on: new practitioners' understandings of the nature and purpose of child observation; why and how they used it; and observation as an aspect of their work within early years settings.

Findings indicated that new early years practitioners demonstrate both informal practice, underpinned by an ethic of caring which guides observant, responsive work with young children, and formal practice, rooted in a developmental view of childhood leading to conscientious recording of predetermined, sequential, learning outcomes. The former is seen as an intrinsic, relational response whilst the latter results from the implementation of external policy requirements (as described above).

Ways of knowing

These formal and informal ways of understanding child observation can usefully be considered in terms of 'women's ways of knowing' (Belenky *et al.* 1997). Belenky and her three colleagues recognised five gender-related epistemological perspectives, from their research involving analysis of in-depth interviews with 135 women from diverse social and educational backgrounds. They argued that views of truth and knowledge contained a masculine bias, perpetuated by a male-dominated further and higher education system, and neglected ways of understanding and educating which were relevant to women's experiences of life and learning. Five ways in which women learn and know were identified as: silence; subjective knowing; received knowing; procedural knowing (which is divided into separate and connected knowing); and, finally, constructed knowing (Belenky *et al.* 1997).

The two types of procedural knowing (separate and connected knowing) are of particular interest here, as they offer a means of understanding the two main categories of understandings that were found in this study. 'Separate knowing' acknowledges expertise encapsulated within extant knowledge and the use of impersonal procedures for establishing truth (Belenky *et al.* 1997: 102). This can be equated with practitioners' conformity to external regulations and reference to developmental norms for observing and making judgements about children's progress. 'Connected knowing' involves a capacity to empathise and understand the experience of others and to know through caring, as illustrated in informal understandings and ways of thinking (discussed above and illustrated below). Thus practitioners' understandings can be characterised as 'ways of knowing' the children whom they observe.

Lenz Taguchi (2010: 172) similarly highlights different ways of seeing and interpreting children's activities. On the one hand there are 'majoritarian' habits of thought, based upon predetermined and dominant standards. Early years practitioners' charting of children's growth in comparison to universal developmental norms could be characterised in this way. On the other hand, 'becoming minoritarian' involves a complete change of perspective, reliving the event as though one were deeply involved in it. Lenz Taguchi (2010) illustrates the concept of a 'minoritarian' view using examples of imaginatively becoming the pen that the child draws with, or the play dough that is moulded. Thus, the observed event is read differently and the child and the pedagogical possibilities within the situation are more fully appreciated. This is an extreme form of 'connected knowing' and one that would require more conscious responses than the intuitive empathy shown in the participants' informal understandings of children.

The tensions experienced by practitioners when working in both 'separate' and 'connected' ways are explored explicitly elsewhere (Luff 2012). Here it is the informal, connected ways of seeing and knowing children, based upon relating to children and forming caring, responsive relationships, that are of interest. In the discussion that follows, this informal way of understanding and working with children is related to the dimensions of 'maternal thinking' (Ruddick 1989) thus valuing the intuitive responsive work of early years practitioners.

Practical thinking

Ruddick (1989: 9) posed the question 'What is the relation of thinking to life?' Her answer is that thinking emerges from collective, purposeful, human activity and that each human practice, including caring, results in distinctive kinds of perception, conduct and perspectives upon the world (Ruddick 1989). Her idea of reasoning derived from action resonate with Dewey's (1929/1987) arguments that knowledge and action are related, with thought leading to practical action; and that meanings are built up through intelligent activity (Dewey 1933/1998).

The informal understandings of child observation demonstrated by the participants in the study on which I draw compare with elements of 'maternal thinking' described by Ruddick (1989), notably: preservation of the child; fostering the growth of the child (physical, emotional and intellectual); and the child's social acceptance. Ruddick defines mothering broadly as the work of caring for children, which is not necessarily dependent upon a biological relationship. The practitioners who participated in this research, therefore, do fit Ruddick's (1989: 40) description of 'a person who takes on responsibility for children's lives and for whom providing child care is a significant part of her or his working life' and so might legitimately be viewed as maternal thinkers who act to fulfil children's needs. Niikko (2004) presents similarities between parents' and kindergarten teachers' views of care and education and identifies common features in their roles. Likewise, here, I argue that the informal understandings of children, enacted in practitioners' work, display elements of maternal thinking. In their daily acts of nurturing and watchful alertness to health and safety, they accept and feel responsibility for each child's survival; they understand their role as promoting every child's development; and they implement the routines of the nursery, thus playing an important part in children's socialisation.

Preservation of the child

From the research data, the notion of the preservation of the child was evident in formal risk assessments prior to outings and any activities considered hazardous. Safety checking (of the indoor premises and gardens), cleaning surfaces with disinfectant sprays before and after serving food, and hygiene and hand-washing procedures, were noticeable throughout each nursery day. There were also multiple instances of practitioners seeing children's vulnerability and responding with care. An example of this protective and attentive understanding is illustrated in these small incidents, between practitioner, Kel, and young toddler, Sophie:

> Sophie slips on the slide. She cries a little and rubs her head and arm then goes over to Kel and points to her head. Kel gently rubs Sophie's head and she is immediately reassured and runs back to the slide, laughing. Similarly when Sophie is barefoot, playing with soft foam shapes on the carpet, she comes near to Kel and points to her toes. Kel makes a sympathetic response, rubbing Sophie's toes and saying 'Remember you've got no shoes!' to which Sophie nods and says, 'Shoes.'
>
> (Transcribed from field notes)

The observant, protective responses of early years practitioners revealed appreciation of the importance of the child to the parent and the significance of caring for the child. Teaching assistant Hollie's scanning of the infant school playground, when she was one of the members of staff on duty outside during the children's break time, displayed, as Ruddick (1989) suggests, 'a cognitive style which I call scrutinising ... watchful and alert for potential danger' (72). The same caring approach was seen within the baby and toddler rooms, where practitioners managed very young children's play and enabled their explorations whilst watching to ensure that they did not injure themselves or one another; teaching strategies for safety and yet, at the same time, giving children freedom.

Even when the participants in this study were tired, feeling unwell or overwhelmed with the demands of the workplace they adopted a positive attitude towards the children. One practitioner, Charlie, apologised that she was too tired to respond to my interview questioning: 'I'm normally much more talkative but it's been very hard work this week!' But this exhaustion was not at all evident in the efficient way in which she then readily changed all the children's nappies and encouraged the use of potties and the toilet with the group of toddlers she cares for. This is reminiscent of 'resilient cheerfulness' (Ruddick 1989: 75), a virtue linked with preservative attention.

Fostering growth

Practitioners' watchfulness went beyond physical care with positive attention directed towards fostering children's growth, the second element of maternal thinking. This was seen in playful, responsive interactions through which practitioners get to know the children and provide the encouragement necessary for them to flourish and reveal their abilities. This resonates with a notion of 'caring presence' (Goodfellow 2008), which can be defined as: 'A state of alert awareness, receptivity and connectedness to the mental, emotional, and physical working of the group in the context of their learning environments and the ability to respond with a considered and compassionate next step' (Rodgers and Raider-Roth, cited by Goodfellow 2008: 18).

There are multiple instances of this 'ability to respond with a considered and compassionate next step' in the work of early years practitioners. This episode, where Mij is playing with two 1-year-old boys, is typical:

> Jesse posts a stickle brick down the front of his vest. Mij joins in and, taking turns, they fill the front of his vest (which is quite loose fitting and tucked into his trousers) with stickle bricks. Mij smiles and Jesse laughs and pulls the bricks out one by one. Jesse then begins to post more bricks into his vest. With Jean-Paul, the game is different. He takes a brick from Mij's right hand and picks up another brick from the floor in front of him. He presses the two together. Jean Paul then puts the bricks onto his head. Mij holds them, helping the bricks to balance there. Jean-Paul tips his head and Mij says, 'Ooo!' when the bricks fall off.

> (Transcribed from field notes)

In reciprocal sociable games, such as these, the children are active in constructing opportunities for learning and the adult is, likewise, active in her responses. This corresponds well to Trevarthen's (2004: 2) view of the child as 'playmate and companion in meaning' seeking communicative contact, which is then 'matched by the motives to share creativity and teach in the adult' (Trevarthen 2003: 239). As with the preservation of the child, the fostering of growth has parallels with maternal care. Within families interactions in which babies lead and parents follow (Parker Rees 2007) are seen as important for promoting holistic development. In childcare environments outside of the home it may not be so easy to provide opportunities for these attuned interactions (Elfer 2007; Parker Rees 2007) but where they do occur they are recognised as a key feature of effective practice (for example, Siraj-Blatchford *et al.* 2002; Manning-Morton and Thorp 2006; Payler 2007). The practitioners in this study demonstrated and articulated a sense of responsibility to nurture children, whilst they are in their care, in order to make their time at nursery worthwhile.

Heshusius (1995: 121) writes of 'a participatory mode of consciousness' when a listener attends and engages fully with another person, putting aside their own concerns. This has similarities with the ways in which Rinaldi (2005: 139) discusses the importance of observation and documentation as a means of allowing 'the subjectivity of each child' to be appreciated in relation to the teacher and others. Likewise, for Noddings (2003, 2005) the ability to be observant and responsive to a child's needs is characteristic of the caring educator. She emphasises that caring relations can be the foundation of pedagogical activity and thought. There are parallels between Trevarthen's (2003, 2004) descriptions of adult and child relationships, Nodding's notion of the educator as 'one caring' deriving rewarding feedback and motivation from the responses of the child, as the 'one cared for', and Goodfellow's (2008) explanation of reciprocal relationships as evidence of practitioners' 'presence', listening to and interacting with children.

Social acceptance

The social development of children has long been a priority of nursery education (McMillan 1919). Webb (1974) highlights the tension in the early years between educating autonomous individuals whilst training for social compliance. In a Finnish context, too, socialisation is seen as a key aspect of education within kindergartens and families (Niikko 2004). Within the current study, four features of an observant promoting of children's social acceptance were witnessed. First, functional independence, as children's attempts at washing, dressing and feeding themselves were supported, noted and praised. Second, group participation, as even for the youngest children there were times when the whole group gathered, such as around the table at set mealtimes and also for singing and story activities. Third, encouragement to play with others, with practitioners sometimes facilitating games between babies and older children; and fourth, gentle insistence upon conformity to rules and routines. This final element was especially noticeable in the school context, where part of Hollie's scrutiny of the classroom and playground was to manage children's behaviour. These features correspond with the third dimension of maternal thought: 'training the child to be the kind of person whom others accept and whom the mothers themselves can actively appreciate' (Ruddick 1989: 104).

Pro-social behaviour was certainly a topic of discussion with parents when children were collected from nursery. Reporting of observed negative behaviour was an area of difficulty that had to be handled with sensitivity, especially when it involved injury to another child (such as biting). Practitioners' roles have been characterised as part of a three-way 'caring triangle' (Hohmann 2007: 43) in which what is seen at nursery is reported and ways of knowing about the child are negotiated. As Cuffaro (1995: 97) says, 'Teaching is too hard to do alone.' Thus dialogues between adults are essential for understanding children in early childhood settings because their care is a shared endeavour, between practitioners and the children's families.

The importance of connected seeing and knowing

The three aims of protection, nurturance and social training, characteristic of maternal thinking, were, thus, in evidence within the informal understandings of observant child care and education practice articulated and enacted by the participants in the research study. Ruddick (1989: 25) argued that maternal thinking should be considered 'no less thoughtful, no less a discipline than other kinds of thinking'. Similarly, respect should be shown for practitioners' informal thinking. This does not mean that practitioners' thinking and actions could not be critiqued but it raises questions about who the critics should be, and highlights the importance of an insider perspective. From my own experience of becoming a participant observer, I have developed and appreciated understandings of practitioners' thought (categorised here as informal ways of understanding) through experience alongside them in the field. I had to acknowledge that their ways of thinking are different from those based upon formal educational and developmental theories which, when coming from the outside, I had expected to form the basis for their ideas about observing children.

Ruddick explains that thinking does not have to be limited to a single discipline and, just as mothers may draw upon ways of thinking from other disciplines with which they are engaged, reflections about care and education could, and arguably should, also be informed by other ways of thinking. Insights from developmental psychology and pedagogical theory can usefully illuminate practice. According to Ruddick (1989: 27), 'interpractice criticism' can offer important insights and influence positive change and, similarly, in early years care and education different theoretical and disciplinary perspectives may inform and enrich 'wise practice' (Goodfellow 2001).

Implications for ECEC

In their connected ways of seeing and knowing children, the early years practitioners in the study display 'natural caring' (Noddings 2003; Niikko 2004): the positive responses of one human being to another through an unconscious obligation to care. Being fully attentive, in the ways that Kel and others achieve in their responses to children (as in the examples above), is essential for work with very young children. Gerber (2002: 63) exhorts those who care for babies to 'Observe more, do less.' She contrasts the actions of a 'caregiver', an adult who takes the initiative, with those of an 'educarer' (Gerber 2005: 49) who is responsive to cues from the child. Money (2005) and Memel and Fernandez (2005), writing from the same perspective, also highlight the importance of sensitive responses for building respectful relationships with babies and children, emphasising that being understood promotes the child's confidence and trust whereas being misunderstood can lead to insecurity and self-doubt.

Caldwell (1991, 2002) writes of the importance of services provided for young children offering both educational and protective, caring components. Smith (1993), following Caldwell, similarly calls for child care to become 'educare', guidance that combines care with nurturing children's development and fostering intellectual potential. This definition of 'educare' goes beyond that proposed by Gerber (2005) as, although careful following of the child's lead is important, the adult also takes responsibility for extending learning through sensitive scaffolding of the child's emergent understandings and abilities.

This is similar to the Early Years Foundation Stage curriculum guidance, which advocates observant caring, within the 'Supporting Learning' aspect of the 'Positive Relationships' theme of the framework (National Strategies 2009: no page). Practitioners are expected to 'observe children sensitively and respond appropriately to encourage and extend curiosity and learning', to discover children's preferences and feelings and to 'tune in to, rather than talk at, children'. The challenge is in balancing this advice with a pressure to focus upon children's learning and achievement. Morton (2009: 39) recognises that: 'The more synchronised the interactions between the carer and the baby, the more a positive relationship is formed'; and she also warns that when focusing on children's skills and abilities and the achievement of developmental milestones carers can miss really seeing the child and appreciating him or her as a person.

Practitioners' observant care indicates that they are aware of the nuances of children's growth, even though it is the achievement of certain learning outcomes that are formally recorded. Selleck (2001: 86) suggests that observation 'opens up possibilities for empathy' and a positive emotional connection with children. This is typified in practitioners' abilities to 'be with' babies, toddlers and children and to establish warm and trusting relationships. Noddings (2003) characterises such responsiveness, receptivity and availability as demonstrating key features of caring. The capacity to be aware of, notice and make connections with each child's experience can also be described as 'presence' (Goodfellow 2008).

It would be inspiring to believe that all practitioners are as naturally caring and responsive to children as those who participated in this study. Alarming examples of lack of care within early years institutions (e.g. BBC One 2004; Gaunt 2008; Marcus 2008; Morris and Gabbatt 2009; Carter 2011) indicate that this is not always the case. Nevertheless, whilst practitioners who volunteer to participate in research studies, such as this one, do not necessarily represent their entire profession, the impulse to care and an ethic of care is evident within wider research (e.g. Niikko 2004; Osgood 2006; Goodfellow 2008) and, where this is fostered and supported within a positive organisational culture, children are likely to benefit from being noticed and affirmed (Elfer 2007).

The important role of the adult care-giver and educator is highlighted in research, which indicates that the quality of young children's educational experiences and the benefits of early years provision depend upon practitioners' knowledge and experience (e.g. Siraj-Blatchford *et al.* 2002; Anning and Edwards 2006). Whilst the informal and connected ways of seeing and knowing children, described above, may provide children with important nurture, more might be achieved, in terms of offering a 'curriculum for thinking' (Nutbrown 2006: 113) within an inspiring environment, if practitioners were encouraged and enabled to reflect upon their practice, and children's experiences. Malaguzzi (1998: 68) offers a reminder that caring has cognitive as well as affective and expressive aspects and thus should be 'understood not merely as a warm, protecting envelope, but rather as a dynamic conjunction of forces and elements interacting towards a common purpose'.

Equally, it is important that the balance does not shift away from care. Rinaldi (2005: 65), writing about documentation and assessment, reminds us that 'listening is emotion'; whilst Papatheodorou (2008), discussing the challenges of implementing early childhood pedagogy in different contexts, also emphasises that early childhood pedagogy is not just a political or intellectual exercise but also has a strong affective dimension. Thus it is important that 'formal' and 'informal' ways of using child observation are combined, in 'wise practice' (Goodfellow 2001) as is achieved in relational pedagogical approaches in, for example, the Nordic countries (OECD 2006).

Conclusion: the place of care

Tronto (1993: 115) suggests that the more powerful people in society, including those in public roles, 'take care of' issues; and it is left to the less privileged to 'care about' and meet the needs of others, including children. Whilst carers see value in their own work, as did the practitioners in this study who expressed their joy and satisfaction in working with children, childcare work is not valued and rewarded in society, with all the participants in this study working for low pay. Their sensitive caring is appreciated by children's parents, who praise their personal qualities and abilities, and by the babies and young children whose well-being and positive responses suggest recognition that they are really cared for (Eide and Winger 2005). Leffers (1993: 72) writes of the importance of 'continual striving to maintain and expand our awareness of our interconnection with others' and this is seen in the connected ways of seeing and knowing, exemplified in the interplay between the practitioners and young children. This sensitive caring is skilled work: 'It needs very observant and astute people to tune into babies from other people's families' (Selleck 2001: 84). Yet it is the emotion invested in caring for children that may undermine the status of the work (Tronto 1993; Moyles 2001; Osgood 2006).

ECEC is typically discussed and debated in relation to theories of pedagogy, developmental psychology, or the new sociology of childhood. Here a new lens has been brought to bear upon the work of early years practitioners, in explaining the caring dimension of their role in terms of maternal thinking and an ethic of care. The ideas presented here merit fuller exploration in a developed review of concepts and ethics of caring in relation to the work and experience of early years practitioners.

Notes

1 This is the name often given to the 'Children and their Primary Schools' report, presented by the Central Advisory Council for Education, chaired by Lady Bridget Plowden. It offered a wide-ranging review of primary schooling and advocated for child-centred approaches to the curriculum.
2 Sure Start formed part of a government initiative to prevent social exclusion, primarily targeted at preschool children and their families in disadvantaged areas. The aim was

to give young children 'the best start in life' through provision of high quality, community-based services. The programme included the setting up of Sure Start Children's Centres offering daycare and nursery education and a range of other services for children and families.

3 The Office for Standards in Education, Children's Services and Skills (Ofsted) is the official body responsible for the regulation and inspection of care and education services for children and young people. Ofsted took over responsibility for registration and inspection of early years settings from local authorities.

4 Eight-year-old Victoria Climbié died in February 2000, a victim of abuse by her great aunt Marie-Therese Kouao and her boyfriend Carl Manning. They were convicted of her murder and Lord Laming headed a public inquiry into the circumstances leading up to her death. The report made recommendations for changes to child protection procedures.

5 Stake (1995) differentiates intrinsic, instrumental and collective case study approaches. Intrinsic cases arise from curiosity and interest in the distinctive features of a particular case; whereas instrumental cases require the study of people or programmes to answer a research question, in order to gain more general understanding of an issue. Collective case studies are instrumental in nature but allow for the study of more than one person or setting to contribute to the inquiry.

6 Level three represents a qualification equivalent to an Advanced standard (equivalent to sixth-form qualifications such as A Level or National Diploma). It involves study at a college of Further Education. This is the level required to take responsibility for a group of children and to supervise others with lower qualifications.

3 Revisiting care in schools

Exploring the caring experiences of disengaged young people

Uthel Laurent, The Open University

Introduction

In the 1980s, Nel Noddings, an American feminist, put forward a case for an educational philosophy built on a relational ethics of care. She envisaged a school where there was no rebellion and where the multiplicity of interests, capabilities and experiences of each student was acknowledged (Noddings 1992). In such schools, caring relations would form the foundation of teaching with the goal of developing morally educated and caring citizens. Despite the criticism levelled against her views from feminist and non-feminist writers (see Tong and Williams 2009), Noddings's ideas offer a useful framework to explore 'caring' from the existential experiences of disengaged young people. In this chapter I seek to apply Noddings's US-based work on relational care to explore 'caring' in English secondary schools. I begin by considering the theoretical basis of Noddings's argument before examining the context of care in English secondary schools. Drawing on data from a case study, I then explore the schooling experience of disengaged young people within a relational ethics of care framework. My key argument is that, notwithstanding institutional constraints, teachers ought to develop a capacity to care for their students which should form an integral part of their teaching. Hence, this chapter aims to shed light on the plausibility of developing caring relations as a possible intervention for tackling student disengagement.

A Critical analysis of Noddings's approach to care

At the core of Noddings's care theory is a focus on caring relationships. Thus, Noddings (1988) concentrates on encounters between two parties (one-caring and one cared-for) aimed at preserving or producing caring relations. This relation is born out of a sense of love and natural inclination rather than a sense of moral duty. Noddings (2003) believes that there are four basic requirements of caring: engrossment, motivational displacement, recognition and response. The one-caring must show engrossment and motivational displacement, and the one cared-for must recognise the care and respond to it. During engrossment, the care-giver listens without bias with a view to understanding the other's situation before suggesting an appropriate action (Noddings 2003). However, caring may not always be straightforward as the care given may depend on the need to be satisfied (Noddings 2010a) or may vary according to cultural interpretations (Smith 2004).

In motivational displacement, carers set aside their goals temporarily in order to help satisfy the expressed needs of others (Noddings 2010b). Sometimes carers may not approve of the other's need and motivational displacement takes a different form. Instead they may suggest an alternative goal and attempt to persuade the cared-for of its validity (Noddings 2010a). At other times, the desire to help the cared-for is constrained and motivational displacement becomes impossible, for example, when expectations to kill someone to protect the cared-for clash with deeply held moral beliefs (see Rogers, Chapter 11 in this volume). Hence, Noddings (2003) maintains that when caring relations become too burdensome and relationships are broken, the carer becomes 'ethically diminished'. In order for the caring relation to be complete the cared-for must recognise the effort of the carer as caring. In this way, both the one-caring and the one cared-for would be satisfied with their care (Noddings 2010b).

Noddings argues that caring relations should be the foundation of pedagogical activities. This focus on school care was a response to the decline in religious influence and the simultaneous waning of moral education in American schools in the early twentieth century. As such, Noddings contends that 'secondary schools, where violence, apathy and alienation are more evident, do little to develop the capacity to care' (2003: 28). To her, the US educational system has become dehumanised, with schools driven by a relentless quest for academic adequacy (1992: xii). Thus, Noddings argues that the main aim of education should be the production of competent, caring, loving and lovable people who will become morally educated citizens (1992: 174). To this end, Noddings (2010b, 2010c) suggests that caring at school should be accomplished through modelling, dialogue, practice and confirmation. Through modelling, teachers demonstrate a caring attitude in everything they do. Open-ended and mutual dialogue should be marked by attention to the needs of students. Confirmation implies picking out the best attributes in students instead of condemning them. Additionally, practice signifies providing students with opportunities to demonstrate care.

Nevertheless, Noddings's ideas have been subject to criticism from feminist and non-feminist writers alike. Critics argue that caring can be potentially one-sided (Hoagland 1990; Smith 2004) and can lead to a situation where carers may be in an exploitative, harmful or abusive relationship (Card 1990; Hoagland 1990; Houston 1990). Moreover, carers can suffer from a 'moral paralysis' when they should be acting to protect themselves (Houston 1990), and there should be the possibility for carers to withdraw from the cared-for without being considered as 'ethically diminished' (Card 1990; Hoagland 1990). Hoagland (1990) also argues that teacher–student relations are ethically problematic. This is because these transitory relations are designed to allow for the independence of the cared-for and do not provide a complete analysis of caring. Interestingly, Heidegger's (1962) notion of care takes this opposite line, being concerned with 'releasing' the other to enable them to be independent.

Noddings (1990) does, however, acknowledge the potential for exploitative relationships and labels them as 'pathological caring'. She argues that the threat of exploitation does not undermine the value of relational caring, and maintains that, except in necessarily unequal relations, the threat of exploitation should not normally be a problem. Furthermore, reciprocity in caring relations would buffer against exploitation as it allows for interchangeability of roles in mature relationships. Thus, caring cannot be conceived as an activity devoid of judgement as there is usually a sense of focus and reasoning associated with the experience of caring (see Ruddick 1980; Tronto 1995a). However, Finders (2001, cited in Smith 2004) notes that reciprocity in unequal relations can become complex as issues of time, intensity and situational variations have to be taken into account. Besides, Noddings (2002) acknowledges that caring relations can have temporal frames. She contends that caring is a contextual activity which requires different behaviours depending on the situation and persons involved.

Arguably, most of the criticisms aimed at Noddings's work have focused on exploitation in mature adults' relationships that are assumed to be equal. However, these criticisms may not be applicable to unequal teacher–student relations as the nature of the exploitation may differ. Moreover, in these relations, caring is still able to flourish as the parties collaboratively attempt to re(solve) issues of concern. Besides, this focus on unequal relations is not uncommon among feminist writers as seen in the works of Ruddick (1980), Held (1983) and Kittay (1999).

The context of English secondary school care

In England, caring for disengaged students has usually operated within an 'inclusive' provision for the well-being of students. This focus on students' care and welfare has been a long-standing governmental aim and, to this end, various educational programmes, policies and initiatives have been implemented over the past sixty years.[1] For example, the advent of universal secondary education was accompanied by early provision for the spiritual, mental and physical development of students by the 1944 Education Act. Furthermore, the National Curriculum, instigated by the 1988 Education Reform Act, included the requirement to teach some form of religious studies, expressly aimed at developing pupils' spiritual, moral, social and cultural well-being. In 1996, Personal, Social and Health Education (PSHE) was made a statutory entitlement for all, followed by the inclusion of Citizenship Education, made compulsory for English secondary schools in 2002. More recently, mounting concerns over child welfare issues saw a shift from this early focus on students' general well-being to a preoccupation with more specialised programmes of interventions targeting specific groups of students including those who were disengaged (Broadhurst *et al.* 2005) or at risk of exclusion (Gillies and Robinson, Chapter 4 in this volume).

With the introduction of further policies such as the Children Act 2004 and the Social and Emotional Aspects of Learning (SEAL) Programme (DfES 2004c, 2005a, 2007a), increasing focus has been placed on professional caring where specialists focus on controlling, monitoring and supporting students with social, emotional or behavioural problems. Alongside these, emphasis has been placed on the implementation of support initiatives in schools intended to reduce student disengagement (e.g. alternative curricula, Excellence in Cities and Education Action Zones).

The specialised focus on professional care has been criticised by many writers and researchers alike. For example, critics such as Furedi (2004) claim that the proliferation of programmes geared at student welfare are having a pernicious influence on individuals, being potentially damaging to children and young people. They argue that the SEAL programme has the potential to foster narcissism and self-obsession (Furedi 2004; Craig 2007), worsen students' well-being, detract from a focus on academic work and turn teachers into therapists (Furedi 2004; Ecclestone and Hayes 2008). Moreover, others argue that, in large secondary schools, students' problems are increasingly handled by unfamiliar adults who do not have a rapport with students, have no prior knowledge of them, or of their lives out of school (Bryk 1988). Besides, these specialists are dissuaded from pursuing expressive relational care through practices that emphasise professional detachment (see Gillies and Robinson, Chapter 4 in this volume). Additionally, some writers contend that interventions to counter disengagement have proved to be inadequate (Broadhurst *et al.* 2005) and futile in meeting their stated purpose (Smyth 2006).

When examined against a relational ethics of care framework, these existing approaches to students' care and welfare in secondary schools are wanting in some respects. First, these programmes are based on compartmentalised modes of study being delivered by form tutors,[2] specific subject teachers or other specialists. The implication is that the majority of teachers who are not expected to teach these courses are dissuaded from engaging in caring relations with students. Moreover, these programmes and initiatives, though well intentioned, are geared towards the acquisition of specific skills and give less attention to the maintenance of caring relations. Nevertheless, there is still the general expectation in some quarters that relational care is a fundamental part of a teacher's job (Ferreira and Bosworth 2000; Schaps 2003; see also Victoria, Chapter 5 in this volume).

Researching care and young people's disengagement

This chapter draws on data from a pilot case study of a secondary school in central England. The project represented a preliminary phase of my ongoing doctoral ethnographic study which aims to explore young people's disengagement from school. There has been much disagreement within the research literature about what constitutes student disengagement (see Libbey 2004; Fredricks *et al.* 2004; Appleton *et al.* 2008; Skinner *et al.* 2009). However, in this chapter I use the term disengagement as a sensitising concept to refer to the ways in which students do not participate in learning processes or involvement in school life or are prevented from doing so.

The research site was a small, mixed secondary school with approximately 500 students. Most of these students were drawn from socially and economically deprived catchment areas with approximately three-quarters of them travelling by bus. Additionally, the majority of this intake was from a white British working-class background with over 30 per cent being entitled to free school meals, an indicator often used to denote socio-economic disadvantage. Data were gathered through interviews held with eight white British working-class girls[3] in Year 11 (aged 15–16 years) who were perceived by their teachers to be disengaged and four teachers who had taught the Year 11 students. Other sources of data included informal conversations with other teaching staff and final year students, school documents such as students' assessment data and term reports, as well as reflective observation notes.[4]

In the discussion that follows I will draw on the accounts of three students – Rachel, Marlene and Elsa – whose narratives exemplify the caring concerns shared by the participants as well as caring moments experienced. Whereas Elsa and Rachel began their secondary schooling in Year 7 (aged 11[5]) and lived with their families in the catchment area, Marlene entered the school in Year 10 (aged 15) and lived with her boyfriend outside the catchment area. I also draw on interview data with Mr Pritchard, the Head of the Science Department, who taught Science to all the Year 11 students.

When caring is neglected

Within a relational ethics of care, caring is deemed to be incomplete if one or both parties are unsatisfied with their care. This section highlights this deficiency in care that the girls experienced through lack of attention to their expressed needs and their teachers' inability to engage in fruitful dialogue with them.

Caring Concerns: Rachel and Marlene

Both Rachel and Marlene expressed concerns about their subject choices at school. Rachel had a strong interest in hairdressing and spoke enthusiastically about her part-time job:

> I work in a hairdresser's. This is what I'm doing when I leave school. I want to go straight to work. I've worked in a hairdresser's since I was 14. At the moment I work on Wednesday, Thursday and Friday from 4–7, and on Saturday from 9–5. I don't want to be lazy. I don't want to sit home all the time doing nothing.

While Rachel spoke with excitement about her job, she complained that she was denied the opportunity to pursue a hairdressing course at school:

> I wanted to go to college[6] to do hairdressing but they said I couldn't go to college because I'm too clever. I couldn't take it because it is not a GCSE[7] subject. They teach you a lot of pointless stuff . . . Getting training is better than going to school.

Thus, although Rachel was focused on her hairdressing career, attempts to discuss this issue with her teachers had failed. Unlike Rachel, Marlene was more ambivalent about her subject choices. She had applied to do Hairdressing and Beauty at college, however, she recounted that:

> I like cooking as well. I was going to do Food Technology for my option but I did Arts instead. I wish I did Foods; I wish I had actually . . . My Nan said I could be a good cook or a chef or something when I am older.

This ambivalence was partly linked to deeper worries about doing subjects that matched her learning style. She reported that 'I prefer more hands-on that's why I get bored in lessons.'

Yet, Marlene was concerned about the way practical subjects were taught. She explained that:

> I like Art. I don't like Graphics. Ms G. can make it difficult in Graphics . . . it takes her half an hour to come to you . . . then she shouts at you because you have done no work but it is her fault . . . because she hasn't come to you.

Like Rachel, Marlene was unable to discuss her concerns with teachers. Marlene voiced her distress when she argued that 'I prefer practical but I have not spoken to anybody about this; if you go to the Head of Year with your concern she just tells you to go back to your lesson.'

The girls' complaints highlight an area of concern that deserves attention from caring teachers. However, a different perspective was taken by the school. For example, with regards, to subject choice, Mr Pritchard reasoned that:

> Basically if you get too many people on your stats [statistics] exclusion,[8] you can be Ofsteded;[9] some of the people in this cohort really aren't engaged in the education system at all; and rather than permanently exclude them they are given alternative curriculum.

Here, teachers' concerns were related to the overall ethos of the school. Hence, it seemed that the selection of students for pursuing an alternative, arguably more vocational, curriculum was tied to wider goals of monitoring and assessing school performance and alleviating factors that affected performance such as exclusion. Thus, subjects like hairdressing were offered to students who had been placed on an alternative curriculum because they were unable to cope with academic subjects. In this regard, Rachel was considered a more-able student who was capable of accessing academic subjects and therefore was not eligible for placement on an alternative curriculum. This reflects the tight accountability regimes under which schools operate where their performance is continually monitored, and any failure to meet 'targets' penalised.

Noddings (2002) sees this sort of denial of opportunity as a destructive form of coercion, since it forces students to do activities that are not connected to their own purposes. Noddings argues that forcing students to take particular subjects in school 'for their own good' suggests that students' own interests, talents and purposes are not highly valued. To her, the best-intentioned coercions may lead to feelings of frustration and incompetence and may encourage forms of disengagement from learning and school. In this sense, seeing about the academic interests of students would allow them to become 'engaged' learners.

Marlene expressed three related concerns: (a) ambivalence with regard to her future career choice; (b) matching the teaching to suit her learning style; and (c) studying more practical subjects in line with her learning style. These concerns merit attention as they affected the way she responded to her learning. Hence, the need for dialogue with teachers was pressing for Marlene. Noddings (1992) acknowledges students' diverse learning styles and advises that there should be open discussion amongst teachers and students about these matters. Noddings (1992) also argues that teachers should accommodate the diverse talents of students in their teaching. Furthermore, in order to cater for the multiple intelligences of students, Noddings advocated the introduction of a varied curriculum instead of focusing mainly on academic subjects. In her view, 'if students' interest and talents are not admired they may never really learn what it means to be cared for' (Noddings 2002: 31). Moreover, Noddings (2010c) alludes to these opportunities for awareness and sensitivity towards the students' interests and needs when she stresses the centrality of 'receptive attention' to caring.

The students' interest in practical or vocational subjects is significant given that the English education system has focused attention on alternative educational initiatives, and particularly on vocational qualifications, as a means of tackling disengagement. For example, Kendall and Kinder (2005) argue that vocational education does not have parity of esteem with academic qualifications, which has resulted in students being given academic courses that are inappropriate to meeting their learning needs. They caution that vocational subjects will only be successful in reducing disaffection if they are fully integrated into the curriculum rather than provided as a differentiated curriculum.

Rachel's response to the denial of opportunity was seen in the manifestation of behaviours reflecting her disengagement from learning and school. For example, she recounted that:

> In Year Seven and Eight I used to like school but I don't look forward to school anymore. I skive [truant] because I don't like school. I hate studying; I really want to do my hairdressing. I go to most lessons and I just sit there and doodle and stuff like that. The teachers sometimes notice but I don't care. As for homework, I've never done that for ages. I don't do anything connected to school. Instead of going to school I would have liked to spend my days working.

As such, Rachel produced little work in lessons, refused to participate in school activities and on occasions truanted. Thus, whilst she was highly committed to her hairdressing career she was disengaged at school.

Mr Pritchard recognised that Rachel was disengaged when he reported that 'the state she arrives in lessons you can tell she's not really in the frame of mind for it', and 'she simply isn't doing anything at home'. However, his assessment of her behaviour was at variance with the view presented by Rachel. To him, Rachel had attributes that would make it difficult for her to pursue a career or seek employment after she completed school. He reasoned that:

> Rachel stands out because she doesn't get involved in anything outside of lessons really . . . I think what to say generally about these kids is that a lot of them lack a focus on what they want to do when they leave . . . those like Rachel will try and melt into the background . . . so you do get that there is an engagement issue; if someone whose got self esteem issues and they find it hard to talk, they would just melt into the background . . . that's a real battleground to engage if they don't get it.

This account suggests that Mr Pritchard was unaware of Rachel's commitment to her career or her out-of-school preoccupations. Hence, Rachel's disengagement was explained by means of a deficit model which focused on inherent behavioural problems. However, both accounts seem to suggest a deficit in the teacher's understanding.

Like Rachel, Marlene's non-school concerns were not recognised by teachers. Marlene was highly preoccupied with her home life as she explained:

> because like family problems: I got kicked out of my dad's; my mom is in a hostel and I have not seen her since three years now. I've got my own house now. I live with my boyfriend; my boyfriend goes to work at nights and it's like my time to do what I want to. I do some homework and cook and clean.

This preoccupation with home life greatly impacted on her learning and generated forms of disengagement at school. She recounted that 'sometimes, I get stressed about things at home or people and then I switch off and won't learn; and then if someone asks me a question I won't answer and it affects my performance'. However, like Rachel, Marlene's behaviour had been interpreted differently by Mr Pritchard:

> Marlene is a strange one; sometimes I look at Marlene and the way she reacts I wonder if she is in an act. I've come to the conclusion that she really is like that . . . I wonder very much about what she's experienced in the last five years.

This lack of focus on the 'out-of-school lives' of students is part of a system where students' care is highly monitored and regulated. However, this inconsistency in students' and teachers' views does not accord with a relational ethics of care perspective.

Within caring relations, teachers would be attentive to students, demonstrating a willingness to listen or observe receptively, with a view to understanding what they are going through (Noddings 2010a). Thus, teachers would be open to them and would get to know them through dialogue (Noddings 2010c). As such, caring should be at the centre of educational efforts, and caring for students should not depend on their academic prowess (Noddings 1992) but should be closely tied to the actual experience, concerns, welfare and legitimate differences among students (Noddings 2003: 180). Hence, caring should not be restricted to educational matters but should extend to other personal concerns relating to out-of-school life, including family dynamics (Barber 2002). Tronto (1995a) also acknowledges this type of care when she states that 'caring for' involves responding to the particular concrete physical, spiritual, intellectual, psychic and emotional needs of others.

Having background knowledge about these students can influence how teachers interact and deal with them, thereby facilitating the learning process (Noddings 2010c). Moreover, such knowledge would allow teachers to confirm the best attributes in these students who are otherwise perceived as disengaged. According to Barber (2002), this background knowledge can only be acquired through building supportive relationships with students and establishing trusting relations with them. Of course, some staff may informally care for students, but they find themselves situated within a system that does not value care, especially as schools are seen as places where academic achievement is the priority.

When caring is fulfilled

Students highly value even the smallest acts of care shown by their teachers. This final example illustrates one student's experience of care received and the significance of this care for her.

Caring Moments: Elsa

Elsa enjoyed socialising with her school peers and this association led to her involvement in negative activities. She recounted that:

> In Year Seven I used to be really, really, good; I used to get on with my work; like ... Year Eight I started faffing [messing] about, following people I shouldn't hang around with ... like trouble makers ... in Year Eight I fell back and didn't even put my head down ... I'm not proud of what I was doing.

This negative behaviour was acknowledged by Mr. Pritchard when he reported that Elsa 'hangs around with the less desirable elements' and that she was 'a concern'. From an ethics of care perspective, the establishment of caring relations serves as a buffer against such behaviour. In this regard, Noddings (1992) suggests that guidance should be provided to students as even within their 'inner circle of friends' they can be pushed into harmful or wrongful acts' (99).

Despite what was perceived as her negative behaviour, Elsa was able to recognise caring occasions at school. She reported that:

> Miss B really motivated me at school ... She helps me a lot ... like when I was in Year Eight, Year Nine and Ten when I was doing bad at school; then it's like she helping me because I was getting letters at home [about my

behaviour] and it was upsetting my mom and I was going to her room to speak to Miss B about home and school.

Moreover, Elsa's response to the care received took the form of a change in behaviour:

I don't really speak to her anymore because I've gotten better in school so I don't get any home letters at home; well yeah you still get the odd letter home but I don't see the point in sitting there and being bad.

Furthermore, Elsa showed a desire to model the caring characteristics of her teacher by seeking a career in care work:

You know Miss B? I was thinking of going into college – how do I say ... like care, care therapy or something ... and then I want to work my way, try and work in schools.

This attention given to Elsa's home and school issues and the opportunity that she had to discuss her problems correspond to aspects of Noddings's relational care, namely attention and dialogue. Moreover, from this perspective, caring was complete as Elsa was able to recognise the care that she received. Noddings (1995a) alludes to care of these sorts when she argues that 'teachers should demonstrate the capacity to care' (679). In this light, Noddings (1988) argues that teaching is filled with caring occasions and teachers should use teaching moments for caring. Thus, teachers should be ideally equipped to engage in caring relations and should demonstrate an impulse to care as illustrated in Elsa's case. However, for such care to be realised, it must be embraced as a core aspect of teachers' pedagogical practice (Noddings 1990), a proposal which may be made possible through teaching training.

Elsa's account showed that caring moments matter a lot to students and are often the memorable or cherished part of their school experience. This teacher–student relation has been shown to be crucial to students' academic and affective development (Barber 2002) and has been found to be positively associated with learning and school outcomes (Lovat 2010) and a decreased level of student disengagement (Merwin 2002; Frydenberg *et al.* 2005). Moreover, support and care from teachers have been found to be related to young people's pursuit of goals to behave in socially acceptable and responsible ways (Wentzel *et al.* 2010).

Conclusion

The accounts of these three girls confirm the view that teachers seem to show care out of a sense of duty and that there might be a potential mismatch between how teachers feel they are giving care and how students experience it. This variance in students' and teachers' notions of care has resulted in little attention being directed to addressing concerns from students' perspectives. Moreover, the girls' accounts demonstrate that due to their focus on other educational priorities, schools may not always be environments where care is able to flourish. Furthermore, the recent preoccupation with values education and social and emotional learning has led to a specific focus on highly regulated professional caring rather than a school-wide focus on pedagogical care. Besides, within the classroom, barriers to this kind of holistic interest in caring for students may be due to constraints such as the emphasis on what is to be learnt (Silins and Murray-Harvey 2000); the focus on improving instruction (Bryk 1988) or the pressure to produce high test scores (Noddings 1995a).

Where caring moments are experienced they tend to have enduring effects on students, which confirms the need to take a deeper interest in students' well-being. Thus, schools should not solely be a place for learning but one where learning and caring are closely associated. Moreover, relational caring should not be confined to one aspect of school life or be relegated to a course of study in moral or affective education but should be provided within interpersonal relationships that are embedded within pedagogic practices. According to Noddings (2003), this 'pedagogical caring' would begin with the caring and not the pedagogy (70).

On a practical level, teachers can begin to demonstrate caring moments by seeking to establish a positive social climate in their classroom and devoting a little of their time to establishing caring relations with students. Moreover, having some background knowledge about students, obtained either through the school or students themselves, can be a step in that direction as it will help in reaching out to students and responding to them with sensitivity. In this way, teachers would be able to express some concern for students beyond merely imparting knowledge. As such, Lovat (2010) argues that the essence and potency of quality teaching lie in the synergy and balance between academic and affection dimensions of teaching and learning (491).

More than twenty-five years on, many of Noddings's recommendations are yet to be realised as many institutional factors inhibit the establishment of caring relations (Noddings 1995a). However, this does not eliminate the establishment of teacher–student bonding as a viable teaching objective, nor does it diminish the need to incorporate some element of caring within current pedagogical practices. Rather, teachers as carers can be 'change agents' in nurturing care in students (Noddings 1995a). As Bryk (1988) puts it, 'It is a teacher's sense of agape that can unite the academic and moral aims of education and engage students in an education of intellect and will' (279). In view of current institutional impediments, the best way forward should be the incorporation of a specific course of study on 'relational caring' within the initial teacher training programme. In this manner, teachers would be encouraged to focus more of their efforts on matters of care and maintain sustained interpersonal relations with students to ensure that they are cared for or perhaps given opportunities to practice or experience care.

Notes

1 See Gillard (2011) for a timeline of key events in the history of education in England.
2 Form tutors are designated staff charged with the responsibility of overseeing the welfare of a group of students. At the primary school, there is one member of staff who takes on

the dual role of class teacher and form tutor. At the secondary school, the form tutor, unlike those in a primary school, does not necessarily teach the students in their tutor group.

3 The focus on girls' disengagement was significant given that much research emphasis had been placed on understanding boys' underachievement (McIntosh and Houghton 2005).

4 I had taught at the school for two years and also drew on my teaching experiences there.

5 In many parts of the UK young people begin their secondary schooling at the age of 11.

6 Most Further Education colleges in the UK often focus more on vocational courses.

7 The General Certificate of Secondary Education is an academic qualification that is awarded in different subject areas.

8 Number of students on the school's exclusion register.

9 The Office for Standards in Education (Ofsted) which is responsible for the inspection of schools in England, mainly assesses school effectiveness in key areas including teaching and learning.

4 At risk pupils and the 'caring' curriculum

Val Gillies and Yvonne Robinson,
London South Bank University

Introduction

Over the last decade or so interpretations of student care in the context of UK educational institutions have undergone significant change. Pedagogic models have traditionally reproduced a Cartesian split between scholarly rationality associated with educational achievement and emotionality as a disruptive force, resulting in what Lynch and colleagues describe as a history of 'carelessness' in the classroom (Lynch *et al.* 2007; Lynch 2010). Powerful critiques of this dualism from feminists and liberal educationalists have pointed to the impact of affect and social relationships on learning, prompting such concerns to be addressed, but through a regulatory focus on pupil well-being. In this chapter, we document the ways in which care in the classroom has come to embody this very particular meaning, prioritising psychological development, professional competence and risk at the expense of relationality and situated ethics. More specifically we explore how a discourse of professional care has come to frame and structure teacher–pupil interactions in UK schools.

Drawing on data from an ethnographic study of pupils at risk of school exclusion we show how a contemporary preoccupation with notions of personal development and emotional learning shape formal policy and practice in inner-city London schools. We highlight the way in which this apparently progressive and inclusive agenda generates a highly regulatory framework, ordering the ways in which teachers and pupils are expected to experience and express care. We demonstrate how therapeutic discourses prioritising emotion management and the raising of self-esteem position challenging young people as psychologically troubled and in need of formal, professionalised caring interventions. More spontaneous expressions of care and caring between teachers and students are constructed in terms of 'risk'. We show how these institutional meanings operate on a day-to-day basis and how they are interpreted, appropriated and often subverted by teachers and other school staff.

The policy context

Current approaches to care in the classroom have developed in response to a series of formative policy changes initiated by the New Labour Government at the turn of the century. The Every Child Matters (ECM) framework was introduced as a Green Paper in 2003 and was quickly enshrined in the Children Act 2004, implementing what is generally recognised to be one of the most significant policy changes of the post-war era (Read 2010; Simon and Ward 2010). Revolving around the themes of risk and rescue, ECM prompted a radical reorganisation of children's services, encompassing almost every government department and frontline professional. Ostensibly ECM was developed in response to the tragic abuse and murder of 8-year-old Victoria Climbié and the subsequent review highlighting service failures.[1] A key feature of the legislation was the introduction of new structures forcing agencies and professionals to share information and work together to protect children from abuse and neglect. However at the core of ECM is a broader moral and political concern with well-being and the rearing of children as a key mediator of disadvantage and other social problems. This is reflected in a widening out of more traditional understandings of risk to encompass a range of poor outcomes for children including underachievement, school exclusion and poor mental health (Read 2010).

The ECM framework also represents a fundamental plan in the emergence of what Parton (2006) has termed the 'preventative state', with initiatives increasingly directed towards predicting and heading off social problems before they have even manifested. This predominantly operates through the identification of 'at risk' groups within the wider population who are then subject to targeted interventions. Under this legislation schools have been given a prominent role in recognising 'at risk' children and implementing the ECMs' mantra of 'early intervention and effective protection'. More specifically the remit of schools has expanded beyond that of educating to encompass child and family welfare, imposed through a legal duty to recognise and safeguard 'vulnerable' children on their register. As a consequence teachers are now expected to work with a range of professionals to monitor children's development and intervene where necessary. As many commentators have pointed out, the focus of this concern does not extend to addressing the pervasive and engrained structural inequality driving outcomes for children (Hoyle 2008; Simon and Ward 2010). While social and economic disadvantage is articulated in terms of risk, ECM centres instead on 'protective' interpersonal factors such as strong parent–child relations, parental involvement with education, availability of appropriate role models and self-esteem (Reay 2000, 2007; Gillies 2008).

Reflecting this preoccupation with risk, vulnerability and child development, a new significance has been accorded to emotions and social relationships in the classroom. In particular, fears have coalesced around the mental health of pupils who are viewed as lacking the 'soft skills' needed to interact and cooperate as good citizens. New social pressures and sub-standard parenting are depicted as having led to an epidemic of disconnected and emotionally stunted young people facing high-risk futures. Aggression, violence, impulsivity and school disengagement are assumed to result from an inability to communicate and manage feelings. Policy makers have been particularly inspired by US psychologist Daniel Goleman's claims (2006, 1999, 1997) that cultivating 'emotional intelligence' or

EQ could dramatically improve pupils' conduct, attainment and well-being.[2] Such assertions have underpinned a range of school programmes and initiatives designed to teach and nurture emotional literacy, most notably the nationwide UK schools initiative, SEAL (Social and Emotional Aspects of Learning). This programme was introduced at primary and secondary level with the aim of providing 'a whole-curriculum framework and resource for teaching social, emotional and behavioural skills to all pupils' (DfES 2005a: 12). Adapted from Goleman's work, the SEAL strategy centres on five core domains: self-awareness, managing feelings, empathy, motivation and social skills. The principles of SEAL are intended to inform and guide the day-to-day running of schools, alongside structured lessons designed to equip students with the relevant competencies.[3]

While ECM and SEAL are generally viewed as liberal progressive frameworks, their characteristic references to inclusion and well-being mask a more regulatory and reactionary ethos operating through a technicalisation of risk in relation to social and emotional relationships (Hoyle 2008; Piper and Stronach 2008). Children and young people are positioned within this approach as potentially at risk, not only from incompetent parenting but also from teachers who mismanage or abuse their duty of care (Lynch 2010). Guidelines, policies and sanctions operate within schools to ensure this duty is properly discharged and that pupils are appropriately protected. For example, teachers attend formal training in how to safeguard children, are expected to exercise their responsibilities in collaboration with social workers, the police and other agencies, and are subject to criminal record checks and other vetting procedures. As our research demonstrates, the requirement for teachers to foreground and assess children's well-being is operationalised through a therapeutic and professionalised ethos of care which can in practice prioritise instrumental risk aversion above a more expressive relationality.

Pupils at risk of social exclusion: the research framework

The data informing this chapter were drawn from an ESRC (Economic and Social Research Council) funded study of pupils at risk of school exclusion.[4] This ethnographic participatory study focused on 12- to 15-year-old pupils attending Behaviour Support Units (BSUs)[5] in mainstream secondary schools located in disadvantaged inner-city areas. Fieldwork spanned over the course of two years with the researchers based in three secondary schools: two co-educational and one single-sex girls' school. Research methods included participant observation, group activity work and interviews with pupils, their parents and key staff in the schools including headteachers, year heads, BSU managers, mentors and teaching assistants (see Gillies and Robinson 2010a and 2010b for a more detailed discussion of the fieldwork). Each BSU operated as a separate onsite unit within the schools designed to contain difficult pupils and remove them from mainstream classrooms. Somewhat ironically they were administered as part of school inclusion policies.

A total of 73 pupils participated in the study: 24 young women and 49 young men. The sample of pupils drawn from the two co-educational schools was predominantly male. At the time of the research, this largely reflected the ratio of boys to girls attending the BSUs. Pupils came from a range of ethnic backgrounds including white, Black African and Black Caribbean, Turkish, Eastern European, South East Asian and mixed heritage. A majority of the sample were from black and minority ethnic communities, again reflecting the general make-up of the units. Almost all the students lived in areas characterised by high levels of deprivation. Family incomes were generally low and housing was often extremely poor. Another important social context framing our research relates to the serious problem of teenage knife crime that areas surrounding all three schools were experiencing. Through the course of our fieldwork three teenagers known to our research participants were fatally stabbed while several of the participants themselves were hospitalised with knife wounds. These contextual factors, whilst highlighting the emotionality of student experiences, also point to the important and constructive role of care and caring as complex and fluid expressions that are not fixed, but are instead located in and outside of the classroom.

Activities in the BSUs centred largely on the SEAL agenda pursued through circle time,[6] anger management sessions, mentoring and project work. This focus on communication, emotional literacy and self-regulation reflected a broader construction of challenging pupils as developmentally delayed and lacking in personal and social skills. School staff tended to draw on therapeutically oriented explanations of difficult behaviour attributing it to the psychological effects of damaging home lives, adolescent turmoil, poor parenting or undiagnosed disorders (such as Attention Deficient Hyperactivity Disorder or Autistic Spectrum Disorders). In this context teachers were expected to demonstrate the professional nature of their role in addressing the troubled lives of their pupils. However, as our research suggests, this discourse of professional care and the medicalised approach to behaviour it underpins, can conceal a considerably more ambivalent and complex reality.

Professional caring in the classroom

As Woodward (2008) has explored in relation to nursing, the very concept of 'professional caring' could be viewed as a contradiction in terms. By prioritising notions of instrumental competence above unregulated expressive relationality, an essential quality of caring as an organic situated process may be undermined. A similar troubled dynamic can be indentified in the context of education, with understandings of caring as integral to good teaching in tension with measures designed to monitor and regulate proficiency. Educational reforms during the 1980s and 1990s introduced a new ideal of 'the competent employee', undermining identities structured around the notion of vocation (Martin 2010). The introduction of a national curriculum, testing and inspection regimes, and the standards agenda worked to reconfigure and circumscribe teaching practice, placing new emphasis on management and accountability, leaving less and less room for spontaneous expressive caring in the classroom (Lynch *et al.* 2007). In line with the introduction of the ECM framework and the SEAL agenda, caring within schools has been increasingly transformed into a performance indicator in its own right. Care and concern have been formalised as professional responsibilities of educators, to be monitored and regulated accordingly, with personal qualities of kindness and sensitivity overlaid by more manageable routines of 'due care' (Clegg and Rowland 2010).

For example, the General Teaching Council for England (GTCE) introduced the 'Code of Conduct and Practice for Registered Teachers' in 2009, with the first listed principle emphasising the requirement to 'put the well-being, development and progress of children and young people first'. The document specifies how this care and concern should be enacted, with teachers (including supply and temporary teachers) expected to:

- use their professional expertise and judgement to do their best for the children and young people in their care;
- take all reasonable steps to ensure the safety and well-being of children and young people under their supervision;
- follow their school's child protection policies and procedures;
- establish and maintain appropriate professional boundaries in their relationships with children and young people;
- demonstrate self-awareness and take responsibility for accessing help and support in order to ensure that their own practice does not have a negative impact on learning or progress or put children and young people at risk of harm;
- use appropriate channels to raise concerns about the practice of other teachers or professionals if this has a negative impact on learning or progress or risks harming children and young people.

Significantly this sets out a vision of professional care in which the themes of proficiency, personal distance, risk evaluation and fitness to practice are stressed in contrast to emotional commitment, compassion and respect for the different experiences and identities of pupils.

The school staff participating in our research drew heavily on principles of professional caring in making sense of their everyday practice, but as our analysis demonstrates, these could be articulated to achieve very different ends. For some, regulations governing responsibilities of care provided them with an objective framework to guide and limit troubling interactions with pupils. The ability to manage turbulent relationships and discharge duties of care with dispassionate skill was highly valued by some teachers, particularly in the context of large classrooms and multiple social deprivations. To be able to formally address concerns about behaviour and welfare while minimising personal anxiety and involvement could promote a sense of efficacy alongside a positive identity as a caring professional. This was often achieved through recourse to psychologised discourses emphasising developmental difficulties, with teachers positioning themselves as addressing and alleviating such problems. 'Troubled' and 'troublesome' were readily conflated through a focus on bad behaviour as a manifestation of emotional disorder or deficit, ensuring the wider social and structural context framing conduct remained unexplored. In fact most school staff carefully policed pedagogic boundaries to ensure the more disturbing aspects of pupils' lives were kept out of classroom discussions and interventions (see Gillies 2011).

Despite the professed emphasis on sharing emotions as a therapeutic, remedial initiative, SEAL-based activities were structured by unspoken boundaries which limited the feelings and thoughts pupils were permitted to voice. As has been outlined elsewhere (Gillies 2011), only certain forms of emotional expression were sanctioned in classroom interventions and these were monitored carefully by the teacher. For example, Kate Blackman,[7] a BSU manager who organised various circle time groups, described how she often had to remove pupils who were too forthcoming.

> In a workshop you might realise, very quickly, that, 'This is not the appropriate support for you.' . . . and that's happened before, where, you know, some girl is talking so inappropriately about stuff, that 'This is not the right place for you to be talking about, you know, sharing your, your home life here.'

As the GTCE's Code of Conduct and Practice demonstrates, new caring responsibilities accorded to teachers have been accompanied by new regulations and guidance stressing the importance of boundaries and professional conduct. Some school staff placed this concept at the centre of their practice, adopting a strong identity around competent professionalism, particularly in the context of relationships with troubled and troublesome pupils. For example, Susan James, a teaching assistant, emphasised the importance of her knowledge, proficiency and ability to maintain professional boundaries.

> When people say, 'Oh, that was, you know, managed so well', I had the training and they introduced Tom Greenfield, who is a doctor and a behaviour management specialist from Australia, and his strategies and methods work. And I always believe the way you start off is the way you must continue, and keep a professional . . . er . . . keep professional boundaries.

Investment in a professional approach to caring could reflect a strikingly technical approach to notions of child-rearing, with parents often depicted by school staff as suboptimal in their practices. For example, a classroom mentor described her preference for dealing with foster carers above parents because of their professional training and greater competence. Parents could be viewed as caring too much about their children, to the extent that it clouded their judgement and precluded rational behaviour, or caring too little, or at least failing to demonstrate the caring actions deemed appropriate by the schools (see Gillies 2010).

Teachers were particularly likely to invoke the spectre of incompetent or disinterested parents to make sense of disruptive behaviour in the first place. Even where teachers recognised the efforts and good intentions of parents, a BSU referral tended to be viewed as evidence of parental failure adequately to care for a child. Interviews with school staff highlighted the extent to which understandings of caring, inclusive teaching practice are currently built around psychologised assessments of parental competence and personal well-being – as the following quote from Jocelyn Reed, a BSU manager demonstrates.

> You've got students who come with a range of public background issues relating to home, so therefore you have students who are 'non-attendants', students who don't like school at all and students who have various home situations which causes them NOT wanting to come into school. Whether because they feel they are going to be intimidated by other students? And those that can't really make friends with . . . they can't socialise. Then you've got the students that come in but they've got behavioural issues, which probably is linked to the way the home is run or there's no order or they just speak to their parents anyhow, and so they think they can come into school and conduct themselves in that way. So you have quite a wide range of students coming in.

Relational care and emotional investments

While strong adherence to ideals of boundaried dispassion and notions of professional good practice could allow school staff to manage risk, experience a sense of competence and reduce personal feelings of emotional distress and anxiety, most also demonstrated a more connected expression of care in their everyday encounters with pupils. Highlighting the extent to which discourses of professional care can obscure ethical dilemmas facing school staff in the classroom, some mainstream teachers described a passionate dedication to the well-being and educational development of academically promising students, while adopting a more clinical detachment in discharging a duty of care towards those less able and more challenging in their behaviour.

For example, Mr Phillips, a year head, discussed his passionate enthusiasm to ensuring those in his class learnt for their own sakes.

> I know most of the kids in my Year really, really well because I MADE myself get to know them well. Every time I get a free period I go in their class and I walk around . . . I go round the playground . . . I talk to 'em . . . I have my dinner in the canteen and some of them sit down and talk . . . so I know what's going on in my Year. I know what the problems are and I know who has got what going on cos they talk to you and they also know that if they've got a problem they come and knock on the door and I'll speak to them. On top of that, they know that if they kick off and I get the Incident Report I will find 'em and I'll come down like a ton of bricks on them. I'll be fair but if they take the piss they'll be dealt with most severely because if they are taking the piss out of me or their teacher then they're NOT learning and I don't give a damn about anything else apart from THEM learning, THEM coming out of here, THEM going to college, doing well and having a beautiful life and if I have to kick their backsides a hundred times before they leave school to do that then I'll do that!

However, the year head was considerably less concerned about those he regarded as lacking in potential, as the following quote from him demonstrates.

> I was told that when I first started teaching, 'Accept the fact that 5–10% of the kids you will NEVER get through to and they WILL fail.' I did my training next to one of the biggest housing estates in the country and really rough . . . 'You know, some of the boys are really frustrating me' and he [headteacher] said 'you've GOT to accept it, 5–10% you will NOT get through to and there are systems in place for them but don't kick yer own ass about it, it's just the way the system works!' It's really hard to deal with that though because you start off all idealistic and I am still a bit idealistic but I know there are certain kids I can't get near and I don't get pissed off with it anymore and just work with the ones that I can.

In the high-pressured environs of a secondary school classroom a teacher's time and attention is limited, with competing demands. The effort required to engage troublesome and/or needy students could be viewed as disadvantaging those more willing and able. Dealing with challenging behaviour in the classroom was often viewed as a distraction which compromised teachers' ability to practice care and commitment. By drawing on a formal discourse of professional care teachers were sometimes able to frame exclusion of difficult pupils from mainstream lessons as a caring act designed to better meet particular 'difficult' children's needs (Clegg and Rowland 2010; Florian and Black-Hawkins 2011).

In relation to the BSU staff expressions of care towards attendees they often went beyond the boundaried accounts associated with professionalism. Teachers, mentors and teaching assistants could develop strong relationships with pupils at risk of school exclusion, sometimes placing them in conflict with mainstream staff. BSU workers commonly assumed the role of advocates for accused students, negotiating with headteachers, appealing against decisions to permanently exclude and constructing pathways back into mainstream education. As the following quote demonstrates, Dave Stirling, a teacher and BSU manager made strident efforts to challenge decisions that might see particular students marginalised:

> Why is the Headteacher going 'Der . . . der' and giving the name of this kid?' And you think to yourself, 'Well, all right, it's because he is about a foot taller than everybody else out there, he is a young black man, he is quite defensive in the way that he responds to authority', and those are the reasons why, I think, that it's . . . you've got locked into this situation where *he* is always the one who is being called, yet there are people around him behaving badly and all this sort of thing . . . and at no point was I making excuses for this kid's behaviour, and neither was his father. However, the idea is, how can you enter a dialogue with the boy, you know, unless you're straight with him, and say, 'Look, I think I understand what you're saying. I understand that there is this situation. Yes, racism exists. Yes, there are racist practices going on in school. Our job really is to unpick those in your favour. This is your

entitlement, your education' . . . it's empowerment, it's advocacy, it's actually standing up for some of these people.

In drawing attention to institutional shortcomings and prejudices rather than personal pathology, Dave articulated an emotionally involved expression of caring rooted in relationality, reflexivity and respect for the individual feelings of the pupils concerned. Yet he also sought to appropriate the language of professional caring as an objective framework to validate his arguments with staff in the mainstream school. He discussed initiatives such as ECM and SEAL as part of a more general 'inclusion agenda', and described how he would quote policy literature in school negotiations to secure better outcomes for pupils at risk of exclusion.

> Along comes this concept called 'Inclusion', in'it! And then you think, 'Oh yeah, this is interesting, in'it. There is actually a group of people out there, or a tendency, if you like, that says it is absolutely correct to *include* people in situations, not to *exclude*' . . . I suppose like everything else, I want to see it actually articulated in reality. And actually, I then began to understand that I could actually be part of that articulation in reality, support it politically. So the arguments about whether this kid should be excluded or not excluded, suddenly became non-arguments. There is no argument. He should be included in education . . . but an interest in all that, and then a legitimisation of that really, through this Inclusion initiative, certainly gives me some kind of actual status in terms of what I'm trying to . . . what I feel like is the right thing to do.

However, Dave's passionate determination to secure justice for his pupils did not endear him to his colleagues in the mainstream school.

Many staff felt he condoned bad behaviour and demonstrated unprofessional practice by defending troublesome pupils, although he was highly respected and valued by the pupils themselves. After 26 years as a teacher (with much of this time spent specialising in behaviour support) Dave received a redundancy notice in the context of cuts to the school budget. This appeared to be part of a more general move to direct greater resources towards improving the GCSE exam results in response to government edicts to raise standards or face closure.

Pushing the boundaries

Some staff members were sceptical of professional caring discourses and felt they were too constraining in work with children and young people. For example, Glen Taylor, a BSU mentor, expressed some resentment towards the boundaries he was expected to maintain in his relations with pupils. Glen often drew on his own personal experiences as a young black man who had experienced marginalisation from education. He commonly employed slang or spoke in Jamaican patois and used humour and physicality to relate to students.

Glen was aware that his methods were at odds with the expectations of the school, but he built strong and productive relationships with BSU attendees and their parents. He felt he should have the leeway to pursue this more expressive form of care.

> To tell you the truth a mentor has individual work because you are working with different minds . . . but the senior people are saying, 'this is the way we want it, this is the way to be supportive'. But if that way is not getting through, you can bring a horse to water but you can't make him drink, so therefore, it could be the actual thing that you're trying to get them to do that is messing them up . . . they say I'm not allowed to cuddle students because I'd be giving off the wrong message . . . or the things that they've gone through, you know, it could be damaging. You know girls having crushes and if they've got insecurities, turning that crush into a rumour and into something else. So really it's covering yourself and them . . . So, I can understand why but it just becomes out of this world.

Institutional sanctions against physical contact with children and young people to express care particularly where a pupil is distressed and in need of comfort, reinforces the emotionally detached ideal through which professional care is expected to be administered. Yet as research by Piper and Stronach (2008) highlights, 'no touch' policies in educational establishments are more often born out of a concern to protect staff rather than children and can be enforced to the detriment of children and young people's emotional well-being. Stronach and Piper (2008: 146) stress the importance of the child's perspective in judging physical contact, rather than being informed by overinflated, adult-led 'assumptions of horror, harm, and abuse'.

Despite his success in connecting with deeply marginalised pupils, Glen's unorthodox practices were viewed as suspect by some of his colleagues, particularly the BSU teaching assistant Susan James. Susan's strong adherence to notions of professionalism and boundaried discharge of due care led her to repeatedly question the appropriateness and safety of Glen's relationships.

> I think it's a very, very clear line. You are *not* friends. Friends support each other to the degree where you have access to that person. We have a very closed shop. You're in here between here and here, and this is a work environment for you to benefit yourself, and we are here for that purpose. I think it gets distorted, and I think the distortion then becomes a problem to the student, because the stability is not there. Because when it comes, when push comes to shove, the student stands on their own, where a friend would be able to defend you right to the end . . . you know, so we're not friends. We don't have a friendship as a friendship, you know, and I think we should make that clear, and just using the same language as the student, you know, I think you've got to be a positive role model, you've got to be somebody who's moving on. 'I understand where you're coming from, the street, and the street

talk', you know, leave that outside, let them come into school, into the Behaviour Support Centre, this is a safe environment, leave that where it is, you know.

Susan's highly instrumental account of the role of school staff to provide a formal, stable and safe environment for pupils contrasted sharply with Glen's more expressive emphasis on providing love as a family member might. While Susan emphasised the 'closed shop' of work hours, Glen admitted worrying about particular young people when he was outside of school and even unofficially 'fostered' a former pupil. Susan found the uncontained nature of Glen's involvement so concerning that she eventually left the BSU to work elsewhere. Glen's tenure at the school was also short-lived. He was suspended when the school re-examined his check from the Criminal Record Bureau and identified a spent minor conviction which they claimed had gone unnoticed when they first employed him.

Care in the classroom: discourse and practice

In this chapter we have examined how meanings and experiences of care in the classroom have shifted to embrace new understandings of professional practice. A boundaried, instrumental exercise of care demonstrating competence and neutrality is expected to be prioritised above more relationally embedded concern towards particular pupils and their well-being. We have explored the specific context of Behaviour Support Units and the extent to which BSU attendees are formally constructed as in need of caring interventions to support and shape their personal development. As a result the complex social and structural challenges framing pupil behaviour are routinely reframed in the language of developmental psychology, with teachers expected to identify needs and address them clinically through SEAL-based activities.

We have also shown how such discourses of professional care in the classroom foreground issues of risk, ostensibly in terms of child well-being, but perhaps more meaningfully in relation to the career security of the practising staff member. In an effort to predict and foreclose potential threats to pupil welfare, risks become magnified in line with professional responsibilities to prioritise safety. Under the new managerialist agenda governing schools, the notion of care becomes reduced to performativity through the monitoring and regulation of pupil–staff relationships, particularly in relation to risk. As a result concern is directed towards the documenting of 'due care' rather than towards seeking the understandings and relationships that would enable more realistic evaluations of pupil welfare. As we have outlined, more involved and informed pupil–staff relationships are likely to be viewed as inherently risky in their own right.

By drawing on our ethnographic research we have explored how school staff made sense of the expectations placed on them and the ways in which care was expressed within and beyond conceptualisations of professional boundaries. Discourses of professional caring in the classroom were often articulated to manage the new burdens of risk and responsibilities now carried by schools. This was characterised by personal detachment and efforts to avoid witnessing or knowing too much about pupils' lives. Some even constructed pupil–teacher relationships as inherently risky, emphasising the duty of staff to safeguard children through maintaining a protective emotional and physical distance. Nevertheless, as we observed, professional structures and risk anxieties were also routinely overcome during the course of everyday interactions, with school staff displaying strong attachments to particular pupils.

As our analysis demonstrates, conceptualisations of care in the classroom are complex and mutable reflecting the different interests and standpoints of staff members. Despite exhortations to the contrary, attention to the well-being of pupils is unevenly distributed ensuring some receive committed support and protection while others are subject to arm's length exercise of professional duties and responsibilities. That these differences often map on to broader experiences of inclusion and exclusion suggests greater attention should be paid to teacher–pupil relationships in order to better understand the production and reproduction of inequality.

Notes

1 Headed by Lord Laming, *The Victoria Climbié Inquiry Report* (2003) inquired into the circumstances leading to and surrounding the death of Victoria Climbié, identifying gross service failures and making recommendations for future best practice.
2 See Goleman's *Emotional Intelligence* (1997) for genesis of ideas on emotional literacy.
3 See Gillies (2011) for a critique of the how the SEAL agenda is operationalised within secondary schools.
4 The project, Disruptive Behaviour in the Classroom: Exploring the Social Subjectivity of Disaffection was funded by the Economic and Social Research Council under grant number RES-061-23-0073.
5 Behaviour Support Units are facilities (often self-contained) within mainstream schools and are designed to address issues around conduct. Pupils are sent to the units for varying amounts of time, ranging from weeks to years. The terminology used to describe these units varied between schools. We use Behaviour Support Unit as a generic term to describe them all.
6 Circle time, as administered in the BSUs we were based in, aimed at giving pupils the opportunity to express and share their feelings with support staff and other BSU attendees. The design and layout of classrooms, as 'circle time' suggests, are usually set out 'in the round'.
7 Staff names have been changed to protect their identity.

5 A discourse analytic study of power as caring relations in Philippine university classrooms

Mabelle Victoria, The Open University

Introduction

Using audio recordings of naturalistic[1] classroom interactions as data, this chapter explores a re-conceptualisation of power as caring relations. The perspective adopted here is derived from Bloome and colleagues (2005) which offers a feminist rethinking of power as 'power with' rather than 'power over'. Intrinsic in their model is the belief that *communities*[2] like the classroom are more than a collection of individuals but also a network of emotional, caring connections between teachers and students. This chapter draws on Brown and Levinson's (1987) social interaction theory to illustrate how Filipino professors[3] use language to show care by the strategic downplaying of power and the use of linguistic devices that invoke solidarity.

It has been claimed that the school is a 'universe of language' (Bourdieu and Passeron 1994: 19); a universe where language serves as the object of the lesson, the medium of instruction and the means with which learning takes place (Bloome *et al.* 2005). Language is not only a way to *say* things; it is a way of 'doing' and 'being' in the world (Gee 2005). We use language to promise, to apologise, to share knowledge, to express affection, to criticise and so on. We use language to present an identity of who we are and how we want other people to see us. When we want to be perceived as 'highly educated' we tend to use discourse associated with being scholarly; when we want to appear friendly, we choose words that convey warmth and informality. Given that language pervades learning and teaching activities, I suggest that a language-focused study using a discourse analytic approach can provide useful insights into the linguistic manifestations of power as caring relations.

Power, caring relations and language

Power is one of the most basic features of human interaction (Johnstone 2002; Vine 2004) and yet has escaped satisfactory definition. In this chapter power is viewed as having two levels. The first level is fixed, it is 'given', vested upon by the institution resulting in an asymmetrical relationship between professors and students. The second level pertains to the discursively constructed and negotiable nature of power (Locher 2004; Rees-Miller 2000; Victoria 2009a, 2009b). For example, as Takano (2005: 656) illustrates, Japanese women in powerful executive positions may use less powerful language to downplay their authority which makes it easier for them to gain support and empathy from their subordinates. At other times, they may highlight the asymmetrical nature of the interaction to demand conformity and deference.

Bloome *et al.* (2005: 162) propose that power can be conceptualised as 'a set of relations among people and among social institutions that may shift from one situation to another' which makes the 'processes that structure relationships among people' as its localisation instead of individuals or groups. In other words, power is seen as 'having the potential to bring people together for mutual benefit, both with regard to social relationships and with regard to other accomplishments' (Bloome *et al.* 2005: 165). Bloome *et al.* point out that in the power-as-caring relations model, personhood and community are re-conceptualised so that the following points are taken to be true:

• that emotional and caring connections to others are essential to every person;
• that a classroom be seen as a community that consists of members who not only share a geographic location, interests, goals and history but, more importantly, a foregrounding of caring relations amongst its members (Bloome *et al.* 2005: 165).

Power in the classroom

Within Philippine Higher Education contexts, professors are said to hold the seat of power in the highly teacher-centred and authoritarian classroom (Licuanan 1994). They are considered as the 'supreme authority' whose words are accepted by the students as the 'gospel truth' (Tiongson 1994: 197). Indeed, they are institutionally sanctioned to give or withhold praise, commend or criticise, and express approval or disapproval.

The professorial authority seems to be Janus-faced: one side magnifies power, thus creating hierarchy, and the other side downplays it, thus invoking solidarity. The asymmetrical relationship tends to create social distance between professors and students. It can be argued that social distance needs to be decreased in order to create an atmosphere conducive to caring relations. In this chapter I show how professors use language to subvert institutional power to pave the ground for the establishment of caring relations. As Locher (2004: 2) notes:

> power . . . reflects the degree of solidarity between interactants. One may, for example, exercise power merely to prove that one is in a more powerful position, thus emphasising difference. Or one may show restraint in the way power is exercised, taking the addressee's face [see below] needs into consideration and thus indicating some degree of solidarity as well.

Paradox of pedagogical and relational goals

The quality of the relationship between academics and students is underpinned by a constant interplay between the pedagogical and relational goals. As Nguyen (2007) suggests, professors are expected to deliver lessons prescribed by the institution; they are, at the same time, expected to attend to their students' relational needs. This creates a paradox: to achieve the instructional goals, academics cannot avoid performing speech acts that can potentially cause hurt feelings or embarrassment such as disagreeing with students' ideas, correcting their errors, giving negative feedback, giving orders and so on. These speech acts that may threaten harmonious relations need to be mitigated with linguistic strategies that show care. The interface between caring relations and pedagogy is made more complex by the power differential between professors and students. To 'do' power means emphasising one's authority, thus creating social distance, and to do 'caring' means evoking symmetry and intimacy, thus minimising social distance.

Power and caring: a linguistic framework

Power and caring are both very abstract concepts. Their conceptualisations inevitably reflect the researcher's disciplinary allegiances and research contexts. In this section I explore how a theory of social interaction can help us unpack how the two concepts are discursively enacted. To achieve this end, I use Brown and Levinson's (1987) theory of politeness as a descriptive framework for the linguistic operationalisation of power as caring relations. Simply put, to emphasise power means to create social distance (power over), and to downplay it means to reduce symmetry allowing more space for social closeness (power with).

Brown and Levinson's (1987) theory of politeness[4] provides us with a comprehensive taxonomy of linguistic strategies that allows us to see how language can be used to discursively downplay or highlight power, and to soften face threat as instantiations of care. The theory has been criticised by various scholars (see Eelen 2001; Gu 1990; Lakoff and Ide 2005; Spencer-Oatey 2000) who question its universal application and cross-cultural applicability. However, I argue that the theory's emphasis on preserving harmony and avoiding conflict make it a suitable descriptive framework for exploring caring relations between students and their professors.

Face and the mitigation of face-threatening acts

Face, a concept borrowed from Goffman (1967), is the heart of Brown and Levinson's (1987: 61) theory of politeness. Roughly equivalent to self-esteem, face is defined as 'the public self-image that every member wants to claim for himself'. It is argued that everybody has face and face needs, namely positive face needs and negative face needs. Positive face needs refer to an individual's desire to belong and to be well thought of, liked and admired by others; negative face needs refer to a person's desire to act freely, unimpeded and not to be imposed upon by others. In Brown and Levinson's approach, to use positive or 'solidarity' politeness strategies means to use language that invokes belonging and solidarity; negative or 'deference' politeness means to use language that orients to the addressees' wants to be left alone and to be free from imposition. The mitigation of the face-threatening act is the key notion of Brown and Levinson's (1987) politeness theory. These face-threatening acts can result in loss of face and an intimidating classroom environment. In such an atmosphere, professors who want to foreground caring relations over pedagogy need to put the instructional task on hold to restore face and preserve harmony (Brown and Levinson 1987: 285). Simply put, I suggest that to be caring means to use language that respects the other person's need to belong, to be admired and liked (positive face), and to be left alone (negative face). A teacher, for example, who considers that a blatant correction of a student's answer is too face-threatening, may choose to give partial agreement (*yeah, but . . .*), repeat the student's answer with a rising intonation to indicate an indirect challenge, or not say anything at all. To soften a directive with solidarity politeness professors might say:

A: 'C'mon guys, we need to work harder this term,' instead of
B: 'You have to work harder this term.'

In A, the speaker uses solidarity strategies which are signalled by the use of informal language (*c'mon guys* which is less authoritarian) and the inclusive pronoun 'we' when 'you' could have been used. The utterance might have been intended as criticism, but with linguistic politeness, the student's self-esteem is preserved. The use of 'you' in B has a distancing and disapproving tone. Utterance A is more caring than B because A demonstrates the speaker's desire to maintain the students' face. To cushion the act of disagreeing, a professor might use A instead of B as the following example shows:

A: 'Well, yes, sort of, but I think that might not be what the author is trying to say.'
B: 'No, that is not what the author is trying to say.'

The deference strategies used in A are partial agreement (*yes, sort of*), a softening hedge phrase (*I think*) and modal verb in the subjunctive form (*might*) to mitigate the disagreement or correction. Even the initial 'well' seems to soften the act of disagreeing by signalling hesitation. I propose that the use of these linguistic devices when performing potentially face-threatening acts such as giving orders, disagreeing, criticising and so on are manifestations of caring relations. They are clear attempts by the speaker to signal that they are taking the other person's esteem needs into consideration. Brown and Levinson's (1987) linguistic taxonomy of face-mitigation strategies is shown in Table 5.1:

Table 5.1 Brown and Levinson's taxonomy of positive and negative politeness strategies

Negative (deference) politeness	*Positive (solidarity) politeness*
Be direct 1 Be conventionally indirect.	*Claim common ground* 1 Notice, attend to H (his/her interests, wants, needs, goods).
Don't presume/assume 2 Question, hedge.	2 Exaggerate (interest, approval, sympathy with). 3 Intensify interest to H.
Don't coerce Hearer (H) 3 Be pessimistic. 4 Minimise the imposition 5 Give deference.	4 Use in-group identity markers 5 Seek agreement. 6 Avoid disagreement. 7 Presuppose/raise/assert common ground. 8 Joke.
Communicate Speaker's (S) want not to impinge on Hearer 6 Apologise. 7 Impersonalise S and H. 8 State the FTA (face-threatening act) as a general rule. 9 Nominalise.	*Convey that S and H are cooperators* 9 Assert or presuppose S's knowledge of and concern for H's wants. 10 Offer, promise. 11 Be optimistic. 12 Include both S and H in the activity. 13 Give (or ask for) reasons. 14 Assume or assert reciprocity
Redress other wants of H's 10 Go on record as incurring a debt, or as not indebting H.	*Fulfil H's wants* 15 Give gifts to H (goods, sympathy, understanding, cooperation).

Source: Brown and Levinson (1987)

Notes: S = Speaker; H = Hearer.

Data collection and analysis

Methods of data collection

The research site for this broadly ethnographic study is the Philippines, a multicultural and multilingual South East Asian archipelago. English and Filipino (also known as Tagalog) are the country's two official languages, with English used as the principal medium of instruction. The data, collected in May 2008 via non-participant observation, consist of 25 hours of audio recordings from four Higher Education institutions. I used two digital recorders to record the classroom talk and took notes during the sessions. I also engaged in brief informal chats with teachers and students during breaks.

Analytic framework: an eclectic approach in the study of language in interaction

Inspiration for data analysis derives from a combination of insights from Conversation Analysis (CA) and Interactional Sociolinguistics (IS). IS is the study of language in use in specific contexts which attempts to explain how interlocutors interpret each other's communicative intention and how they negotiate meaning in interaction (see Gumperz 1999, 2001; Swann and Leap 2000; Tannen 2005). CA focuses on the micro-structural aspects of talk based on the dynamics of turn-taking which accounts for the successful management and orderliness of everyday language (see Sacks *et al.* 1974; Eggins and Slade 1997). It is argued that a turn-by-turn analysis of spoken discourse can enable the researcher to 'discover and explicate the practices through which interactants produce and understand conduct in conversation' (Drew 2005: 73). The analysis done here and the transcription conventions[5] applied are not as detailed as is required in a 'pure' CA study. I have borrowed the basic mechanics of CA as a way to demonstrate the participants' joint efforts in meaning making.

Linguistic devices to express caring relations

This section illustrates how professors delicately balance their pedagogical and relational objectives. First, I explore how a female professor mitigates the potentially face-threatening speech act of giving an order (e.g. giving homework), thus instantiating 'power with' rather than 'power over'. Second, I illustrate how different professors and students build caring relations by using the linguistic devices of in-group identity markers, language-switching and story-telling.

Balancing act: giving orders and showing care

In the following are extracts taken from an undergraduate class taught by Professor Neri (P. Neri in the extracts). The excerpts were taken from four hours of observation over two consecutive days. Prof. Neri was talking about a writing assignment she wanted the students to do over the weekend. It can be inferred from the Professor's use of redressive language that she considered giving this particular homework threatening to the students' negative face (the need to be left alone and be freed from imposition) requiring a four-step process. In the extracts, I use *S* for a single student speaker, *Ss* for multiple student speakers.

Step 1: Paving the ground for giving homework

1	*P. Neri*	so, question, 'am I going to write a *ten-page* essay for my
2		argumentative essay to persuade?' the answer is no, ok?
3	*S*	ok, twenty? (in a light-hearted tone)
4	*Ss*	(laughter)
5	*P. Neri*	(laughs) NOT twenty, twenty is already a research paper
6	*Ss*	(laughter)

Line 1 illustrates Prof. Neri's use of linguistic resources to attend to the negative and positive face wants of her students. By using active voicing 'am I going to write . . . ' with the personal pronoun 'I' she displaces her identity as teacher and assumes the role of a student which helps in claiming common ground. Her humorously taking on a student voice demonstrates her awareness of her students' concerns. Her choice of the word 'ten' (*ten-page essay*) is negative politeness output 'to minimise the size of the imposition'. Prof. Neri proceeds to deliver her directive:

Step 2: Softening the directive

7	*P. Neri*	I want you to write MAY::BE between a three to five page
8		essay, depends on how heavy your topic was. some
9		people have very difficult topics, some people have
10		easier ones ok? erm so we will start
11		doing the writing next week so I want you to start getting
12		getting the books so that Monday I want you to have the
13		books with you. the only way to write at all is for you to
14		have the books first ok? so tomorrow
15		read pages 158 to 160 that's what we will discuss. I
16		hope we'll end a little bit earlier cuz it's any way a Friday
17		erm ok?

In line 7, Prof. Neri says that it is not a *ten* but actually a *three to five page* essay that she wanted the students to write – so the 'hypothetically' huge imposition in line 1 has been minimised. It is hedged with *maybe* and *I want* which she also used for lines 11 and 12. In line 15, she gave an unmitigated order (*read pages 158 to 160*). It can be inferred that she considers the reading assignment not face-threatening at all. However in line 16 (*I hope we'll end . . . Friday*) she uses positive politeness strategy to 'give an offer or promise'. According to Brown and Levinson (1987: 125), speakers may stress their cooperation with the hearers by claiming that whatever it is the hearers want, they want for them too. Solidarity politeness strategy 'assume or assert reciprocity' is also contained in line 16 by 'fulfilling H's want for some X' (Brown and Levinson 1987: 129). So Prof. Neri is satisfying her students' need to belong (positive face) by giving them gifts of sympathy, understanding and cooperation. She is also putting emphasis on 'power with' and not 'power over'.

After line 17, there was a question from the students about the assignment due date (not included here). Prof. Neri then continues:

Step 3: Negotiating symmetry

21	*P. Neri*	It's just one short essay, three pages,
22		which I assume we will finish MUCH faster than
23		the ten-page we did today right? ok ? and I want you to start getting
24		your sources so that on Monday we have time to take notes in class ok
25		YOU CAN actually start taking notes erm at home on Saturday and
26		Sunday while I labour checking your test papers ok coz I still have not
27		finished the (coughs)
28		the short seat work I gave so maybe two or three more and then your
29		actual essays. I normally spend my weekends checking, ok ? (laughs)

One of the ways in which we can tell when speakers are being careful to give an order is the length of the utterance (e.g. *lend me £20.00* vs. *I was wondering if maybe you could . . .*). In Step 3, Prof. Neri could have said a swift 'use the weekend to get your essay references ready for Monday' to tell students what she wanted them to do. But from lines 21 to 29, we see a mixture of solidarity politeness and deference positive politeness: *just* in line 21 is her attempt to minimise the imposition; use of the inclusive pronoun *we* (lines 22, 23 and 24) to appeal to solidarity and to avoid the use of the pronoun *you* which is an intrinsically face-threatening act. Using an inclusive 'we' form when 'you' or 'me' is meant, invokes cooperative assumptions which mitigates the act of giving a directive (Brown and Levinson 1987: 127). In lines 26 and 29 above (*I labour checking your test papers, I normally spend my weekends checking, ok?*), Prof. Neri seems to convey the message that 'we are in this together, I am also giving up my weekend to do school work'. In Brown and Levinson's terms, it is a solidarity strategy 'assume and assert reciprocity' implying that 'I'll do X for you, so do Y for me' (Brown and Levinson 1987: 129).

Step 4: Navigating between pedagogical and relational goals

The following extracts were taken the day after the extract above. Prof. Neri refers back to the essay mentioned the day before.

1	*P. Neri*	that, I would like you to do on Monday.
2		I'm LETTING you off early, in fact
3		half an hour early ok (.3) so that there will be no excuse not to have
4		any materials for- on Monday okay you have you have plenty of time
5		so get your notes first so by next week you already have an outline.
6		we'll revise your thesis here so that you don't have to worry about it
7		at home. write your essay Friday Saturday Sunday at home ok,
8		so okay that's our game plan for next week.

The extracts illustrate how Prof. Neri's institutional power as teacher interfaces with 'doing' power and 'doing' caring. Line 3 embodies Prof. Neri's authority with '*so that there will be no excuse*'. Notice that this voice of authority, while carrying force, is still mitigated by the use of a general and agent-less construction. Instead of saying '*you won't have any excuses*', Prof. Neri uses '*there will be no excuse*'. Line 7 carries the most direct order, an unmitigated '*write your essay Friday Saturday Sunday at home ok*' which can be considered as an impingement on the students' negative face want to act freely. In line 8, '*so*' is used to mark 'pseudo-agreement' when in fact there was none (Brown and Levinson 1987: 115) and '*our*' implies cooperative effort when the plan seems to be just Prof. Neri's. It can be argued that the whole utterance '*that's our game plan*' is Prof. Neri's way of emphasising power; quite similar to the use of tactical summaries in negotiations where one of the parties presents a summing up move that's favourable to their cause and unfavourable to the interlocutor (Charles and Charles 1999: 74). The use of 'game plan' can be interpreted as Prof. Neri's use of metaphor to call upon solidarity that they are on the same team. It might also have been intended to connote fun (instead of burden) which is what *'game'* brings up.

The point I wish to make is that it took Prof. Neri four stages, over two days, to give her students homework that needed to be done over the weekend. Her discourse strategies reflect the constant navigation between prioritising pedagogical goals and relational needs of the students. It becomes clearer when we bring more contextual information into our interpretation. The course took place in May, the height of the summer season in the Philippines when people usually flock to the beaches and countryside. Prof. Neri was aware that getting the students to give up a weekend to do homework was a huge imposition. So, she had to use a mixture of linguistic strategies to show caring relations without relinquishing her professorial power.

Establishing social cohesion in talk

In this second illustration, I show how different professors downplay their institutional power through the use of in-group identity markers, language-switching and story-telling. I suggest that these resources help professors convey the message that they do not just want to teach a lesson; they want to make sure that it is in a caring manner.

Extract 1: Use of in-group language

In the following extract, the class has just finished discussing a poem about reminiscing. Professor Lagdameo (P. Lag in extracts) was trying to connect the poem to the 'lived experiences' of his students.

1 *P. Lag*   what do you call that a <u>memory</u> <u>candy</u> or <u>something</u> your <u>happy</u> <u>candy</u>
                your <u>thought candy or something</u> ,
2   it's something he can pull out of his
3   memory bank when he's getting low or feeling bored,
4   <u>think back,</u> <u>do you guys do that?</u>

Here, Prof. Lagdameo used several markers of positive politeness: in-group language or slang (*memory/happy candy*) thereby claiming common ground; use of *'you guys'* which presupposes familiarity and invokes camaraderie, use of vague language (*something*) which relies on the 'inevitable association with shared knowledge' (Brown and Levinson 1987: 111). In a study of social cohesion in business meetings Pullin Stark (2007) found that the use of vague language helps in the establishment of informality and decreases the distance between chairpersons and meeting participants. 'Candy' as used by Prof. Lagdameo is a popular term amongst Filipino teenagers. By using their terminology, Prof. Lagdameo signals to the students that they share perspectives and he is interested in their world.

As Prof. Lagdameo continued with the discussion, he asked the class to share their pleasant memories of Boracay, a popular holiday destination for the students. Prof. Lagdameo knew his students' interests and lifestyles so he was able to pursue topics that are 'closer to home'. The professor managed to turn the lesson from simply discussing a poem to showing interest in his students' life outside the university premises. I highlight below the linguistic devices that Prof. Lagdameo used to create symmetry:

- Contractions/Slang: It's *kinda* like . . . / you *gotta* . . .
- Informal vocabulary: he was actually just *goofing* around
- Tagalog expressions: *Pwede na! /Grabe no*? ((That'll do. Horrible, isn't it))

The importance of slang and contractions as an indicator of social relationship is taken up by Morand (1996: 547). He argues that there is a big difference, for example, between 'How' ya doin'?' and 'How are you doing?' The former sounds friendlier and more intimate while the latter can seem more formal and distant. He adds that one of the former presidents of the United States was coached to use phonological slurring (*gonna* instead of *going to, tell 'em* instead of *tell them,* etc.) to appear less remote to his electorate.

The use of in-group language by Prof. Lagdameo is also a message that says 'I am one of you, guys, look I speak your language'. This concept becomes clearer when we think of communities of practice like lawyers, academics or accountants. You signal that you are part of the group by using linguistic repertoire associated with that specific community.

Extract 2: Language-switching to establish solidarity

The following extract is from a female professor in a nursing school. Professor Paderez (P. Pad in the extract) has just given a lecture, in English, on how to handle medical emergencies. Then she suddenly switches to the vernacular.

6 *P. Pad*   *Mahirap talaga.* ((It's really difficult)) Anxiety is normal.
7   Your anxiety fires you up to study *di ba?* ((don't you think?))

Prof. Paderez's use of '*mahirap talaga*' is a solidarity strategy 'give sympathy to hearer' (Brown and Levinson 1987: 102). Ending her utterance with the tag question *di ba*? seems to add sincerity to the act of sympathy-giving because it was said in the native language.

Extract 3: Language-switching to mitigate disagreement

Although the focus of this chapter has been on professorial discourse, I have included an extract between two MA students to show how language-switching can be deployed as caring relations. The exchange below was between Rene, a male student, and Sister Concha, a female student and member of a religious order. Rene was questioning how priests, who have supposedly taken the vow of poverty, could afford to buy cars.

1 *Rene*   *makita mo yung pare bago ang kotse* =
             ((you see the priest he has a new car))
2 *Sr. Concha*   =*depende po yun* // ((it all depends *po*))
3   we have what we call the 'rules of the religious life,'
4   the diocesan priest has no vows they only
5   have alliance to the bishop so they are
6   free to accumulate wealth.

What is of analytical merit is how Sister Concha prefaced her disagreement with *depende po yun* before switching into English. Her use of *Tagalog* immediately invokes solidarity and instantiates shared linguistic and cultural background. The switch allowed her to use the respect particle *po* to convey deference and humility. The language switch works as a form of verbal shadowing (Rees-Miller 1995: 211) which softens the impact of the disagreement, mitigates threat to face and establishes a sense of 'we-ness' saying 'look we can argue together but we're still friends'.

In line 3, Sister Concha switches to English, the official language of education, which allows her to create social distance and mitigate face threat but that was after using *Tagalog* to frame her utterance. The language switch enables Sister Concha to create a 'friendship frame' that invokes closeness with deferential distance.

Extract 4: Use of stories to negotiate asymmetry

Teachers have more specific 'subject' knowledge than students and as a result they have more discursive resources. In most of the classes observed, teachers used narratives (fairy tales, movie plots, personal anecdotes, and current events) to encourage student participation. Through stories, lecturers were able to create a space where contributions were not assessed according to right or wrong; since they do not require specialist knowledge, they tend to mitigate hierarchical differences (Holmes 1995). Story-telling and social talk show the speakers' desire to spend time and effort on being with the addressee, thus indicating a mark of friendship. The narrative space changes the institutional atmosphere from formal and distant to intimate and personal.

Another professor, Prof. Lin (P. Lin) used her personal experiences to create a 'friendship frame'. In the example below, a student was expressing frustration about having to take an Algebra class.

1 *Rey:*   Miss, why do we have to take Algebra?
2 *P. Lin:* Well, I know it's not easy. I used to hate numbers but I realised
3   later on that it is an important part of our lives.
4   When I was your age . . .

After line 2, Prof. Lin proceeded to give accounts of how she overcame her dislike for numbers. Self-disclosure then becomes a way of establishing a caring connection with the students. I should note that this episode did not take place in the Algebra class. However, Prof. Lin set aside her lesson plan to attend to a student who was visibly worried about his Algebra class.

Conclusions

To sum up, this empirical study has used a discourse analytic approach using Brown and Levinson's (1987) politeness theory to illustrate how the discursive manipulation of institutional power can illuminate our understanding of caring relations in Philippine higher education classrooms. I illustrated how Filipino professors used linguistic devices to do 'power with' by mitigating face-threatening speech acts, reducing social distance and negotiating symmetry. The findings show how they used in-group language and language-switching to close the power gap, and story-telling to widen the knowledge base and overturn the participation structure from expert–novice to that of co-participants.

Drawing on interactional sociolinguistics and a conversation analytic approach enabled us to get a close-up view of language in action, within a particular context. A fine-grained analysis of naturally occurring data allowed us to freeze-frame fleeting moments of the interaction to explore 'care in language'. Using a linguistic analytic framework helped us unpack the dynamic quality of caring language; foregrounded in one utterance and omitted in the next. To enact care in language entails an awareness of power relations to make sure that it is used to *connect*, not *constrain*. A word of caution is in order here – although caring relations through the use of linguistic devices has been privileged as the analytic focus of this chapter, spoken language is just but one aspect of a complex set of social and relational practices that feminist ethics of care involves (see Philip, Chapter 12 in this volume).

It is hoped that this empirical research has shed some light on the interface between caring relations and power: using 'power with' as caring is not just an '*enabling condition*' (Bloome *et al.* 2005: 166, my italics) to facilitate the transmission of knowledge between teachers and students; 'power with' is a *pre-condition* which creates an affective space for learning and teaching to take place.

Notes

1 Naturally occurring, not elicited by the researcher.
2 Community is a heavily contested term. The author's definition tends to reflect disciplinary allegiances and research contexts.
3 An umbrella term for academics (lecturers, tutors, etc.) who teach tertiary-level classes.
4 'Politeness' here means showing concern for other people's feelings, being respectful and avoiding saying or doing anything that may be considered offensive by the other person one is talking to. It also refers to positive concern and non-imposing behaviour towards others (Holmes 1995: 4–5).

5 Regarding conversational analysis used in this chapter: transcription conventions are:

.	falling intonation at end of tone unit
?	high rising intonation at end of tone unit
,	slightly rising intonation at end of tone unit
!	animated intonation
-	unfinished utterance, e.g. false start
=	latching, no perceptible pause after a turn
(laughs)	single brackets describe current action, transcriber's comments
(( ))	double brackets contain English translation of Filipino words: e.g.

      A: *Isulat mo ito.*
          ((Write this down.))

Part II

Caring amongst communities and networks

Part II Summary

Caring amongst communities and networks

Maxine Birch, Nina Nissen, Tracey Reynolds, Andrea Doucet, Natasha Mauthner and Linda Bell

In this part of the book we explore key themes relevant to care, communities and networks. These include the separation or connectedness of care with work, consumption practices, communication (including newer digital technologies), neighbourhood, and relations between communities and 'self-care'. We continue to focus on piecing together relational aspects of care as each chapter explores particular spaces where caring activities and the development of identities occur. Each space discussed in this part is constituted by many factors: geographical, virtual, gender, 'race'/ethnicity, generational or life stage. Other important contextual factors include attitudes towards health and health practices, political ideologies and patterns of consumption.

At the start of this part Maxine and Nina draw on two ethnographic studies to show how alternative health care practitioners promote and foster self-care activities. In their chapter (6) they propose that this alternative framework keeps relational aspects of care at the core of the self-care activities encouraged. This is compared to the relational self found at the heart of ethics of care. Similarities are therefore illustrated between theorists such as Gilligan (e.g. 2011) and Held (e.g. 2006) who recommend care ethics to resolve individual and global moral dilemmas with the commitments from alternative health practitioners who adopt ethical lifestyles and seek to care for others in line with wider global concerns such as environmentalism, feminism and health.

Tracey's chapter (7) follows with an investigation into the provision of community care and the 'care work' performed by black men within the culturally specific space of 'black neighbourhoods'. She examines the gender and racialised relational aspects of care. She considers how intersecting gendered and racialised identities influence the care activities performed by black men. Tracey similarly proposes that wider structural constraints such as racial inequality and social exclusion experienced by black and minority ethnic people living within these neighbourhoods provide the context to the caring relations and community care performed by these men.

Andrea and Natasha's chapter (8) brings forward the importance of digital spaces and blogs as relatively new forms of social networking around care work. They focus on a case study of mommy blogging, which is a growing set of practices taken up by mainly middle-class mothers (in the USA, the UK and

Canada). Their chapter builds from, and revisits, the concept of 'maternal thinking' from the philosophical writing of the late Sara Ruddick (1983, 1995) and examines how mommy blogging intersects with her three central maternal demands/ responsibilities. They argue that the practices of mommy blogging are underpinned by overt and covert linkages between care, work, and consumption. They also point to how new digital practices expand, challenge, and raise pressing questions about what maternal care is in a digital and neoliberal age.

Linda's chapter (9) describes a cross-cultural project in which UK and Iran-based female researchers collaborated to explore the everyday lives of women as mothers in the city of Tehran (Iran). This project included a specific focus on caring, as well as examining health issues, employment and family lives. The chapter includes material taken from diaries kept by women participants, focusing on two case examples. Linda explores her anthropological voice to question and reflect on her presentation of the relational aspects of how these Tehrani women were 'caring for' and 'caring about' others, in the context of a patriarchal political and social environment. In doing this she challenges some ethical assumptions which can be made by Western researchers about life in different cultural contexts.

The authors of each of these chapters discuss how the different communities and networks that are represented draw out meanings of 'care' for their participants. This opens up the possibility of identifying and valuing the separate relations involved in caring, for example, within families, communities and networks, alongside offering evidence which suggests the interconnectedness of care with other social processes such as work or consumption. For example, Andrea and Natasha (Chapter 8) highlight how the activity of mommy blogging inter-meshes care, work, and consumption, in addition to the responsibilities of maternal care, outlined by Ruddick and others. They ask, following Lynch (2007), whether care as a separate form of 'love labour' can be identified. This is graphically illustrated by their phrase 'tea and Tupperware' when pointing out the encroachment of neoliberalism and capitalist consumption which poses increasing challenges to this separate valuing of care within communities. Linda, in her chapter (9), suggests that in a society where a patriarchal model tends to focus women's attention on maternal forms of caring, at an everyday level the ways in which Tehrani women 'care' and develop their identities as mothers can also be expressed through other social processes, for example through neighbourliness and via wider forms of citizenship. Using Lister's (2002) notion of 'sexual citizenship', for example, can disrupt the 'public' expectation that may be associated with citizenship, while suggesting broader opportunities to care within communities. In a similar way but within a different context, Tracey in Chapter 7 describes how the culturally prescribed understandings of black masculine identities are a critical feature of black men's caring. The men in her study expressed commitment to their neighbourhoods, with community activities being linked to their strongly felt obligations to ethnic communities and kinship networks. Maxine and Nina also explore this focus on community in their discussion in Chapter 6 of the holistic approaches to care developed by alternative health practitioners. They suggest that in their aspirations to 'being holistic' the alternative health care practitioners in their studies approach care on many levels. Reflecting Held's (2006) work, Maxine and Nina demonstrate how self-care and care for/about others and the environment connects people within social and professional networks and links to wider political and global concerns.

As particular associations have been drawn from all the different spaces discussed in this part of the book, aspects of caring for and about others have been located within notions of communities and networks. In so doing, we show how the processes that connect different caring practices and identities in these spaces may foster and/or constrain the individual within wider caring relations.

6   A different way of caring?

An exploration of alternative health care relationships

Maxine Birch, The Open University
Nina Nissen, University of Southern Denmark

Introduction

In this chapter, health care relationships with an emphasis on self-care (caring for oneself) in alternative health are explored. The care relationship is observed in two very different alternative health practices, western herbal medicine (WHM)[1] and self-discovery groups,[2] which illustrate a common objective to care for the whole person. This notion of the whole person is central to the values of holistic practice which encourage practitioners to consider multidimensional understandings of people and their environment. Critical for both groups of practitioners[3] is to instil ideas and practices about the importance of personal responsibility for health and well-being in their care recipients. Providing professional care for another depends on the development of self-care resources and activities, grounded in specific and individualised interventions that promote individual well-being and improve health problems. These interventions combined with values of holism can also result in the adoption of socially and ethically responsible lifestyles. Accordingly, the particular alternative care relationship and its emphasis on self-care explored in this chapter echoes many aspects espoused in the feminist care ethics framework.

At the heart of care ethics is the negotiation between people in caring relationships. Caring relationships are viewed as essential for life to flourish so that individuals, groups and communities are enabled to reach their potential and achieve a sense of well-being (Held 2006; Sevenhuijsen 2002). Ethical concerns arise within networks of relationships where varying dimensions of care are negotiated and balanced 'for the self, for others and for relations between these' (Sevenhuijsen 2002: 132). This perspective does not imply notions of care as altruistic acts or involve judgements on selfish or selfless acts, but looks at the complexity of care as sets of feelings, activities and resources that enable a caring relationship to support one another (McCarthy and Edwards 2011). Therefore a caring relationship 'involves cooperative well-being of those in the relation and well-being of the relation itself' (Held 2006: 12). The empirical data on alternative health care relationships presented here lead us to consider some interesting associations between Held's notion of cooperative well-being and notions of well-being in holistic practice. We suggest that cooperative well-being is engaged when self-care activities promote a relational self so that feelings, activities and resources for caring are negotiated and balanced for the self and others.

In general the concept of holism refers to taking a multidimensional view, a picture of the whole. The association of holism with health represents the interdependencies and connections of all parts of the body, the whole body. Holism also infers another aspect: it places the whole person within her or his own personal contexts of family, community, culture and environment. Notions of holism are therefore complex and descriptions of what constitutes a 'whole person' and the identification of their personal context can vary within each therapeutic practice and healing modality. Pietroni (1990) states that holism is not linked to any particular practice but signifies an approach to health and healing. Consumers of alternative and complementary health practices note that holism, being treated as a whole person, is a positive, beneficial experience and a key reason for consulting alternative practitioners (Bishop *et al.* 2007; Long *et al.* 2000; Paterson and Britten 2008). Holism is frequently associated with alternative health practices and is aligned with understandings of health as the unity of mind, body and spirit. In alternative health, holism is often applied to describe notions of balance, harmony, well-being and healing, and a holistic approach promises to restore this sense of unity. The influence of humanistic philosophy and the awareness of human potential, the growth and popularisation of psychology and psychotherapeutic traditions have also influenced the ways that understandings of holism in western societies stress different aspects of the whole body and person. The individual and sense of self become defined through notions of balance, harmony, well-being and healing. Being healthy or feeling content are said to arise from an inner, innate self-healing ability. Therefore, in order to examine self-care as a component of the alternative health caring relationship it is important to explore how these practices construct a whole person and its corresponding location of self.

Holism and care ethics are grounded in the notion of a relational self, set within interdependent networks of relations with others and the wider environment. The concept of individualism can help illuminate how this relational self is promoted through self-care. Foucault defined individualism as having three important components: first, the values attributed to being a singular and independent individual within groups or institutions to which he or she belongs; second, the positive valuation of private, personal and family life; and third, the intensity of the relations to self, where the notion of self is an object of knowledge that becomes 'a field of action' whereby transformations of self can be constructed (Foucault 1984: 42). This notion of individualism underpins Foucault's discussions of historical and cultural cultivations of the self that promoted and developed activities to take care of one's self. The care of the self is historically located as a social practice. We suggest that the social practice of self-care in alternative health practices today is observed alongside the acceptance of holism. Holism becomes a way of life as the personal quest for health and pursuit of the good life becomes central (Crawford 2006). We go on to propose that the values of holism foster self-care activities that cultivate a relational self. This relational self is distinct from descriptions of increasing individualism and the perpetuation of a narcissistic self. Alternative health offers a 'field of action' where activities and resources of self-care construct a particular shaping of individuality, and where a relational self is strengthened. This permits a sense of autonomy where an individual can construct new meanings within her or his personal biography, while these meanings, at the same time, emphasise the interdependence and connections with others. Therefore, as recognised in Beck and Beck-Gernsheim's (2002) theory of individualisation, self-care becomes a biographical resolution for tensions within society whereby alternative health care practices align autonomy and self-direction within a new patterning of social relations. We therefore suggest that both holism and care ethics emphasise self-care activities as an inherent part of social and ethical relations and an emerging life politics.

The studies

Two ethnographic studies carried out in the UK – a study of self-discovery groups (Birch 1997) and a study of the practice and use of western herbal medicine (WHM) (Nissen 2008) – included a narrative analysis of practitioners' accounts of working in alternative health settings. The two groups of alternative health practitioners – 'therapists' and 'herbalists' – at first appear very distinct, but on revisiting their accounts many similar narrative patterns and resonating themes emerge. In particular, meanings of self-care and holism underpin both alternative health practices. After introducing the practitioners, we focus on their narratives to discuss how the similarities and resonances found between the two studies link with a feminist care ethics framework that has the potential to offer wider social changes as championed in Held's (2006) work.

The practitioners

The first group of ten therapist practitioners, six female and four male, were accessed via alternative health networks, directories and health centres. Three popular psychological approaches were found to underpin the therapist's approaches. First, transpersonal psychology that draws on the works of Carl Jung, second, psychodynamic bodywork based on the works of Wilhelm Reich and third, process-oriented psychology founded by Arnold Mindell (Birch 1996). These approaches are considered and often associated with ideas about human potential and personal growth. The therapists all offered different blends of psychotherapeutic work combined with bodywork and different philosophical and spiritual regimes to offer a journey of self-discovery. A vital part of their approach was to develop group work for the purpose of obtaining a more satisfying and fulfilling life, improving a sense of self and well-being. All the therapists were self-employed and had established businesses for individual counselling and group work in this alternative health context. The therapists had developed their way of working over many years, drawing on varying accredited training courses and personal experiential development work to establish credibility in this setting. Their self-employment within counselling and group work was often a second or third career.

The second group, six women herbalists, were drawn from a survey of registered WHM practitioners (Nissen 2010). Collectively, these herbalists represent a plurality of approaches to the practice of WHM. These include the adoption and adaptation of women's healing traditions which are articulated as explicitly feminist while others reflect the current shifts in WHM towards academic training and calls for evidence-based knowledge in the context of professional accreditation and statutory regulation. Cutting across these differences are shared ideas about the practice of WHM as support and care for the whole person, and the aim of facilitating personal transformation. The six herbalists were self-employed and largely work from their own home-based clinics on a part-time basis. Only one practitioner worked full-time in clinical practice. Four of the herbalists combine their private herbal practice with teaching WHM and/or herbal research. Three of the herbalists have been in practice for twenty or more years, one for seven years, one for two years and one qualified during the course of the study.

Establishing self-care within alternative health care relationships

In the beginning, a professional relationship of care is established between the practitioner and the recipient of care. The practitioner has acquired, either formally or informally, the legitimacy to deliver a specific type of alternative health care. In these studies 'client' was the term preferred by the therapists and 'patient' by the herbalists; we adopt this patient/client distinction throughout the discussion to reflect the practitioners' own words. Crucial to both alternative health practices is how patients/clients are positioned as active participants. This active component is already observed in the initial selection of alternative health care and in engaging with a particular professional and her/his healing modality. Most patients/clients are recommended or referred to a practitioner by word of mouth through a layperson's social networks where the assessment of a particular alternative modality and/or a practitioner's expertise, quality and legitimacy are based on individuals' personal experience of a therapy or a particular practitioner. During extensive first consultations between the practitioner and the patient/client, often lasting one hour or more, the basis of the patient/client as an active participant in their own care is first developed. Both practitioner and patient/client jointly seek to identify the reasons why an individual is seeking help, their expectations and how an individual's needs are best met. In this way a collaborative relationship is established. The active participation of patient/client is further emphasised through the alternative health practitioner's position as a facilitator of care. This is, for example, summarised in one therapist's rejection of the term therapist: 'I always say I am not a therapist; people take their own responsibility for their reactions. It is a learning self development support group and people can use it for their own journey.' The same is witnessed with the herbalists who describe the aim of their practice as 'supporting' their patients 'in their own healing and transformation'. As one herbalist elaborates:

> I very much see my role as kind of helping them to make sense of the situation, helping them to figure out what's going on with themselves, so they can take back that kind of control over their body, their health, their circumstances.

This understanding of facilitation is demonstrated when practitioners acknowledge the patients/clients as experts in knowing their own bodies and lives and gradually encourage the patients/clients' own self-care. Herbalists for instance encourage their patients to 'listen to their bodies' or to 'listen to their hearts' as a way of exploring and understanding present life experiences and responses, and to facilitate self-discovery and self-knowledge. In so doing, herbalists address women's embodied selves where both the material body and the self constitute the context in which women's 'own healing and transformation' can be imagined, and a desired self be aimed for and achieved (Nissen 2008). Similarly in the therapy study, each groups' ethos is underpinned by the belief that the discovery of a 'real self', an inner self, connects with the realisation of authenticity – 'how to be true to one's self'. By expressing emotions it is promised that each participant can 'tap into a natural healing ability', 'heal past hurts' and 'realise future potential'. The holistic approach observed here associates inner resources with the personal responsibility to work towards balance and a sense of well-being. Other studies on complementary and alternative health practices also observe the common belief that health comes from within and inner healing abilities are said to be elicited through a holistic approach (Long *et al.* 2000; Hughes 2004).

This call to an 'inner voice' and the accessing of an interiority is however not only critical to an individual's self-discovery and self-knowledge but also central to practitioners' notions of holism that are shaped by ideas of balance and connections where caring for oneself, others and the world become intertwined. The following comment by a herbalist talking about women's health illustrates this point:

> It's about supporting women in the broadest sense, from an individual woman's health and well-being in society to the preservation, nurturance and healing of the Divine Feminine as a principle in Nature and therefore within us all.

This is echoed by a therapist who facilitated a women's self-discovery group:

> there by linking our subjective and personal life ... that is our emotions, ideas, loves, hopes and fears with the objective and collective life of our soul which is linked to nature. This may enable us to gain deeper understanding both into and beyond our individual lives in particular as women of today.

As such, personal knowledge about the body and one's life engages with ideas of the inherent wisdom of the body, where an assumed self-regulating capacity of the body is mirrored in understanding health as harmony and balance and a vital force or 'energy' connects the bodies of individuals with the universe (O'Connor 2000).

Over time, the professional attention of therapists and herbalists is replaced by patients/clients' increasing adoption of everyday self-care practices, shown to constitute a vital part of this alternative health environment. Self-care is an integral part of herbalists' therapeutic approach and encompasses ideas about diet, nutrition and exercise, as well as activities that focus on self-actualisation and self-fulfilment (Nissen 2008). The therapists promote that the realisation of a true self and therefore well-being depends on continuing self-knowledge of how to look after the body and the mind. Creative activities, healthy eating, yoga and meditation are actively sought by both therapists and clients (Birch 1996). As these 'embodied practices' (McGuire 2008) become woven into patients/clients' everyday lives, their need and reliance for professional support gradually becomes secondary to care for oneself. In this way the patient/client is further positioned as authoring her own healing and transformation while practitioners' ideas and values are literally embodied 'forming/informing the body' (McGuire 1995: 29) and embodied selves. Yet these embodied self-care practices should not be confused with the encouragement towards individualised healthier lifestyles prominent in biomedical health promotion (Nissen 2008; Schneirov and Geczik 2003). Instead they are connected with processes of acquiring the skills of taking care of oneself and the commitment to oneself as worthy of attention and care. This self-worth becomes increasingly linked and connected to the well-being of others. It is now that the holistic theme of connection – with others, with the environment and with spiritual concerns – begins to broaden meanings of health within self-care practices.

Holistic lifestyles and new ways of working

For the practitioners the belief in personal responsibility for health, well-being and personal change is consistently realised through daily activities that constitute holistic lifestyles. Holism is not just an approach to health but a way of being in the world. For the alternative health practitioners being holistic is a form of life politics, where the imperative for holistic health aims to achieve the best outcome for each individual while also extending towards attaining a greater social good. Alternative health becomes political in the sense that 'actors self consciously practice in the present and future changes they seek' (Melucci cited in Schneirov and Geczik 1996: 628).

The discourse of holistic health is also documented in health movements that gathered currency in the UK during the 1980s. Various groups developed holism to challenge the dichotomies of art/science, masculine/feminine, healing/treatment in an attempt to broaden the knowledge and practice of health care. The holistic health movement embraced other disciplines in order to broaden and complement scientific medicine and emphasise experiential and intuitive knowledge (Power 2000). Holistic health calls for a continuum of understandings to fully appreciate the contextual related individual in modern societies. In this way holism becomes a political movement in challenging the knowledge and organisation of health care. This understanding of movement is reinforced when the care relationships, in particular through the promotion of self-care, encounter and connect with different networks. In this way being holistic becomes a networked activity that can connect different alternative health practices and develop new or strengthen existing connections with other networks, such as environmental, feminist and spiritual networks, that also focus on creating a more sustainable and just social world. A social world where democracy, individual and community diversity, act local but think global and a politics are fostered. But most importantly one where socially responsible economies are developed to avoid extreme wealth or poverty and waste.

In both the ethnographies drawn on here the practitioners' rich narratives tell how each one entered this work in alternative health. Practitioners relate a series of events and life experiences that are shown to construct a 'path' or 'journey'. An important part is the personal positive experience of alternative health treatments (see also Nissen 2010). One herbalist for instance describes 'flowing into' herbal medicine. Other practitioners mention the importance of meeting others who have found solutions through engaging with alternative practices. A therapist's journey began through yoga: 'Yoga teachers and doing my yoga teacher training made me really look at myself.' Frequently there is a sense of 'being on the right path' which resonates with the notion of a 'life force' that directs and determines events in this alternative world. As one participant in the therapy study said 'the negatives turn to positives'. These observations resonate with McClean (2005) and Lee-Treweek (2010) who also note this movement from client to practitioner of crystal and spiritual healing practitioners, as well as Searle-Chatterjee (1999) who found that feminist and environmental activists were motivated by past personal experiences in their activist politics.

Having embarked on this journey of self-exploration and self-fulfilment, underpinned by values of holism that are shaped by ideas of balance and connection, practitioners demonstrate the integration of these professional ideas and ideals with their personal lives. New models of working can be identified in this alternative setting where working from home is common practice and the negotiation of time for other commitments means that work is more often than not part-time. In both studies practitioners practised from home, blurring boundaries of work and home. A continuum of work/home environments that move from using the lounge as the 'group room' or 'consultation room' to creating a distinct 'work' space within the home was frequently noted. A portfolio of work emerges where the home practice is complemented with time spent at alternative health centres, teaching or in research. These strategies and commitments resonate with Gibson's (2004) study, which highlights that alternative health practitioners, especially women, situate their work in the voluntary sector which is characterised by its community orientation. Gibson further suggests that practitioners' values and practices support the blending of economic activities and personal belief towards a social ethics of healing that includes broad notions of care. In doing so, practitioners prioritise a notion of livelihood over traditional notions of work as economic activity, and notions of healing and care take priority over claims to cure.

Furthermore, practitioners' ways of working are firmly embedded in social and professional networks that are underpinned by beliefs in the importance of 'connection', both spiritual and practical, and the centrality of values of mutual support that combines care for oneself with care for others, the environment and/or the universe. Herbalists in this study were noted to be part of an extensive network of practitioners, which included other herbalists, alternative practitioners of different therapies that are perceived as complementary to herbal medicine, as well as sympathetic GPs and nurses and also health food shops. When relevant, patients were referred for other or additional treatment or biomedical testing. This was reciprocated by practitioners of other healing modalities and also GPs and nurses when approached by patients for contacts of alternative health practitioners. In addition, herbalists formed local practitioner groups that served as mutual support networks and provided peer supervision and ongoing training and professional development.

The complex networks described by the therapists also demonstrated how chance meetings with others have a cumulative effect whereby participants of self-discovery groups were themselves practitioners in other alternative health practices and also became facilitators of self-discovery work themselves.

> I suppose it was a series of accidents really, I came across friends who were involved in this sort of thing and it was so good to be with real people and not function at a superficial level. In my nutritional work I have seen people transformed by just changing what they eat. Like when I go to my (discovery) group or at my medicine wheel group it makes you feel different. You know there is more to life than worry, work and family problems.

The boundaries between patients/clients and practitioners were constantly blurred and different alternative health practices could merge and blend to produce another approach. The practitioners all espoused ecological and environmental concerns that frequently resulted in belonging to active 'green' grassroots movements. Many also expressed connections with feminist ideals and support for women's health movements. Involvement within alternative health settings reveal that care relationships offer opportunities to encounter and engage with other diffuse and decentralised networks relating to health and the environment.

In this way, care and self-care become a complex system of values, activities and relationships that are characterised by intentions of developing egalitarian partnerships and the desire to address shared social and environmental concerns. In turn being holistic compels a commitment to foster and guide others in care for self, others and the environment. Self-care strategies and techniques promote subsequent improvements in well-being, self-worth and self-knowledge for both practitioners and patients/clients at all times. Care is therefore expressed as the cooperative well-being between the delivery and receipt of care, for those involved, and its holistic practice constructs opportunities to realise a different sense of self so that caring becomes an everyday, embodied and transformative experience with particular aspirations for the future. Furthermore, when individual actions and experiences are understood as having social, cultural and political consequences, the practice and use of alternative health can be seen to promote not only personal transformation but also social change, changes also espoused by feminist care ethics (Gilligan 2011; Held 2006).

The connections of holism become firmly embedded in the care ethics notion of 'co-operative well-being' (Held 2006: 12). This places the autonomy of an individuated, developed self and self-aware, reflexive individual within a network of relations where 'co-operative well-being' becomes imperative. A positive caring relationship requires each individual to engage in self-care as this becomes integral to caring for others: 'Persons in caring relations are acting for self and other together' (Held 2006: 12). In this way the personal self-care activities and resources become linked to wider societal concerns. When the caring relationship becomes the focus, rather than the individual, cooperative well-being creates a mutual transformative force. It is this cooperative well-being that also transcends gendered constructions of care. The capacity to care has been traditionally associated with women and many feminists have identified care as a critical component of constructing gender differences and inequalities, still argued to be in evidence today (Miller 2011; Wright *et al.* 2009). However a new consequence of care within an increasingly individualised modern society (Beck and Beck-Gernsheim 2002) and the emergence of life politics as the combined attention of self and institutional reflexivity (Giddens 1991) suggests that care perceived as sacrifice or restriction 'living for the family' has shifted towards the demand 'to live a life of one's own' (Beck and Beck-Gernsheim 2002: 56). This does not infer the continuation of a narcissistic preoccupation with self-interest but rather an empowering of women's autonomy, an autonomy that has been previously denied. This fits well with discussions of self-care in alternative health practices and research that strongly indicates that women in particular compose the majority of users and practitioners of alternative health (Flesch 2010; Sointu 2011). The women patients/clients in both studies reported on the value of space for themselves, a time for personal reflection and gathering of self-worth. The close associations between holism and well-being are argued to resonate well with women's experiences (Sointu and Woodhead 2008; Sointu 2011). 'The search for well-being asserts "ownership and entitlement" for care and discourses of well-being develop self-worth' (Sonitu 2011: 363). Therefore notions of holism and well-being support the value of caring, reinstate the significance of relationships and consequently reassert the importance of women's caring roles within a culture that can marginalise such concerns. It is interesting to note that the male therapists all ascribed to feminist views and the call for re-evaluating the cultural position of care. This shift towards valuing care and qualities traditionally associated with women is also observed in the development of alternative ideas and movements observed in North America (Magnuson 2008; Ray and Anderson 2000). In both studies the practitioners all talk about their personal ethical life politics, where the goal is to enable and empower others on a journey to achieve well-being. This also combines with the practitioners' own personal rejection of materialistic and consumerist values. Viewing alternative health care relationships in this way can illustrate how the personal is reconnected with the political and how caring relationships become mutually cooperative. Alternative health and being holistic becomes political through personal choices and actions in changing relationships and lifestyle behaviours that work towards a greater 'good'.

Concluding thoughts

Care is a fundamental and universal basic need for humans to survive, a concept that can link all of humanity and underpins care ethics and holism. The holistic vision of maintaining and building connections together with living a holistic way of life unites caring actions and serves to exemplify the values of caring in a society that has tended to marginalise such values. Care ethics establishes care as a 'way of being in society as well as a way of making connections' (Daly 2002: 253). It encourages the 'capacities that constitute our humanity and alerts us to the practices that put them at risk' (Gilligan 2011: 177). A holistic approach developed in alternative health practice reflects Held's (2006) work where care connects people within families, friendships, social groups and neighbourhoods, political and global concerns. Alternative health care practitioners approach care on many levels and this is integral to aspirations of 'being holistic'.

The transformative potential of taking personal responsibility for well-being within the collective common value base of holism connects the well-being of self with others that profess the success of alternative health practitioners. At an intrapersonal level it is the personal responsibility of all to engage with self-care, to develop an inner potential to maximise health and promote well-being. At an interpersonal level care is constructed as the active participation of both care-giver and receiver. This expands into wider societal concerns as holistic practices involve caring for others and the environment. Just as holistic thinking challenged dichotomies in understanding health during the 1980s, understandings of care that relied primarily on distinctions of paid/unpaid, formal/informal, women/men, are argued to be ineffective in the twenty-first century. Care no longer implies personal sacrifice but can be seen as positive expressions of intimacy, sources of meaning and social solidarity (Fine 2007). The alternative health care relationships observed in these two studies celebrate and confirm this expression, meaning and connection. Drawing on a care ethics enables these multifaceted aspects of care to become visible, offering a potential vision of what a caring society could be like in the future.

Notes

1 Western herbal medicine (WHM) refers to the practice of herbal medicine that uses plants largely native to Europe, within a philosophical tradition arising from European thought. The practice of WHM is characterised by a person-centred approach to health care where the patient rather than the disease is the focus of the practitioner's attention (Nissen 2008).
2 Self-discovery groups refers to different groups that use a mix of psychotherapeutic traditions, eastern bodywork, and philosophical and spiritual regimes to offer participants the promise that to know yourself more will help create a more satisfying life, improve well-being and heal past difficulties (Birch 1997).
3 We use the terms 'herbalist' or the 'therapist' when talking specifically about each study; the term 'practitioner' is used with reference to both studies together.

7 'Men's business'?

Black men's caring within black-led community organisations

Tracey Reynolds, London South Bank University

Introduction

The chapter addresses the role of black men in care provision and the care work they undertake within their local communities and black-led community organisations in Britain. Black men's involvement in community care, and the gendered and racialised nature of their caring has, thus far, received limited attention in the literature. The analysis draws on a feminist ethics of care and debates on fatherhood and care to explore how gendered and racialised identities intersect and influence the caring activities undertaken by black men. Throughout the chapter the men are presented as an essentialised racialised category.[1] The reasons for doing so are twofold. First, in the British context, there are relatively few theoretical studies on gendered caring, which also take account of 'race' and racism. Second, this construction of an essentialised category is a vital first stage towards ensuring that black men's voices are collectively represented in contemporary British care research. This is important because existing debates tend to characterise black men and their caring relationships as deviant from white, middle-class norms (Williams and Hewison 2009).

The empirical material that follows emerges out of a number of my research projects on Black-Caribbean men's and women's family and community networks. For this chapter, I focus particularly on the relational and contextual aspect of black men's care work. I explore how black men's desire to provide protection and support for community and family members within 'black neighbourhoods'[2] plays a crucial role in their participation and care-giving. I also investigate how the care work performed by black men in neighbourhood settings are underpinned by wider systems of structural racial and gender inequalities in society.

The chapter opens with a background to the research. I then attempt to position and contextualise black men's community caring within (black) feminist and fatherhood debates. In the following sections the significance of ethnicity/race, family/community networks and socio-cultural contexts underpinning black men's perceptions and experiences of care are critically assessed. The chapter concludes by asking if a feminist body of literature on care can provide a basis with which to challenge the often negative, exclusionary and marginalised images of black men in society.

Research background

The research material presented in this chapter is drawn from a number of separate but interconnected projects that I undertook between 2003 and 2009. Three of the projects were commissioned by statutory agencies – a local authority, a housing association and a parenting support group – and took place during 2007–09. The studies were conducted in socially deprived neighbourhoods spread across the London boroughs of Lambeth, Brent, Haringey and Southwark. Common strands connecting each of these projects were that they all took place in 'black neighbourhoods'. This term refers to those neighbourhoods, or locales, that have historically high patterns of African-Caribbean settlement. The projects also recognised Black and Minority Ethnic (hereafter referred to as BME) people's contested and contextual understandings of belonging, identity and community. In addition they highlighted the complex range of social and economic issues affecting BME communities and the way in which local organisations operated at neighbourhood levels in terms of care provision to its BME community members (Reynolds and Miah 2007; Reynolds 2008; Reynolds and Briggs 2009). Qualitative, in-depth and one-to-one interviews took place with a total of 43 participants. For the purpose of this chapter I have drawn on interviews with 17 black men working or volunteering across black-led welfare-based community organisations. They provided a range of services focused on children and youths, the elderly and vulnerable adults, training and support to the unemployed and parents whose children were at risk of school exclusion. Qualitative data on black men's participation and engagement in black welfare-based community organisation were also collected as part of a larger study on Caribbean Families and Diaspora Youth during 2003–06.[3] This analysis explored how social capital is reproduced and generated within Caribbean family and community networks by individual members, including black men (Reynolds 2006).

Framing racialised and gendered care

There is a scarcity of studies exploring black men's caring within community organisations; particularly understandings of how their gendered and racialised identities underpin their community care work. Contributing to black men's invisibility in community care is the valorisation of 'black community mothers', who are viewed as carrying the social and emotional burden of caring within black communities (Hill Collins 1990; Reynolds 2005). In black feminist scholarship, with regards to this issue of gender relations and caring, the extent to which black women provide a fathering role within family and community has long been debated (Clarke 1957; Reynolds 2002a). The literature points to the interdependence between the dual roles of carer/economic provider, which has made it possible for black women to undertake caring practices and roles traditionally associated with fathering and masculine identities (i.e. 'breadwinner') (Reynolds 2001b; Reynolds 2002b; Foner 2009). Rarely, if ever, in this literature is the question asked whether black men can provide caring roles traditionally associated with women. Similarly, in the more general fathering literature where men's caring relationships and practices have been more closely examined, black men also occupy a marginal or invisible space. Black men are either absent from debates or deficit understandings and stereotyped models of black fathering exist, such as, for example, the 'no-good', 'deadbeat', 'feckless' black fathers (Reynolds 2001a, 2002b, 2009; Williams 2009; Fatherhood Institute 2010).

In recent years a growing number of studies emerging out of the UK have attempted to challenge this invisibility by documenting black men's history of providing care within their extended kinship and community networks (Goulbourne and Chamberlain 2001; Reynolds 2009; Williams 2009) as well as highlighting the various ways in which black men have worked in partnership with black women to respond to the cultural and ethnic specific needs of their communities (Goulbourne 1989; Sudbury 1998; Reynolds 2003). Yet despite inroads made by the literature to redress the imbalance, it would be fair to say that stereotyped images of black men exist that continue to portray them as 'hyper-masculine', 'hyperaggressive' and 'hypersexualised' (Connor and White 2011). The persistence of such negative images leaves limited scope for understanding black men's caring relations within communities.

One of the challenges for researchers, policymakers and practitioners is how to relate issues of community care with broader conceptual understandings of gendered racialised relations. A moral dimension is crucial to understanding caring relations within community and family networks (Williams 2005). Yet, contrasting approaches exist in terms of understanding these moral perspectives of care. On the one hand, caring is understood as 'local and subjectively influenced' (Kuhse *et al.* 1998: 453), and is viewed as important in maintaining intimate connectedness between individuals. Informal care practices provided by family and kinship members usually fall within this camp. Yet, on the other hand, caring is recognised as a universal objective principal where it is not necessarily a requirement that intimacy and a personal relationship exist between the care-giver and care-recipient (Sevenhuijsen 2000). Formal care in the public sphere provided by statutory, charity and community organisations falls within this camp.

The large body of feminist literature on care points to the gender inequalities underpinning caring practices performed by men and women (for example, Ruddick 1995; Ve 1989; Finch and Mason 1993; Noddings 2003; Philip, Chapter 12 in this volume). With regards to black welfare-based organisations this claim is borne out. Sudbury's (1998) study of black women's organisations in the UK found that whilst it was women who undertook the lion's share of caring activities, the male carers worked in positions that were viewed as having higher status, power and authority. These men usually assumed leadership roles working at the helm of organisations, and with minimal involvement in the hands-on, practical and day-to-day care work. She also noted that these men's higher status within black welfare-based organisations was usually disproportionate to the total number of men working or volunteering there.

Gendered forms of caring lead to gender differentiated experiences of care-giving between men and women (Finch 1989; Finch and Mason 1993; Sevenhuijsen

2000; Wolf 2004; Doucet 2006a). Gendered labour divisions in society, and the different meanings attached to culturally prescribed models of masculinity and femininity, result in different understandings of men's and women's care roles, responsibilities and relationships (Coltrane 1996; Doucet 2000). Indeed, Doucet's (2006a) seminal study *Do Men Mother?* clearly acknowledges this point. She argues that men are caring within the confines of constructed masculinity, and so in those instances where they are performing similar or identical tasks to women they still adhere to culturally prescribed notions of masculinity. In the main, men's nurturing style within care-giving focuses on playfulness, physical activity and protective care. Whilst women's care-giving centres on the more practical-oriented work. In her study Doucet also saw evidence of the greater responsibility women have for organising and directing daily care activities. The women concentrated more than men on building emotional bonds and networks of support. There were also notable gendered differences in the way that men and women accessed, built and maintained networks within their local communities (Doucet 2006a).

With regards to my own research exploring black men's care relationships within black-led community organisations, it was similarly noted that a gendered division of labour existed in the caring activities undertaken by these men and the women working in these organisations. The men generally undertook caring activities conventionally (and stereotypically) regarded as male-oriented tasks, such as working as mini-bus drivers and porters. The men were involved in other activities where they were given responsibility for coordinating outings and day trips for the service-users and clients. They were also important figures when it came to organising any sporting activities, musical events and festivals. Although men were the minority gender within the vast majority of these black-led organisations, they tended to quickly gain positions of leadership within a few short years of joining the organisation. These men tended to be put forward as the organisation's representative at high-profile events and conferences in far greater numbers and frequency than the women who also worked or volunteered there. They were also more likely than the women to be called upon to perform public tasks on behalf of the organisation, such as giving public speeches. Of course there were situations whereby men and women performed identical tasks within these organisations. However, it became clear that there existed an unequal distribution of care work between them. During team meetings and group meetings with clients to discuss issues around care provision, it was observed that the female staff and volunteers frequently arrived early to prepare any materials and equipment required. It was the female staff or volunteers who generally offered to make the cups of tea and coffee, and it was common for them to be left with the tidying and washing up once the meeting ended. The unequal distribution of caring tasks observed in many of these organisations could be said to mirror the gender inequalities that exist in wider society.

The gendered divide around care was most marked during the men's discussion around the struggles they had in balancing care demands of the community with related obligations to family members, and other commitments. The struggles the men highlighted in their narratives concerned what they saw as an imbalance created by care demands on their personal time. The time pressures experienced in caring greatly reduced the time spent on other family obligations and social/leisure activities, and some men resented this. Importantly, the men recounted that they were able to compartmentalise their lives in a way that women were not able to do. Consequently, community care was viewed by these men as an additional aspect of their identity and social life. For black women, however, a care-giver role is an embedded part of self-identity. Studies by Hill Collins (2004) and Reynolds (2003) assert that black women's community lives are strongly tied to their personal and family lives across the differing contexts of the USA and Britain.

Conceptual understandings of care within the feminist ethics framework, whilst a useful analytical tool in understanding gendered relations, is problematic when it comes to incorporating issues of 'race' and racial identity and the extent to which these issues impact on cultural, social and economic conditions that inform black men's caring experiences. What the research evidence reveals is the gendered division of caring work that takes place within black-led community organisations. This community setting provides a context for black men to express patriarchal notions of power, authority and leadership, which is otherwise denied them in wider society and other spheres of public life because of their racial subordinate status.

Community caring through family and fathering

Ethnic-specific community networks encourage bonds of trust and reciprocal support to develop among black (and minority ethnic) individuals (Reynolds 2006; Goulbourne *et al.* 2010). The men interviewed stated that they valued the trusted relationships and support resources that emerged through black-led community organisations. The case study of Gus, an elderly Black-Caribbean male, gives us some indication of this. Gus, age 79, volunteers twice weekly at a black elderly day centre, which his wife attends. Gus is the main carer for his sick wife suffering with severe arthritis, and it was this issue that led him to access and seek voluntary work within the centre. Gus states:

> I was finding it hard to manage her [wife] on my own, and the stress was building my [blood] pressure but I didn't want social services because I didn't want them poking around in my business, and the next thing [being] that they want to put my wife in a [elderly sheltered] home. I don't trust social services and keep them at a distance and out of my business. My experience of those people working at the Town Hall [social services] has always been very negative. They don't respect black people and our ways, despite what they may say. They think they are superior and know what's best for me and my wife . . . I am an old man but I am also a proud black man and come from a [Jamaican] nation of proud black men and we are warriors and fighters . . . As a black man I like to think I can manage on our own and we don't want to ask for help. I don't know if it's an ego thing being a man? I'm sure that has a lot to do with it. But it could also be because as black people we know the system

is always going to be stacked against us. We have had a long history of fighting for our rights as a race people . . . My doctor, an Indian man, put me in contact with [organisation] he told me 'Gus, it will be alright, just go and see them, they will look after you, they are your own people.' And it was a blessing when we started coming. I trust them and we are a team and look out for each other. By helping out and doing my own little bit for them I don't feel that I am just taking from them but I'm contributing something too.

(Gus, age 79, interview black elderly organisation, Southwark, 2009)

For Gus working in the organisation his wife attended was regarded as a reciprocal process; he traded his practical support, such as escorting other service-users on shopping trips and visits to the local library, for the emotional support he needed, as his wife's condition deteriorated. As Gus recounts, providing a caring role within this organisation allowed him to maintain his sense of dignity, and, what he terms, 'his male pride'. Indeed, Gus was one of a number of men interviewed who also highlighted that black-led community organisations acted as a safe environment for them to expose their vulnerabilities and allow them to ask for care support for family members.

Gus's example mirrors a general reluctance expressed by others interviewed in approaching mainstream organisations for assistance because they were afraid of encountering racial prejudice, which they felt would ultimately undermine their 'male pride'. Traditional forms of masculinity inhibit men's abilities to trust other people with their emotional or personal experiences (Connell 2005; Whitehead 2002). Consequently, even within the relatively safe confines of a black-led community organisation, many male participants felt their vulnerability would be exposed by admitting they might require assistance in providing care to others. In many respects, working or volunteering assistance in any organisation, which they could also access for care provision, reduced the stigma they associated with requesting care from community care agencies.

The concerns Gus shares about turning to social services departments for care assistance also reflect wider views shared by many people across BME communities concerning more formal and mainstream care services offered by statutory agencies. The research evidence points to a general mistrust of the mainstream services among minority and migrant groups. There exists a common perception that people from BME communities will experience ineffective care provision and incidences of racial discrimination (Afshar *et al.* 2008; Lievesley 2010). This has created differences in the way that white-majority and BME communities access care services. Principally, the white UK population are more likely to draw on mainstream services (such as local authority and statutory agencies), as well as national charity organisations (e.g. Age UK), for primary care provision. They turn to the smaller-scale community-based organisations within their local community as their secondary source of provision. In contrast, BME individuals are more likely to use their own family and/or ethnic-specific voluntary services in their local neighbourhoods as their primary care providers. Mainstream services are typically regarded as being their secondary source of service provision (National Council for Voluntary Organisations 2009). Critics have argued that racial disadvantage is perpetuated and BME communities continue to experience an unequal access to resources because of the fact that mainstream services have more resources and funds available whilst voluntary organisations tend to struggle for survival (Lowdell *et al.* 2000). At a policy level it is also recognised that social care services have been unsuccessful in their attempts to successfully engage black and minority ethnic men over the years (Williams and Hewison 2009).

The example of Gus, who is highlighted above, and his experience of community care in caring for his sick wife, was one of a number from the people interviewed that highlighted their involvement in community caring work (either paid work or volunteering) stemming from caring tasks performed with family members. In the vast majority of cases it was men's fathering role that acted as a catalyst for community care. In recent times there have been important, if ambivalent, changes in defining normative family roles and practices for fathers (O'Brien 2005). Idealised notions of fatherhood increasingly valorise fathers' participation in child care and their adoption of parenting values traditionally associated with motherhood. Parenting values customarily ascribed to the role of mothers and women in family life – for example, 'caring', 'nurturing' and 'emotional availability' – are now being employed to examine fathers' roles and responsibilities (Clarke and Roberts 2002). There is strong evidence in my research that the gendered processes of care and changing definitions of fatherhood have influenced these black men's understandings of fatherhood, family and community life.

The following case study of Donovan, a youth worker and volunteer, highlights this relationality between fatherhood, community care and the socio-cultural worlds that these men occupy. Donovan is a non-resident father of four children. He also volunteers on a black mentoring programme aimed at black youths involved in youth crime. During our interview Donovan spoke of his involvement in campaigns against youth and gun violence primarily involving young black men within the local community. He readily admitted that his interest and his involvement in this community initiative stemmed from being a father to three teenage sons (and one daughter) who lived within a neighbourhood experiencing some of the highest rates of gun and knife crime in Britain. Donovan was particularly concerned with how the threat of increasing gun violence in urban black neighbourhoods could potentially impact on his own sons' lives. This prompted Donovan to participate in the mentoring programme and become a member of a coalition of parents that actively campaigned against this issue. Donovan enjoyed a high-profile role within the organisation and, as a result, he was a well-respected figure within his locale. In this community care role he was regularly invited to give public speeches to representatives from national and government agencies concerning how to address youth and gun violence. Donovan was one of the many examples of fathers that discussed their caring activities within their local neighbourhoods. A common theme in many of the fathers' accounts was that fatherhood encouraged a sense of obligation and responsibility to become involved in community care. It is also important to acknowledge that their involvement in community care was also borne out of other self-interest motivations. In Donovan's case, highlighted above, his community care was focused around preventing his children becoming victims of gun violence, which was a very real threat in his local neighbourhood.

For other fathers, however, it was simply a desire to become a better parent or improve their parenting skills that led to their involvement in community care networks and associations. Such is the case of Randy. At the time of our interview Randy was acting as parental guardian to his grandson whilst his daughter, a lone mother, was working abroad for six months. Randy recounted that he wanted to update and familiarise himself with the schooling curriculum. First, so that he would be better able to assist his grandson with his school homework. Second, so that he could confidently and with ease speak to his grandson's teachers at the bi-annual school's progress meetings. These reasons acted as a catalyst for Randy volunteering to read to children at the local black-supplementary school his grandson attended every Saturday morning.

Black fathers' participation in their children's social activities enabled them to further establish community bonds and interests. This in turn sometimes encouraged an association and engagement with their community organisations. These men's experiences reinforce the claim by Weller (2006) about the importance of children in developing their parents' social networks within local neighbourhoods. Gender divisions, however, play a crucial role in determining the level and nature of these social networks. The research evidence suggests that fathers have lower levels of access to community resources than mothers. In addition, fathers do not access community resources in the same way that mothers do (Doucet 2000, 2001, 2006a).

Mothers' high rates of community involvement are established through their participation in community activities and as a result of having primary responsibility for organising and coordinating children's educational and social activities within their locales. Fathers, in contrast, feel 'out of place' in these female-dominated spaces and as a result encounter social exclusion from local community programmes (Doucet 2006b). This research finding resonates with my own study of black men's caring as it relates to family and community. Some of the male participants explicitly referred to the fear and public perceptions associated with embodied black masculinities – aggressive, hypersexualised and criminal – and that this makes them feel even more physically 'out of place' in (white-majority) female-dominated spaces. In the following account, Vincent, a mental health manager and father of three children, offers an account that compares his experiences in the school playground, dominated by (white-majority) mothers, with his experiences at the black-led Pentecostal Church he regularly attended, which was similarly dominated by (black-majority) mothers:

> In that situation [school playground] I'm usually the only black person in the playground and being black, male and 6ft 4 I really stand out. They [mothers] don't know what to say. They're usually very predictable and I always get the

same comments, 'my goodness, you're big, you're so big, how tall are you?' or 'Isn't it marvellous you collect your children from school'. I just smile and don't say anything much but inside I'm fuming and thinking 'what does it matter how tall I am' and 'why would I not be with my children?' 'Stupid woman!' But at least these ladies make some effort and to talk to me, whereas some of the others just keep their distance and they're wary of me . . . The other day this little girl was chasing around the playground and she fell down right in front of me and my natural instinct was to help her up . . . I went to pick her up and her mother rushed over and dragged her away from me; she didn't even say 'thank-you' or make eye contact. What did she think I was going to do in a playground full of parents? . . . at our Church I'm one of the few men that go every Sunday but it's really funny because I'm aware I'm surrounded by women, but I never feel self-conscious about it and I don't feel I stand out but I must do, right?

What Vincent's example reflects is that black men's gendered and racialised experiences of broader structural inequalities, as well as social exclusion, underpin their caring work.

A common strand in the discussion that connects these men's experiences was the statements that they felt 'safe', 'less exposed' and 'less vulnerable' accessing and care-giving within black-led community organisations. Continually highlighted in their accounts was the feeling of mistrust and disconnect from mainstream services. The men anticipated racial discrimination which then, in turn, inhibited them from accessing these services and other forms of caring networks found within their local communities. In many ways this finding confirms the importance of perceptions and experiences of racism in influencing black individuals' access to, and participation within, local community organisations (Campbell and McLean 2002).

Conclusion

This chapter demonstrates that black men are involved in caring despite the limited attention given in the literature to understanding black men in this role. Gendered and racialised identities impact the type and forms of care work performed and replicate broader structural inequalities within society. What I have attempted to show with the accounts presented is that culturally prescribed understandings of black masculine identities are an essential feature of black men's caring. Belonging and commitment to their neighbourhood, ethnic community and kinship networks was also an overriding aspect of their community activities. The men interviewed highlighted feelings of obligation and responsibility to family and community. They also expressed a desire to 'give back' to their 'black neighbourhoods'. Participating in black community programmes presented an opportunity for these men to examine and define their identities and place in a rapidly changing world.

Nonetheless what is clear from the analysis is that wider structural factors associated with racial inequality and social exclusion impacted on the care work performed by black men. Their engagement with these black-led community organisations challenges the notion that black men (alongside black women) are passive victims of exclusionary practices and, as active participants of local community organisations, they must be considered as being important agents for change.

Notes

1 From an ideological standpoint this move towards essentialising black men is a deliberate attempt on my part at understanding how conceptualisations of 'race' and ethnicity are utilised in interpreting these men's experiences. The process of reconstructing these men into a homogenised and racialised category, however, does not mean that differences and diversity are not present among them. Variances in care experiences occur as a result of, for example, social class, age and cultural factors and these intersect with 'race', ethnicity and gender to inform their care relations.

2 Throughout the chapter I use the terms 'black neighbourhoods' and 'black community'. Historically, as a concept the term 'black neighbourhood' emerged out of African-Caribbean migration patterns and settlement to the UK, particularly in urban neighbourhoods within Greater London, the West Midlands, Greater Manchester and West Yorkshire. In policy terms 'black neighbourhoods' are generally characterised as being poorly resourced neighbourhoods, where there are high indices of poverty and deprivation. Factors that correlate with poverty and unemployment – such as, for example, underachieving schools, large concentrations of social housing and high rates of mental ill-health – are also portrayed as being significant characteristics of these neighbourhoods. However a plethora of empirical studies also demonstrate that emerging out of, and in response to, these social issues, 'black neighbourhoods' have also acted as critical sites of political struggle and resistance. Community bonds in this neighbourhood created public spaces for the development of day-to-day strategies and networks of survival and self-reliance. Through such urban spaces social solidarity was formed (Goulbourne 1989; Reynolds 2005; Goulbourne *et al.* 2010). The term 'black community' is a more generic term referring to the collective and ethnic identity forged by African-Caribbean migrants and subsequent generations as part of a more widely constructed diasporic identity (Reynolds 2006).

3 Project interviews took place in the UK cities of London, Birmingham, Manchester and Nottingham as well as several Caribbean countries (Jamaica, Barbados, Guyana, and St Kitts and Nevis). However the research material presented in the chapter draws only on those interviews conducted in the UK.

8   Tea and Tupperware

Mommy blogging as care, work, and consumption

Andrea Doucet, Brock University
Natasha Mauthner, University of Aberdeen

Introduction

The *New York Times* magazine (Belkin 2011) recently published a cameo piece on one of the world's most successful mommy bloggers, Heather Armstrong.[1] The *Times* noted that over 100,000 readers flock to Armstrong's site each day and read about her two young children, her husband, her dogs, her former depression, and her life as a liberal ex-Mormon living in Utah in the United States. Armstrong is the only blogger on the latest Forbes list of the 'Most Influential Women in Media' (ranked at No. 26, just 25 slots behind Oprah). She allegedly earns over $50,000 a month from her blog. How does she do this?

> By talking about poop and spit up. And stomach viruses and washing-machine repairs. And home design, and high-strung dogs, and reality television, and sewer-line disasters, and chiropractor visits. And countless other banalities of one mother's eclectic life that, for some reason, hundreds of thousands of strangers tune in, regularly, to read.
>
> (Belkin 2011)

Armstrong recently defined mommy blogging in the following way:

> If you ask me what I do I will gladly tell you that I am a mommy blogger. I write about life as a mother and wife, what it's like to live in suburban middle America, how I sometimes wish I could get in the car, drive to Montana, and assume a new identity because I can't take one more episode of Barney . . . A giant group of women have started their own websites to chronicle their experiences as mothers, and yes, this often includes entire pages about our children . . . I believe . . . that one day our children will look at the thousands upon thousands of pages we have written to them, the love letters, the detailed descriptions of what it felt like to watch them walk into their first classroom, and they are going to be so proud that we were brave enough to do this. Because we've declared that this is important work, hard and sometimes frustrating work, and we didn't wait around for permission from someone else to say so . . . I work harder at this job than I have at any other in my life.

The hours are long, and I don't get to go on vacation. I always pack a laptop when I travel, and I travel for several days at a time at least every other month. As a business, I have to keep up with a never-ending flow of email, Twitter responses, Facebook requests, and whether or not a pitch from an advertiser works with my brand.

(Armstrong 2009: xvii–xviii)

From Armstrong, we learn that mommy blogging encompasses work, care, and consumption. As work, it is a 'job' where 'the hours are long and I don't get to go on a vacation' (Armstrong 2009: xvii–xviii). As care, it is a chronicling of what many care theorists have argued over several decades: that it is 'hard and sometimes frustrating work' (Armstrong 2009: xvii–xviii). Finally, mommy blogging is increasingly connected with consumption; it is a 'business' and a 'brand' linked with advertisers.

In sum, Armstrong exemplifies the main argument of our chapter: that care work, especially mothering, is increasingly becoming a site where care, work, and consumption are deeply intertwined. An excellent example of this is how mothering practices and subjectivities are being articulated in digital forms in Canada, the United States, and the United Kingdom through the use of new social media and the rapid proliferation of mommy blogging. Building on long-standing debates on the need to disrupt binary and boundary lines between production/ reproduction, we argue that mommy blogging further disrupts these boundaries while also adding consumption to this mix. That is, the particular forms, practices, and purposes of mommy blogs are contributing to the rapid transformation of theoretical concepts of care and to a further blurring of the boundaries between care, work, and consumption.

This chapter is rooted in two bodies of literature. The first is the burgeoning scholarly literature on mothering and consumption that spans many areas of the care of children, including the broad range of products and marketing aimed at mothers from before conception has occurred and up until young adults leave the family home (e.g. Clarke 2004, 2007; Pugh 2005, 2009; Taylor *et al.* 2004). A related body of research on families and consumption is work on the 'commercialization of intimate life' (Hochschild 2003; Casey and Martens 2007) who point to how corporate capitalism is constantly encroaching on personal life, especially caring within the family. While scholars have indeed been slowly incorporating consumption practices into theoretical and empirical work on care, we would nevertheless argue that mommy blogging is a rich, but still largely ignored, site for the exploration of contemporary definitions and meanings of care. The second body of scholarship that informs this chapter is the cross-disciplinary work on the practices and subjectivities of care (e.g. Gilligan 1982; Kittay 1999; Hollway 2006; Tronto 1989, 1993, 1995b) and our respective engagement with this work in our writing on mothering and fathering (e.g. Doucet 2006a; Mauthner 2002). Even more specifically, we draw from Ruddick's (1983, 1995) work on maternal thinking and maternal care.

The chapter is organized into four sections:

(i)   First, we reflect on our methodological and somewhat accidental location within this topic.
(ii) Second, we briefly review mommy blogging in the United States, Canada, and the United Kingdom, how it has evolved over time, what forms and purposes it takes, and who engages in these practices.
(iii) Third, we work with a conception of maternal care that builds on Ruddick's threefold conceptualization of caring responsibilities; in addition to the three responsibilities of maternal care, as outlined by Ruddick and others, we highlight how mommy blogging inter-meshes care, work, and consumption.
(iv) Finally, as symbolized in our title metaphor of 'Tea and Tupperware' we point to some of the tensions that arise out of this intermingling.

Our story and mommy blogging

How did we come to research mommy blogging?

We come to this project along joint and separate paths. Some years ago, we developed the idea for a project we tentatively called 'consuming parenthood'. It grew out of observations we made, in our own lives as mothers, of the extent to which consumption was becoming deeply embedded within parenting practices. Building on our existing and respective work on motherhood and fatherhood (e.g. Doucet 2006a, 2009; Mauthner 2002, 2010), we began to design a study that would explore the rise of consumption practices, and their entanglement with reproductive and productive activities. Faced with a paucity of research on these questions, we turned to the emerging genre of mommy blogs as sources of information and possible forms of data. In addition to this shared beginning, we also each bring a distinctive set of experiences and interests.

Andrea

I have been perusing mommy blogs for about five years. My research project on breadwinning mothers included an online forum, which led me to slowly, but peripherally, participate in this burgeoning online community. I read blogs, I commented on them, I conversed on Twitter and Facebook. I became acquainted (and even 'friends') with some of the bloggers who were writing in ways that resonated with my work. I also wrote a few blogs from my work on stay-at-home dads and breadwinning moms.

I did not set out to do research on mommy blogging. But in the process of blogging, I was in fact starting to take part as a participant-researcher. While participating, three things struck me as empirically intriguing and theoretically compelling. First was the proliferation of conferences aimed at women bloggers and mommy bloggers (e.g. Blog Her, Blissdom, CyberMummy) and I observed that mommy bloggers were willing to advertise products on their websites in exchange for sponsorship to attend these conferences.

Second, I noticed the increasing volume of adverts on high traffic sites. Clearly, there was a growing fit between marketers and mommy bloggers. Third, and finally, I noticed that announcements were arriving in my e-mail inbox for courses, webinars, consultants, businesses, and 'social media bootcamps' that were explicitly set up to help bloggers reach wider audiences and to achieve some financial success; in short, I noticed a growing attention to monetizing one's mommy blog. From these three observations, I wondered: What is happening to our understandings of maternal care in this age of social media?

Natasha

From my vantage point, our project on parenting and consumption represented an opportunity to further explore a long-standing research focus on information sharing in a digital age (see Mauthner 2012; Mauthner and Parry 2009; Mauthner *et al.* 1998; Parry and Mauthner 2004, 2005), as well as theoretical ideas around the relationship between human and technological practices (see Mauthner 2012).

My research on digital information sharing draws on a socio-material framework in which the human and the technological are understood as constitutively entangled in everyday life (see Orlikowski 2007). Using this framework to understand the phenomenon of mommy blogging provides fruitful possibilities for building on earlier feminist work on the significance of domestic technology for gendered practices within the home and keeping women tied into domestic spheres and roles (e.g. Jackson 1992; Wacjman 2010). It also allows us to take these conversations in new directions by exploring the role of technology through a socio-material lens in which technology is neither taken-for-granted nor treated as separate from the practices of care (including reproduction, production, and consumption) that it helps produce.

Together, we began to ask questions about how women's mothering practices and identities are constitutively entangled with, and reconfigured through, their engagement with the blogosphere. Thus, we found ourselves in the mamasphere.

Virtual ethnography and community immersion

The methodological approach that guides this chapter can be defined briefly in three points. First, our thoughts are rooted within a burgeoning field of methodological practice that has as its object the study of online cultures through computer-mediated communication (CMC). This large and heterogeneous field, which has exploded in the past ten years, embraces distinct and overlapping forms of inquiry, all with varied methodological, epistemological, and ontological assumptions. While 'virtual ethnography' is the most commonly used term (Hine 2000, 2008), other forms of inquiry, and/or varied ways of describing this field include media ethnography, cyberethnography, and digital ethnography (e.g. Domínguez *et al.* 2007; Carter 2005; Mann and Stewart 2000).

Each of the approaches mentioned above maintains a dialogue with established traditions of ethnography. Some argue that while this field has some unique characteristics, virtual or online ethnographies are similar to other kinds of anthropological ethnography (Beaulieu 2010; Hine 2000, 2008). There are also researchers who argue for the need to draw clear distinctions between the study of real or virtual cultures, and online/offline communities (Markham and Baym 2009; Sveningsson 2003).[2]

Our own approach is more in line with the former, in that we believe that all research fields involve shifting and mobile 'objects' and subjects, and that what matters in research is more likely to be one's informing epistemological and ontological underpinnings rather than the field per se (Mauthner and Doucet 2003, forthcoming). We join writers who have challenged categorical distinctions between virtual and actual, abstract and concrete, hyperreal and real, although we also recognize the particularities of the digital subjectivities that appear online (Stewart 2011a). As Shields (2003) argues, the virtual is constituted by a great deal of 'slippage ... between a past, future and present, from virtual to actual' (34). There is also 'liminality' in that the virtual is always in an ontological state of 'becoming' and of people 'transforming themselves from what they were into what was, a moment earlier, only a possibility' (Shields 2003: 34).

Our methodological positioning is informed by the view that we are not studying the field, but rather, that we are part of this culture. We are thus in agreement with Driscoll and Gregg's (2010) recent plea for 'sympathetic engagement' with online culture and an 'ethnography of online intimacy and community' (16). In the words of Driscoll and Gregg, our object of study is *'the fabric of the community itself'* (2010: 7, emphasis added) rather than the 'cultural artifacts produced' by and in it. We did not set out to study mommy blogging; rather, we became immersed in 'the fabric of community' and these reflections emerge from that immersion.

Mommy blogging(s)[3]: a basic overview

The term 'mommy blogger' is a contested term. On the one hand, it has a slightly pejorative meaning; on the other hand, it has been reclaimed by some mothers who blog and by those who write about them. For example, in a 2009 anthology, co-edited by two academics with contributions from bloggers and academics, Friedman and Calixte ask: 'Why as feminist academics ... do we insist on referring to the authors of the parenting blogosphere as mommy bloggers?' (2009: 26). As they explain and we concur: 'the term has organically emerged as the *de facto* terminology of reference'.[4] They also argue that while the terms *mommy blogging* or *mommy blog* were solidly critiqued in some quarters as being self-indulgent and petty, 'a powerful reclamation of the term has been mounting by mothers who blog' (Friedman and Calixte 2009: 25).

In addition to some debate over the use of this term, there has also been some discussion about what mommy blogging entails, who does it, and why. A straightforward definition is provided by Canadian professor of English and digital humanities, Morrison:

'Mommy blogging' is a phenomenon of the blog world, attracting vast numbers of authors and readers. Sometimes referred to as a 'baby blog' or a 'parent blog' the writings most commonly covered by the label 'mommy blog' consist of everyday experiences written up by people – women, generally – for whom parenthood is a key identity component, and then published online via a content-management system (CMS) technology that provides for interaction and feedback.

(Morrison 2010: no page number)

How widespread is mommy blogging? To date there are no social scientific statistics on the scale and extent of mommy bloggers to report, although there is some market research available. For example, Technorati's 2010 annual State of the Blogosphere report, which particularly focused on women in blogging, noted that mommy blogging is big business for brands and corporations looking to find a niche in social media (Technorati 2010). In fact, it has been estimated that about 3.9 million American women with children currently write blogs; by 2014, that number is predicted to jump to 4.4 million (e-Marketer 2011).

The presence of mommy blogging in both Canada and the United Kingdom has also been growing with the latter accelerating considerably since 2010. This is evident in the 2011 launch of Brit Mums, a blogging community that resembles leading North American sites in its mix of topics ranging from the daily details of parenting to politics and charity works. According to the UK newspaper, *The Independent:*

A new breed of 'cybermums' is using the Internet as an office, PR agency and campaign HQ to launch businesses and charities from their front room. The so-called mummy bloggers are establishing literary careers, making their names as social activists or simply earning extra money through social media. Rather than just discussing issues affecting fellow mothers, the bloggers actively use the net to change women's lives. And the trend is growing. The number of such blogs in the UK has shot up from 100 to 2,500 over the past two years, and they are getting more than 10 million page views a month.

(Manning 2011: no page number)

The evolution of mommy blogging is closely tied up with the wider, burgeoning world of blogs which are, in turn, connected to changes in technology and new social media. According to Stewart (2011a), a high-profile blogger and academic:

The internet and Really Simple Syndication (RSS) have broken down the publishing industry's stranglehold on audience and distribution, and given millions of people access to public, narrative performances of personal life that would have been unimaginable twenty years ago. Blogs, in particular, have made it possible for people to cluster in virtual community with others who share common interests or lifestyles.

(Stewart 2011a: no page number)

Generational changes have made a difference as well, with high percentages of young people, often described as the millennium generation (ages 16–32), spending a great deal of time online (Technorati 2010). To date, there are no reliable statistics on age, class, race/ethnicity, and sexuality.[5] Most evidence is in the form of conjecture within academic collections where '(m)ost would concur that these voices belong mainly to white, middle-class heterosexual women' (Wilkins 2009: 153; see also Stewart 2011a; Lopez 2009). Class is, however, implicit in that one needs some resources to learn the technological side of blogging and certainly education can matter. As Canadian blogger Conners notes, 'the mamasphere is generally understood to be comprised mostly of women with access to and the ability to use the relevant technology – computers and the Internet – which is to say, women with a certain minimum level of education and some economic means' (2009: 107). Stewart also notes: 'The mommyblogging conversation is dominated by discourses of middle-class status and heterosexuality and also of whiteness' (Stewart 2011b; see also Lopez 2009).

Within the recent scholarly and popular writing on mommy blogging, and from front-line speakers at recent mommy blogging conferences in the United States and Canada, there has been some effort to highlight more diverse voices (Stewart 2011b). In their recent chapter, Calixte and Johnson highlight intersections between queer black feminism and mommy blogging and they argue that 'the mamasphere provides a feminist space to challenge hegemonic ideologies around motherhood' (2009: 58). A recent book by a leading political blogger and mommy blogger, Bamberger, claims to 'include the voices of women, diverse in geography, ethnicity, age and political persuasion' (Bamberger 2011). Similarly, the most recent women's blogging conference, BlogHer 2011, showcased the blogs and achievements of a wide array of women of different races/ethnicities, sexual orientations, and other forms of identification (Stewart 2011b).[6]

What do mommy bloggers blog about?

The field of mommy blogging, or what some call the 'mamasphere' (Tucker 2009) is, and does, many different things. Both scholarly and popular sources indicate that there are many reasons why women blog, and accordingly there are different kinds of mommy blogs, some which clearly straddle several aims. What is notable is that with the introduction of Web 2.0, digital technologies have widened and become more accessible to many parts of the population. Parallel to this, as mothering and consumption have become more entangled (Casey and Martens 2007), the purposes of mommy blogs have moved from smaller more personal ones to more consumption-oriented ones.

As is well detailed in recent scholarship (both academic and popular), mommy blogs constitute sites for autobiographic expression and new genres of life writing (Morrison 2010, 2011); they can be venues for empowered mothering (Miller and Shepherd 2004; Lopez 2009; Friedman and Calixte 2009), vehicles for political change (Bamberger 2011), and sources of support and connection for mothers on a variety of general and specific issues, ranging from pregnancy, attachment parenting, breastfeeding, green parenting, and post-partum depression.

From our observations of mommy blogging, we have identified several key motivations. These include: writing as a source of expression, and/or as a way of generating an income, or writing as a platform for larger writing projects (Conners 2009; Piersall and Armstrong 2011); connection and support for one's mothering practices and beliefs; connection and support for one's 'mompreneur' business; or as an online journal meant mainly for family and close friends (Morrison 2010, 2011; Stewart 2011b).

Some mommy blogs are explicitly or implicitly political, although the question of what it means to be political is a constant course of debate. On the one hand some have argued that the simple act of writing and reading about mothers' experiences 'can be tremendously affirming and empowering' (Douglas, cited in Tucker 2009: 8). On the other hand, others have argued that mommy blogs need to go some extra distance to engage with larger macro-level issues that affect all mothers (Tucker 2009; Bamberger 2011). However, in spite of differences in definitions of the 'political', there is an emerging consensus that mommy blogging can be seen as 'an act of empowerment' (Lopez 2009; Wilkins 2009).

Whatever their form or purpose, commentators agree that something has changed in mommy blogging over the past few years. According to Stewart (2011a) 'Mommy blogs are now business platforms for many, rather than narrative platforms'. As was well detailed in a *New York Times* overview:

> Whereas so-called mommy blogs were once little more than glorified electronic scrapbooks, a place to share the latest pictures of little Aidan and Ava with Great-Aunt Sylvia in Omaha, they have more recently evolved into a cultural force to be reckoned with. Embellished with professional graphics, pithy tag lines and labels like 'PR Friendly,' these blogs have become a burgeoning industry generating incomes ranging from $25 a month in what one blogger called 'latte money' to, for a very elite few, six figures.
>
> (Mendelsohn 2010: no page number)

Mommy blogging as forms of maternal care

We now turn to Ruddick's (1983, 1995) classic work on maternal thinking and maternal care. At the heart of it is a threefold conception of maternal care as articulated in the demands and responsibilities of what she termed 'preservation, growth, and social acceptability' (1995: 17–25); Andrea's research on primary care-giving fathers and her question 'do men mother?' (Doucet 2006a) builds on Ruddick's three maternal demands, but she also re-frames these as three responsibilities: 'emotional', 'community', and 'moral'. In what follows, we provide a brief overview of these forms of care – demands and responsibilities – pointing to how mommy bloggers enact and also transform each, thus pushing our thinking on maternal care into several new directions.

Mommy blogging and emotional responsibility

A first maternal responsibility is rooted in a vast body of feminist work on the ethic of care where care is defined partly as 'knowledge about others', which the carer acquires through 'attentiveness to the needs of others' (Tronto 1989: 176–8; see also Gilligan 1982; Noddings 2003). Attentiveness requires presence and the possibility of 'being there' for one's infant or child. How is mommy blogging linked to the emotional responsibility for children? Quite simply, web-based work – mommy blogging or home work sites that are partially or fully linked to mommy blogging – allows mothers to 'be there' for their children while also articulating maternal identity, connecting with other mothers, and possibly earning an income.

Social and political contexts are important here. For example, the United States is the only advanced industrialized country that does not offer paid statutory maternity leave and parental leave (Kamerman and Moss 2009). Working from home presents an ideal opportunity for new mothers to be with their children while building a home-based business. While Canada does offer generous maternity leave and parental leave (up to one year total), this leave is tied to full-time employment benefits, which excludes at least one-third of Canadian women (Doucet *et al.* 2009). The United Kingdom also offers maternity leave (O'Brien 2009) but, like Canada and the United States, it does not offer universal nor affordable child care to mothers. Thus, mothers in all three countries still face challenges with balancing the early demands of child-rearing with paid work. Mommy blogging as a source of income, or being a 'mompreneur' with a blog, are actively embraced by some women as ways of balancing mothering with some form of paid work.

Mommy blogging as a form of community care and connection

A second maternal responsibility is that of community care and responsibility, which connects mothers' care work in the domestic realm to the community; it involves social networking, coordinating, balancing, negotiating, and orchestrating those others who are involved in children's lives (Doucet 2006a). This concept of community responsibility appears in varied guises and with differing names in a wide body of feminist work on families and households (e.g. Di Leonardo 1987; Collins 1994; Hansen 2005).

The work of Bell and Ribbens (1994) remains especially relevant in this discussion, as they were perhaps the first to provide an important corrective to the well-known argument of Oakley (1981) on the isolating character of mother work. Contrary to that view, they posited that mothering networks alleviate the isolation of care work while also broadening the spatial dimension of care from domestic to community sites (see also Doucet 2000, 2011; Mauthner 1995; Marsiglio 2008).

We argue that mothering and care work now also occur in a third site, which is the digital space and activity of mommy blogging. This third site constitutes a dramatic spatial shift in mothering in that women connect, converse, and commune with one another through their computer screens rather than, or in addition to, real life spaces. Thus, many women take up blogging as 'a way to find a community of like-minded people and develop more meaningful relationships than those found in a chat room or an online message board. The writing itself (is) perhaps secondary to the friendships' (Gumbinner, cited in Conners 2009: 107).

This conception of community-based care work encompasses one of mommy blogging's key forms, namely a community of writers and readers (Wilkins 2009). For Stewart, mommy bloggers' stories, including those 'that were once societally unspeakable can be voiced, and likewise heard, validated, and amplified', and they 'become part of the shared conversation of mothering that circulates among those engaged in the practice' (Stewart 2011a: no page number). Morrison also underscores the community aspect by pointing to the intrinsically relational quality of the practice of mommy blogging: 'Most personal mommy blog authors acknowledge the importance not simply of writing in their blogs, but of receiving feedback from readers, and participating in what they describe as a community' (Morrison 2011: no page number).

Mommy blogging and the 'moral' responsibilities of mothering

Returning to Ruddick's work once more, her third aspect of maternal care and responsibility refers to what we call the 'moral' responsibilities of mothering, which relate to people's identities as 'moral' beings and how they feel they *ought to* and *should* act in society (Doucet 2006a, 2009; Mauthner 2002, 2010). There are at least two ways to view mommy blogging in relation to these moral identities and responsibilities. On the one hand, mommy blogging can be viewed as a way of keeping women tied to secondary labour market positions while also taking on most of the responsibility for the domestic sphere. On the other hand, there is good evidence that mommy bloggers are re-articulating what it means to be a mother in the twenty-first century. A recurring statement that appears in both scholarly and popular writing is that 'mommy blogging can be a radical act' and a venue for 'empowered mothering' (Miller and Shepherd 2004; Friedman and Calixte 2009; Lopez 2009). As Wilkins argues, mommy blogs contest narrow or hegemonic conceptions of mothering, and 'are often consciousness-raising' (2009: 152).

In our view, this issue of mommy blogging and empowerment remains an open question. Indeed, one of the central questions that we continue to pose in our ongoing work on mothering and consumption is if and how mommy blogging is reshaping meanings and practices of twenty-first-century mothering, specifically in relation to caring, working, and consuming. Does mommy blogging lead to a greater sense of empowerment, as many mommy bloggers state, or is it just more of the same where women remain primarily tied to care work with weak connections to the power and economic rewards of steady paid work? Moreover, does mommy blogging reproduce class differences, privileging women who have the time and resources to learn how to maximize their potential as mommy bloggers?

Mommy blogging as work and consumption

In addition to the three responsibilities of maternal care described above, mommy blogging also extends out from these central care concerns and raises the issue of how inter-tangled care, work, and consumption are within this set of practices. Mommy blogging as interspersed work and consumption takes at least three forms. First, some bloggers get paid small amounts of money to post guest blogs on other sites. Second, high-traffic blogs often host adverts on their site which generate variable amounts of income depending on how these adverts are viewed and used by readers; the same companies that place adverts might also sponsor these same women to attend blogging conferences and to promote their company products. Third, there is a growing overlap between so-called 'mompreneurs' and mommy bloggers, whereby women run small businesses that sell products and have a blog as part of their brand and approach.

Tensions can arise in this intermixing between care, work, and consumption. First, some mommy bloggers are criticized for seeking and accepting revenue. The arguments they make in response to these criticisms are akin to long-standing socialist feminist arguments about the importance of valuing motherwork (e.g. Luxton and Vosko 1998). The point is well made by Conners who does earn revenue from her blog; she writes that

(such) objections demand that mothers 'sacrifice' the creative and discursive work that they do on their blogs in the name of some non-profit-driven (and so presumably more virtuous) craft and authenticity. The demand seems to be that mommybloggers should *not* put a value upon their written work, in much the same way that mothers generally are expected to *not* put a value upon the work they do in the home. Most mothers stand to really benefit – as both bloggers *and* mothers – from earning revenue from their blogs inasmuch as such revenue might go toward the childcare or household support or technology that facilitates pursuit of their craft.

(Conners 2009: 94)

Another tension is between any 'authenticity' that mothers are trying to portray and the changes that may occur as they become vehicles for corporate culture. Conners maintains that 'the mamasphere has risen to the challenge of negotiating the difficult terrain of commercial interest and identity-driven content' (2009: 92). Others disagree. Douglas (2009: 112), a leading mothering author, journalist, and blogger argues that 'the pressures of marketing and financial incentives, coupled with more old fashioned problems such as mother-blame and defensive judgments, have resulted in a mamasphere that may not work in aid of mothers'. In her chapter 'Web 2.0, Meet the Mommyblogger', Douglas examines how market forces manipulate the need for popularity and consensus within mommy blogs, and argues that 'the result is a very potent form of bullying that may result in mothers being exposed to greater judgment than before' (Douglas 2009: 112).

Douglas also poses excellent questions about the compromises and tensions that arise when care and consumption are mixed, and even more specifically when marketing enters what can sometimes feel like an intimate domain. She asks: 'Ultimately how much of the world of Web 2.0 is about marketing and how much is about moms having conversations with other moms? And to what extent does the growing presence of marketers affect online conversations between moms, both on the social networking sites themselves and in the once sacrosanct space of moms blogs?' (Douglas 2009: 115).

Conclusions

Over 30 years ago, when the late Sara Ruddick began to craft her major treatise on the radical potential of maternal thinking, she focused specifically on the daily practices and concurrent identities of care work. One of her moral, philosophical, and political aims, which remains central to care scholarship, was her view that the moral perspectives developed through maternal practices could form the basis for a peace politics and a broad social critique. As she puts it, 'maternal thinking is a "revolutionary discourse" that has been marginal and peripheral but that, as a central discourse, could transform dominant, so-called normal ways of thinking' (Ruddick 1995: 268) and lead to a 'world organized by the values of caring labour' (1995: 135).

This chapter raises the issue of how to sustain such a commitment to the 'values of caring labour' at a time when the boundaries between care, work, and consumption are increasingly being blurred. We concur with Hochschild, who argued nearly a decade ago that there has been a slow and steady slide towards the pervasive 'commercialization of intimate life' (2003). Recent scholarship on neoliberalism and everyday life (e.g. Braedley and Luxton 2010) also pick up on this trend, noting, as Connell does, that: 'Neoliberalism has settled in . . . To understand the world we live in now, perhaps our most important task is to understand the market agenda and trace its consequences' (Connell 2010: 22). In this chapter, we have tried to 'trace' some of this entanglement of care, work, and consumption in the case study of the increasingly commodified practices of mommy blogging.

Our case study of mommy blogging leads us to four questions. First, how separate are care, work, and consumption practices? Have these always been closely connected?[7] Or are digital technologies actively and pervasively changing what each of these categories means, and how they intersect together? Second, is it possible to pull at least some care work out of this integrated mix and to argue that there *is* a form of care work, or 'love labour that is a distinct and non-commodifiable form of care labour'? (Lynch 2007: 550). Third, is it possible to salvage any of the allegedly radical potential of mommy blogging in an ongoing global recession where state services are being pulled back and workers are seeking new self-generated and entrepreneurial ways to make a living? Finally, how do we make sense of arguments for the 'radical art' of mommy blogging, when some of the bloggers who make this claim are also deeply tangled up in this web of care, work, and consumption? In this chapter, we have pointed to how the constant encroachment of neoliberalism and capitalist consumption pose real challenges to any remaining vestiges of the care-oriented parts of mommy blogging. We close with this view, as eloquently expressed by writer and blogger Lawrence:

For me a blog used to be like someone's home. Reading someone's blog was like being invited into someone's home for a cup of tea and a chat . . . I think that blogging can be an incredibly powerful tool when it comes to building community, even if there are a few blog ads running down the side bar. It can be a way of furthering the mothering conversation when we are just too tired at night to pop into one another's living rooms and jam. But I don't want blogging to be just another guerrilla marketing technique. I don't want to be invited to a friend's home, only to discover that I was *really* invited to a Tupperware party.

(Lawrence 2009: 138)

Notes

1 Armstrong writes under the pseudonym, *Dooce*, a feminized form of 'dude' (Belkin 2011).
2 Related to this is the argument for distinct methodological approaches such as 'netnographic methodology' (Kozinets 2010) or cyberethnographic research methods (Rybas and Gajjala 2007).
3 In a recent book chapter, leading Canadian blogger Catherine Conners cites another well-known blogger Liz Gumbinner who points to how the community is quite divided: 'There isn't mommyblogging, there is mommybloggings' (cited in Conners 2009: 106).
4 The weight of the term 'mommy blogger' is emphasized in the huge difference made by the deletion of one space. As Friedman and Calixte pointed out in 2009, the term 'mommy blogger' yielded, at that time, only 2000 'hits' while 'mommyblogger' had more than 80,000 Google items in 2009. We note that in 2011 its relevance continues to grow, with the term 'mommy blogger' pointing to nearly 700,000 entries while the term 'mommyblog' has nearly a million entries. We use mommy blogger here for purposes of writing clarity.
5 Statistics on bloggers are slim and collected mainly by marketers. In terms of the age of bloggers overall: 65 per cent are age 18–44. In terms of social class (income and education), bloggers are more affluent and educated than the general population. In terms of time, professional bloggers blog more than ten hours a week and 11 per cent report that blogging is their primary source of income (Technocrati 2010).
6 In addition, we have also observed that a leading American online parenting magazine, *Babble*, which also hosts high-traffic parenting blogs, visibly promotes a diverse group of American women and a few men as their top bloggers.
7 One could argue, for example, that Tupperware parties have, over the past 50 years, been an excellent example of the entanglement between care, work, and consumption (Vincent 2003). Thanks to Linda Bell for pointing this out to us. We would, nevertheless, maintain that mommy blogging both deepens and widens these connections.

9 Researching 'care', family and neighbourhood in Tehran, Iran

Linda Bell, Middlesex University[1]

Introduction

This chapter explores issues raised by a mixed-methods study with mothers of young children in Tehran, Iran. These include perspectives on 'caring' encompassing: participants' responsibilities and attitudes towards child care, family, neighbourhoods and the State, within a highly gendered Islamic society; and the researcher's reflections on working in a cross-national team and the 'ethics of care' involved in undertaking research in these circumstances.

In 2004 I was approached by an Iranian, UK-based colleague to propose a topic for research collaboration with Iran-based colleagues. As I have long-standing interests in family lives, particularly mothers' experiences, I suggested a possible project involving Iranian mothers. We and two Iran-based colleagues initially prepared collaborative work over the Internet, using some of my previous PhD research material gathered in England (Bell 1995, 1998). This raised issues first about how far the proposed project might be seen as a comparative, cross-cultural study. As Iran is an Islamic state, the obvious comparison we could make might appear to be between the experiences of Iranian women and British Muslims, yet the social, welfare and political context would be vastly different. As I found out more about the current situation of women-as-mothers in Iran and how this had developed in the recent past (especially prior to and since the Islamic revolution of 1979), a direct comparison of women's present-day experiences in both countries seemed even less likely, if not unfair (see also Abu-Lughod 2002). Yet there were interesting comparisons to be drawn. Meanwhile I needed to reflect on what my 'moral' attitude was towards working with people who lived and worked in a country with an apparently poor human rights record and where the position of women appeared very restricted compared to that of women in Western societies.

My own PhD study in the 1980s/1990s in the UK had revealed women operating within networks that might be seen as 'maternal worlds' that were to an extent segregated by gender, but were also operating in different time frames from men and from women without children (see Bell and Ribbens 1994; also Ruddick 1989). During my ethnographic research, respondents kept diaries 'solicited' for research purposes, so some of these processes were revealed in more depth; such diaries (as discussed elsewhere) raise methodological as well as ethical issues for researchers and research participants (Bell 1998). My research showed mothers often depended on other local women like themselves for social support including child care, especially in circumstances where local kin were not available to them

(Bell 1995, 1998). The opportunity to see whether similar processes were operating in Iran, albeit in different social and political circumstances, was therefore an interesting one. We subsequently decided to try to use diaries in the Iranian context, alongside other methods.

I begin this chapter with a short examination of relevant studies about women in Iran (including material on home/employment roles), following this with an outline of some material generated by this Iranian study. This includes survey material and qualitative, diary data allowing us to hear the voices of Tehrani mothers as they actively 'care' for their children and families. Finally I reflect on my own position in this Iranian study and explore how consciously choosing a 'marginal' position as a researcher may allow awareness of how such positioning impacts on representing the voices of research participants.

The chapter as a whole thus engages with key debates around the 'ethics of care' (see Sevenhuijsen 2002), and maternal practice(s) and thought (Ruddick 1989). I consider how to interpret and fairly represent the voices of women (particularly mothers) living in a society considered patriarchal from a 'Western' researcher's perspective; also how to theorise the 'self' as relational rather than autonomous when attempting to understand and utilise relationships and boundaries in research contexts (see also Tronto and Fisher 1990).

Women in Iran: literature and background

Many researchers have discussed women's status in Iran; rather than focusing on mothering per se, some have investigated employment versus home/maternal responsibilities. For example, Bahramitash (2003) has discussed how female employment in Iran has increased since the 1979 Revolution, especially during the 1990s. Recent Iranian government statistics (from 2006) quoted by Bahramitash and Esfahani (2009: table 4) suggest that as a share of the whole Iranian population (aged 20+), women in employment rose from 8.1 per cent in 1986 to 13.3 per cent in 2006. These authors further suggest that there are important differences between rural and urban Iranian women especially since 1979, with a larger increase in employment amongst women living in urban areas (by 2006 14 per cent of urban women were employed compared with 11.5 per cent of rural women). However, as percentages of the total Iranian population these figures still appear low in Western terms (and some, e.g. Moghadam 2009, have questioned whether these figures are accurate). Other official Iranian statistics (Bahramitash and Esfahani 2009: table 4) show that in 2006, 30 per cent of urban Iranian women and 22.8 per cent of rural women were registered as unemployed. Bahramitash and Esfahani (2009) however present an optimistic, pro-employment account, suggesting this may be a temporary situation due to increased female education: they suggest educated women have simply outstripped the current job supply in the public and service sectors where they are mainly employed. They give economic reasons why women's employment ought to increase in the future and play down the relevance of Islam and other ideological factors in women's low participation in the labour market; this seems however to ignore the reported significance of 'maternal' and family responsibilities to Iranian women themselves.

The potential impact of employment on Iranian women's health was also investigated by several researchers including Ahmad Nia (2002). As she points out, two different but familiar hypotheses, *negative* or *positive*, may suggest, on the one hand, 'role strain' and work overload due to employment combined with home responsibilities; this may be perceived to impact negatively on health (see also Hattar-Pollara *et al.* 2003). However paid employment may be considered to lead to greater self-esteem with positive benefits for women. Ahmad Nia (2002) suggests in her study of employed and non-employed women in Tehran that paid work therefore produces a 'counter-balance' of both positive and negative factors. Ahmad Nia clearly identifies a dominant gender-role ideology in Iran, emphasising that 'For Iranian women their traditional roles as wives and mothers are shown to be privileged by them. In their own views, their traditional roles come before their paid work role' (Ahmad Nia 2002: 763). Like Ahmad Nia, Hattar-Pollara and colleague's (2003) study of employed women in another Middle Eastern[2] country (Egypt) suggests where women undergo stress in relation to home/work life balance this is mainly because 'traditional gender roles continue to be reinforced despite [women's] gainful employment, the participants end up shouldering the demands of and stress in their various roles alone' (Hattar-Pollara *et al.* 2003: 128).

In an earlier study of Iranian women, Ghorayshi (1996) suggests a complex relationship between paid work and women's family lives. Whilst they might gain personally from undertaking paid employment, women were arguably doubly unequal, in terms of numbers participating in employment as well as their employment status (this was noted over a decade later by Bahramitash and Esfahani 2009). Participants in Ghorayshi's study apparently relied on personal contacts and relationships in order to carry out their various tasks at home and in the workplace; however, this was not so very different from women in my own UK study who relied on family members to provide child care, albeit in a different social context (see also Wheelock 2002). Mohseni Tabrizi and Seyedan's (2004) Iranian study of social origins of women's depression, also presents wider social factors such as Iranian women's unequal access to valuable family resources, gendered divisions of labour, family power relationships and women's social and economic status that have significant impacts on women's mental health; this has further implications for 'care' in their families and communities.

This background literature suggests several areas of interest relating to 'care': further exploration of how Iranian gender-role ideology may impact on women as mothers is potentially important, and in our project we attempted to reach this issue through a focus on social support as perceived by Tehrani mothers themselves. We recorded in depth their own views about what kinds of support they experienced and required, trying not to make culturally inappropriate assumptions. It was crucially important in this respect that our team comprised UK and Iran-based researchers. Simultaneously we considered it was important to get a broad overview of mothers' experiences from a relatively large sample so our study might be comparable with other research. We took into account whether or not women were employed outside the home in order to explore issues raised by earlier research, but did not assume this would be the only reason for women to seek social (practical or emotional) support.

The project: methods

The project used mixed methods, first involving a large-scale questionnaire-based survey: 600 women living in eight different districts of Tehran took part and completed questionnaires (the sample was constructed by colleagues living in Tehran and divided across three broad areas of the city: n = 199 [North], n =199 [Central], n = 202 [South]). These areas also reflected class differences between localities, from the more affluent North to the poorer Southern districts (although this methodology also raises issues about possible conflation of women's 'social class' identifications with locality/residence). We explored women's support and health needs, social/economic issues (e.g. employment, time factors) and the relevance of socio-cultural issues including family ties in defining and maintaining child care and other social support. Questionnaires were distributed by Iranian researchers to mothers who attended specific health care clinics.

It was important for this study to explore whether Tehrani mothers obtained or offered support and 'care' from within or outside the household, from friends, wider kin, from 'weaker' local ties or institutional contacts; consequently a focus on area of residence/locality was likely to be important. For the qualitative part of this study, 22 survey respondents from across the eight identified localities were interviewed in more depth and they kept diaries for a 15-day period in May/June 2005. These women were distributed across 'upper class' (n = 6), 'middle class' (n = 8) and 'lower class' (n = 8) localities. We issued guidelines for diaries in advance, so they were loosely structured and intended to record all day-to-day events (7 a.m. to 10 p.m.) and any day-time telephone or face-to-face contacts in women's own words. Diary guidelines were produced in English then translated into Farsi. The women's own narratives were then written in Farsi and translated back into English by bilingual members of the research team. As part of the interview, questions were asked about mothers' social networks and these responses were plotted onto network diagrams, which had been developed from previous work by Wallman (1984: 61).

Women as mothers in Tehran: caring and coping

When I consider what underpinned how Tehrani mothers in this sample 'cared', 'caring' can include 'caring for' (e.g. in relation to children) but also 'caring about' (the family, friends, neighbours, etc.). These two aspects of 'care' do, of course, overlap, as Sevenhuijsen (2002: 135) notes, 'caring is a social activity in itself and . . . the moral orientation of care is crucial both for the provision of basic needs and for processes of social cohesion'. Ruddick's (1989) notion of 'maternal thinking' is also useful here, based on mothering practices that she suggests '"protect" children (universally), "nurture" them (in culturally/historically specific ways) and thirdly "train" or "shape" children's development in "acceptable" ways

. . . [that vary] enormously within and amongst groups and cultures' (21). Tehrani mothers therefore 'cared' and 'coped' with everyday life in ways that made sense within their own social environment and which (following Ruddick) visibly reflect their 'maternal' preoccupations within a highly gendered society. I next discuss briefly some project data that shed light on Tehrani mothers' ways of 'caring', derived from background survey information and from women's diaries. I then present two 'case examples' (taken from diary narratives) to illustrate complex aspects of Tehrani mothers' lives, 'caring and coping'.

Women surveyed ranged from 18 to 45 years (mean age 30): 96 per cent reported they were married; 21 per cent said they were employed outside the home.[3] About a fifth of families shared a home with parents or parents-in-law and this was especially likely in the Southern area ('lower class'; a statistically significant result). Network diagrams produced with the 22 women interviewees shed further light on who was significant to these women. Women identified between 7 and 15 other close relatives who visited their home. In contrast most only identified 1 or 2 close friends (8 women identified 'none') although half could name at least one other household that they visited (5 of the 'upper' or 'middle' class interviewees identified more than 10 households that exchanged visits).

About 40 per cent of mothers surveyed (n = 245) used some form of childcare support; of these 57 per cent did so 'regularly', and 41 per cent occasionally. Over half those using child care given by relatives or friends relied on their own mother; for over a quarter their mother-in-law provided child care. A sister was more likely to care for a woman's children than her spouse, friends or neighbours. 'Upper class' women's neighbours were even less likely to help with childcare support. We also found graduates knew fewer people in their neighbourhood and were less likely to receive help with childcare support. 'Middle class' women were more likely to offer childcare support to someone not considered to be a friend compared to those in upper and lower class areas. We asked survey respondents who made decisions about childcare support: 91 per cent of mothers said they were involved in this decision-making – 38 per cent made the sole decision, 50 per cent did so jointly with their spouse, 3 per cent jointly with spouse and other family members, 2 per cent with their mother; 48 husbands (7.5 per cent), or in very few cases the woman's father or eldest son, apparently made these decisions. Although some women in 'lower class' areas said they were not involved in such decision-making, 'upper class' women were more likely to decide alone:

I decide by myself because my husband is at work [till] late in the evening.

Another 'upper class' woman said:

Just myself because I am more familiar with my child's emotional needs and sometimes I get help from my friend who has a child the same age as my child.

In the survey, women were asked how strongly they agreed or disagreed with several statements relating to 'caring about' their families or people in the local neighbourhood. Women from lower social class districts claimed they knew more people in their neighbourhood compared to those in upper class or middle class areas. They were also more likely to consider themselves 'local' to their neighbourhood (especially if they lived near relatives). We found 'upper class' women were less likely to say they trusted people within their neighbourhood than middle and lower class women.

Case examples

The following case examples reflect two individual mothers' experiences, including comments given in their own words. These examples draw out some of the complex issues involved in the social activity of 'caring for' others. I would comment that each diarist is presenting a picture of themselves they wish others to see. Guidelines supplied probably encouraged women to focus on the 'everydayness' of their activities, but we also get a glimpse from time to time of 'deeper' responses showing what mattered emotionally to these women (see also Bell 1998 on managing aspects of personal 'intrusion' when gathering diary data).

'Maryam'

Maryam is a mother of two daughters aged 5 and 13 living in the central area of Tehran in a 'middle class' neighbourhood. She says she is employed outside her home for about 20 hours a week. She records in some detail the times of her daily activities, many of which are focused on her children or housework. For example, day one is summarised as:

7.00–7.45 a.m.	Breakfast with family
8.00–9.30	park with children
10.00–10.45	watched TV
10.45–11.30	preparing lunch
11.30–12.00	having lunch
12.00–1.00 p.m.	cleaning and washing dishes
1.00–2.00	gone to mosque for prayer. Meeting a few neighbours in the mosque
2.00–3.00	bath children
3.00–5.00	attended religious function at neighbour's
5.00–7.00	cleaning house. 6 p.m. meeting mosque religious person
7.00–8.30	doing work on the computer
8.30–9.30	doing prayer
9.30–10.00	having dinner with family.

Maryam records leisure activities spent mainly with her family such as 'went to the funfair with my husband and children'. She refers to having 'students' and also notes visits to an education centre so we can assume she is a teacher. For example Maryam says she had a 'telephone (call) from my student's mother, I gave support and counselling'. However, she does not record regular times when she is employed outside the home, but we can work out from her narrative that she spends perhaps 7 or 8 hours (across these 14 days) on work-related activities at home.

She presents herself in her diary as a 'caring' person and records telephoning various family members nearly every day (mother, father, sister, sister-in-law, and husband whilst he is at work); she meets each of these people at least once during the diary period. She also telephones a couple of friends and records meeting neighbours regularly, especially at the mosque. She appears to be quite religious and makes a number of comments about her child entering a 'remembering the Koran' competition. Her final diary entry records rather sadly that,

> My child did less well than I thought in the 'remembering the Koran' competition, so because of this I do not feel good.

She refers to an overnight family visit to saints' shrines accompanied by her sisters and brothers-in-law, which seems to have been unexpected:

7.00 a.m.	Heard that we are going on a trip to Raineh (north Iran)
7.00–9.00	started preparing for the trip
10.00	we set off with two of my sisters and their husbands. We arrived at our destination and started looking for a hotel.

Like many women who kept diaries, Maryam records voting in the presidential election which took place during the diary period.

'Farah'

Farah is a mother of one daughter aged 5. She lives in a lower class district of Southern Tehran. She says she is not employed inside or outside the home. Farah enjoys sports including aerobics and swimming, and refers to regularly visiting the local sports centre with her daughter.

> We went to 'Ghianouri' sport centre as Mr Rafsanjani [former President] was opening the centre.
> 3 p.m. my friend was in the neighbourhood, she came to see me and we talked about my sport.

Farah's daughter is clearly a source of pride and her husband seems to share some child care with her:

> My daughter is very intelligent she knew all her colours when she was one year old and knows all the numbers.
> 1.00–2.30 p.m. I went swimming, she stayed with her father.

Farah clearly wishes to pass on 'appropriate' gender-based role(s) to her daughter:

> I went to do cooking, she [daughter] helped me. She likes helping, it gives her feeling that she is grown up. She likes to be the mother in the house.

Like Maryam, Farah records telephoning family members, including her husband, nearly every day whilst he is at work; she speaks to her mother regularly and also speaks by phone to her aunt, grandfather, brother and grandmother as well as to one or two friends. There are regular meetings with her family, some of which involve domestic work:

> I decided to go to my mother and help her with her sewing work.
> We went to my father. They were not in. We waited for them to come home. In their absence I did some cleaning around the house, hoovered, cleaned the cooker and spoke to my father's sister.

Farah suggests that meetings with other family members are less frequent but welcome when they do occur:

> someone rang the door bell, it was my brother, it was some time that he has not seen my daughter (because of life's problems), she was so happy to see him.

Other 'family' events are mentioned in Farah's diary and are a way of meeting family members and also neighbours:

> My mother-in-law and sister-in-law with me and my daughter went to someone's house for match making for my husband's brother. My daughter was shy and was a good girl behaving.
> 2.00 p.m. we went to the funeral of one of our distant family. My daughter was pleased to see the young ones.
> 4.00 p.m. we went to the cemetery for the seventh night after the death. All the family were there so we talked a lot (nowadays we only see each other on special occasions). I saw my father's sisters which I was very happy about.

Women participating in this study produced diaries which identify many aspects of being a 'good' and 'caring' woman in Iran today. It is striking exactly how Sevenhuijsen's (2002) notion of caring as a 'social activity' is embedded within these narratives. Ruddick's (1989) discussion of the various practices underpinning 'maternal thinking' is also relevant, and when interpreting this material, we can never doubt that it is derived from a highly patriarchal society. This raises interesting questions about how notions of caring and citizenship derived from the work of Sevenhuijsen or Tronto (Tronto and Fisher 1990) could be applied in this setting.

In the two examples above, we see Maryam and Farah following 'traditional' gendered roles within their families and neighbourhoods. Farah's comment about her daughter 'who likes to be the mother in the house' reveals the extent to which many expectations in this society remain highly gendered; yet her sports interests may also surprise Westerners. Maryam's comments about having voted in the presidential election seem intended to show us she is a 'caring' citizen alongside being a caring mother, and as someone who is loyal to her religious beliefs. This data might also be interpreted broadly in terms of the concept of 'sexual citizenship' identified by Lister (see Lister 2002) which 'defies and disrupts the public–private divide, which has traditionally underpinned citizenship' (2002: 191).

An 'ethics of care' is underpinned by a relational ontology, as Sevenhuijsen (2002) suggests. In the above material I have tried to bring out relational aspects of 'caring' that are evident in this project material. I am aware that in discussing their diary accounts I have (re)presented 'Maryam' and 'Farah' in specific ways, comparing or contrasting their (urban) lives in ways that may or may not make sense to them. My own 'distance' from these women, having never even met them, also points to my own marginality in this context (as I discuss below). Despite what I say above, I may have selectively chosen to focus on aspects of their lives that 'make sense' to me in a 'Western' context, although I have also attempted to take account of Ruddick's (1989) work, with its emphasis on potential cross-cultural nuances of 'nurturing' and 'training' maternal practices.

Reflecting on my own position as a researcher on this project

As an anthropologist, I might expect to work as a 'professional stranger' in others' lives (see Agar 1996). In practice this can entail active awareness and reading of boundaries in a positive sense, and acknowledging that I might be someone who is said to be neither 'at home' when 'at home', nor when in 'the field' (see e.g. Ellen 1984). This viewpoint has an uncomfortable, yet familiar, ring to it, encompassing ideas of feeling somehow personally guilty about what has been done or not done, about wanting to 'care about' informants in a socially active sense, as I might care about other significant people in my life. This set of personal and professional dilemmas goes to the heart of an ethics of care applied to 'doing research', especially from a feminist perspective (e.g. Tronto and Fisher 1990).

Despite criticisms of the idea of anthropological marginality (see e.g. Shokeid 1988), believing yourself to be marginal in certain settings may still be useful because it reveals the extent to which the self can be constructed within relationships; this suggests its fragility, yet also invites the researcher to develop a strong sense of identity. Acknowledging where you are placed/placing yourself – inside *and* outside – may be uncomfortable, but consciously choosing a marginal position might therefore be considered 'dangerous' but also 'powerful': it is not about being naively ambiguous but knowingly political.

At the beginning of this project I was obliged to acknowledge my explicitly 'marginal' position, knowing virtually nothing of Iranian society; I had to redress that balance immediately by finding out much more about Iran and by making contact with my Iranian colleagues. The question of 'anthropological neutrality' thus arises; can an anthropologist (especially a feminist one) 'ignore' difficult cultural and political questions without being accused of complicity? Would I subsequently have to 'betray' my research participants by making, for example, criticisms of their lifestyles? Could I assist others to 'research ethically' (and therefore 'with care') *inside* the society (and, most importantly, truly collaboratively with my Iranian and British colleagues) in these circumstances?

When I was asked to visit Iran early in 2005 to progress the project, arranging this involved several stages: getting approval to visit Iran from my own university and visiting the Iranian embassy in London to get a visa. I admit that overall this was a tense set of processes and I felt I was under scrutiny. Meanwhile Iranian colleagues had succeeded in getting ethics approval for the study, to be based in Tehran. Besides conducting a project on a topic of interest to Iranian colleagues, my own intention in taking up this work became to explore how far it was possible to research this topic where women were explicitly perceived to have a 'different' status to men. I had already committed myself to wearing appropriate Islamic dress, required in public for all women in Iran. To this extent, I agreed to present myself in public as a cultural 'insider' in order to observe and participate as fully as possible in the project alongside my colleagues.

During 2005 I visited Iran twice and work developed as I have described. We began the project 'face-to-face' with a small focus group for women at the university, which I attended. Some of the dialogue was interpreted for me at the time, but I still remember the burst of responses that emerged when group members were asked about their husbands' participation in the home. Questionnaires (using focus group themes) were prepared and translated into Farsi, and piloted in English and in Farsi before I left Iran. Questionnaire distribution and other fieldwork was then carried out by Iranian colleagues and despite my lack of language skills I was disappointed that due to my short visits I was unable to participate directly in research with Tehrani mothers; I therefore remained marginal on some levels although I also felt very involved in the project. This left me feeling guilty to some extent and, later on, I felt guilty again when political changes in Iran made joint publication of project data difficult. I wanted to tell these women's stories because I 'cared', even though I had not in fact met the study participants and my 'fieldwork' was mainly limited to my relationships with project colleagues and university staff.

I could scarcely have been prepared for the emotional impact of visiting a very different culture in which things seemed very different, yet also very much the same. Work at the university was reminiscent of that in all universities, there were problems over resources, computers broke down, women colleagues described themselves as feminists, we held research meetings and produced reports. I 'fitted in', people were kind, my *hijab* and *manteau* (coat) (bought in England) were admired and I learnt a little of the language. So did I feel marginal? Yes and no. I learnt to smile happily whether people were laughing or arguing. Some things were translated for me, other ideas were picked up through observation that I might have missed if my grasp of the language had been better. What impact did this marginality have on the research project? I trusted the fact that (some of) my colleagues were bilingual, and that we all shared research data. However, because I was obliged to focus on what I saw and felt, instead of on language, I learnt a great deal on my own account, particularly about taking different perspectives on feminism; I feel that this could certainly have influenced the project. After two visits I felt very 'at home' in Iran despite the political upheavals and I also felt (and still feel) quite protective towards the people I got to know there; I hope to return one day.

In 2006, after my second visit to Iran in November 2005, when rapid political changes were occurring there, I presented some preliminary project material at a seminar in the UK. I focused, as in this chapter, on the question of how these Tehrani women had presented themselves in their diaries. I noted that, as in my UK study, Tehrani women did not tend to describe themselves in interviews as reliant on other women like themselves for social support (this reliance only emerged in my UK data through diaries and observations). Family members such as mothers, mothers-in-law or sisters (also husbands and fathers) seemed very significant in Tehrani mothers' lives; 'maternal', 'caring' responsibilities seemed paramount for these women, yet citizenship also mattered. However I was not really surprised to be taken to task in that UK seminar for not denouncing the position of Iranian women in general as 'unequal'. I continue to present these data in ways I feel would at least be acceptable (and therefore 'ethical') to these Tehrani participants. I do not consider we were simply being 'anthropologically neutral' in seeking women's own perspectives, because I am still convinced that in any project participants tend to present what they think researchers want to hear; therefore we should take care about what they have to say to us. Perhaps these are the voices (rather than simplistically 'oppressed' accounts [partly?] imagined by Western researchers) that need to be heard.

Notes

1 With many thanks to Dr Fery Ghazi who coordinated the overall project, women research participants and colleagues at the University of Social Welfare and Rehabilitation (USWR), Tehran, Iran.
2 I use the term 'Middle Eastern' since, unlike Egypt, Iran is not considered to be an 'Arab' country.
3 This is a high percentage given the official statistics quoted earlier in this chapter.

Part III

Caring for and about families

Part III Summary

Caring for and about families

Linda Nutt, Chrissie Rogers and Georgia Philip

Where the previous part examined concepts and relations of care through the context of 'communities' and networks, this part does so by thinking about the term 'family' – encompassing both blood and non-blood ties. In different ways, each of the following chapters engages with and problematises the idea of family, drawing on rich qualitative data to also illustrate ways in which this process is lived out for individuals. The settings of caring for foster children, mothering intellectually disabled children and sustaining fathering relationships after divorce or separation all enable an exploration of care in relation to ideas and expectations about 'family'. Each of the chapters therefore provides insights into how 'doing' and 'displaying' family (Morgan 1996, 2011; Finch 2007) in non-standard contexts can shape caring practices and relations in complex and often challenging ways. The chapters illustrate the complexity of emotional responses involved in caring relations and also draw out important practical, relational and moral aspects which the authors' suggest are often overlooked.

The part begins with Linda's discussion of her qualitative research with UK foster carers. Chapter 10 discusses and unpicks the emotional and practical difficulties in responding to, caring for and caring about children who have effectively been abandoned and for all intents and purposes been left 'unloved'. It highlights the importance of particularistic ties and emotional and moral commitments made by foster carers to 'their' foster children. Linda also suggests that these may be at odds with more formal professionalised or 'bureaucratised' conceptions of care. The carers in Linda's study are seen to renegotiate their life paths by changing leisure activities, work commitments and such like, in relation to their caring roles, but also to explain or justify their own actions, and those of foster children, in relation to caring (and moral) identities. In Chapter 11 Chrissie then continues this exploration of conceptions and experiences of caring relations and responsibilities by looking at the challenges faced by mothers caring for intellectually disabled children. Again, using data from qualitative interviews, Chrissie examines the particular experiences and emotions involved in caring in this context. She also considers whether feminist theorisations of care and ethics might improve understandings of and social justice for mothers, children and wider networks in these circumstances. The part concludes with Chapter 12 by Georgia, which is based on qualitative research with divorced or separated fathers.

Using a case study approach, Georgia highlights the relational and moral aspects of fathers' caring practices and relations and draws particular attention to the ways that gender shapes the complex and painful process of parenting after divorce. The chapter demonstrates her use of the feminist ethics of care as a theoretical framework and argues that this provides unique and important opportunities for analysing family and parental relationships more widely.

There are a number of themes uniting the chapters in this part and the first of these relates to the theorisation or conception of care. All three chapters consider what it means to care, and how empirical data on caring relate to conceptions of care found in theoretical or policy contexts. All three authors are interested in how ideas including dependence, altruism, self-sacrifice, obligation or responsibility are understood in contexts of caring where 'family' is also involved or at stake. Linda in Chapter 10 focuses her engagement primarily on the experience of foster care, from the perspective of both male and female foster carers. Her suggestion is that such experiences, and particularly the points of tension between a 'professionalised role' and a powerfully felt 'particularistic tie' are important to acknowledge.

Both Chrissie and Georgia in Chapters 11 and 12, respectively, focus more directly on the theorisation of care found within feminist moral philosophy. In different ways, both authors explore the 'fit' between conceptions of care found with feminist ethics and their respective research data together with the issues it reveals. Both are arguing for the importance of appropriate frameworks for understanding experiences of caring and both offer some evaluation of this literature. Chrissie considers feminist moral philosophy in relation to disability and mothering, noting the differences and tensions in conceptions of caring relations found here. She argues that there are three spheres that mothers with intellectually disabled children exist within. They are the *emotional* – where love and care are psycho-socially questioned; the *practical* – where day-to-day care is carried out; and the *socio-political* – where social intolerance and aversion to difficult differences are played out. It is via maternal narratives that Chrissie explores these spheres theoretically in envisioning a more just and caring society. Georgia demonstrates how the feminist ethics of care shed crucial light on the moral and relational aspects of fathers' narratives, and on the importance of gender in shaping the process of caring for children after divorce or separation. Her broader argument is that the conceptualisation of care within feminist ethics advances understanding of fathering through its ability to attend to the multifaceted and complex nature of caring practices and relationships.

A second theme common to the chapters in this part is their interest in the significance of intensive, practical and routine caring work. Most recently, this dimension of caring relations has been described as 'love-labouring' (Lynch *et al.* 2009) and all three chapters engage with this in different ways. In addition to their shared concern with adequately theorising the complex and multifaceted nature of care, the authors here also point to the implications or consequences of being directly and deeply involved in everyday caring. In Linda's Chapter 10 it is the daily routine care for children undertaken by foster carers, which reveals the tensions between the institutionalised conception of the role and their own, powerfully felt perception of what it means to care. In Chrissie's exploration of mothers' narratives, in Chapter 11, the particular intensity of practical and emotional caring labour is highlighted to reveal the demands, challenges and dilemmas involved; the rewards and costs of caring for an intellectually disabled child, in 'partnership' with other agencies. It is found that partnership is in fact benevolent rhetoric. Chrissie suggests that, whilst important, the emotional and practical challenges are sometimes overshadowed by wider public discourse leaking into and feeding social intolerance towards difficult differences. In the final chapter (12), Georgia also draws attention to the significance of 'dailiness' (Apthekar 1989) for sustaining fathering relationships after divorce. She suggests that this 'ordinary' aspect of caring for children is frequently taken for granted or underestimated by fathers prior to divorce or separation, in terms of its importance as a foundation for both emotional closeness and parental authority. Through these different examples, the chapters in this part resonate with Ruddick's moral philosophical conception of care as a social practice which produces a 'discipline' or a way of thinking (Ruddick 1989).

Finally, the chapters in this part are all relevant to current policy and practice debates. In relation to each field of research – foster care, families and disability, and post-divorce parenting – the three authors engage with the policy context, offering a combination of critique and suggestions for future direction. In Linda's work in Chapter 10 it seems that local authorities measure foster children's 'success' in terms of improving health, educational attainment and employment and yet this was at odds with the care and love narratives produced by foster carers themselves. Currently therefore it seems policy discourse and practice is too focused on the practical 'benefits' that the foster child seemingly requires rather than on the significance and 'love labour' (Lynch *et al.* 2009) involved, and on the whole family as a unit needing support. In Chapter 11 Chrissie's work implies there are overwhelming day-to-day challenges in mothering a disabled child that are felt both practically and emotionally, but for policy intervention the needs are greater than this too. Policy intervention ought to take place via a politics of recognition and social justice (McLaughlin *et al.* 2008; Nussbaum 2006), that ultimately leads to interdependence, ridding policy discourse and then practice of the binary position between dependence (a burden and difficult) and independence (self-sufficient). Finally, in Chapter 12, Georgia suggests that interventions aimed at divorcing or separating parents can be developed with or without an interest in gender equity and can too easily produce yet another adversarial context for mothers and fathers. Her argument is that policy in this area needs to be more attentive and responsive to the investment and 'work' involved in sustaining family relationships.

10 Foster care in ambiguous contexts

Competing understandings of care

Linda Nutt, Independent Researcher[1]

Introduction

Theories of care tread a fine line between celebrating care and identifying its costs to individual carers. This chapter, based on in-depth interviews, will discuss these issues in the context of local authority foster carers in the UK. These interviews offer insights into competing norms of care, in particular:

- a more 'public' and professional understanding of care with regard to children and young people who are subject to bureaucratised regulation and protection within the formal childcare system;
- a more personalised understanding of care that depends on a particularised and emotional bond between an individual adult carer and an individual dependent child or young person, that is seen to have the potential to bring about powerful change in the child as well as offering personal fulfilment to the adult.

In subscribing to, and living through, this more personalised understanding, foster carers have also presented an understanding of self that was highly relational, to the extent that the costs to themselves were seen to be insignificant in comparison to the potential and experienced benefits to both the young people and to themselves.

The research on which my discussion was based was rooted in a constructionist, sociological approach; this meant that – unusually for research on foster care – the focus was upon the carers' personal diverse experiences and perspectives rather than evaluations of 'best care' for the young people. It did not explore the perspectives or needs of the fostered children themselves, although this is undoubtedly an important topic in its own right, which has its own considerable literature (Dowling 1996; Triseliotis 1980). Of the 27 foster households in my study, 7 had fostered ten or more children, and 3 at least five. The 46 foster carers represented different nationalities, cultures and class whilst including all types of fostering from emergency placements to 'quasi-adoption'. They comprised a full range of ages, lifestyles, geographical areas, own family constitutions and single carers of both genders. This chapter considers how they comprehended and explained their framework of care in which the most salient dividing line was between the differing perspectives of 'public' authority, where young people were positioned as 'bureaucratised children', and their own 'private' care. This private care, in the domestic familial setting, had allowed them to identify and prize the significance of a particularistic (an intimate, emotional, individualised) tie between child and carer (Nutt 2006). Moreover, in the process, some of the more common themes of the gendering of care became blurred. I will therefore commence by considering the position of male foster carers in my study before elaborating the underpinnings and meanings through which my interviewees narrated their lives as foster carers.

Men and fostering

Sometimes the ambiguities and ambivalences of care are highly gendered, but with these foster carers, men as well as women, were actively involved in, and affected by, the rewards and costs of caring. Thus, although in most foster families it was predominantly the female carer who took the lead, 20 male carers were interviewed for this research. Five considered themselves as taking the lead role, particularly in all formal negotiations with the authorities. It is significant that all 20 males had views about caring. The majority did not distance themselves but spoke about their own feelings. They were not solely concerned with their paid employment and their careers; work was important but when making work-related decisions they took into account their caring responsibilities for the fostered children.

Although the majority perceived themselves as occupying a supporting role, foster care had significantly compromised their lives. Mike had made arrangements both to leave work early to care for the foster child thus permitting his wife to attend official appointments and to take holiday leave to give witness in court. Simon related changing shifts and giving up overtime opportunities to attend meetings. Both Brian and Harry changed to early shifts to be at home during the day to support their wives' care for foster children. Though Harry noted that this was not always enough:

> Like taking them to hospital, I got to come home, leave work, take Celia [his wife] up there, come back again and then go back to work. Or I'll probably take a day off [work], instead of losing the money. You know, easier.[2]

In different ways they had all made employment and social changes, adapting their work days and their home lives for the sake of the foster children. None of them suggested that any of these arrangements had been altered for birth children. They had organised them because looking after foster children offered them a special relationship. Mo had refused promotion in order to be available for Jodie. He described his idea of heaven as 'her smile': given her profound disabilities this had to be an emotional 'heaven' because of her sentimental value. The male carers in the study described a sense of connectedness with the children and a belief that foster children needed close intimate ties with both male and female carers.

From parents to carers

Whilst fostering has been a common practice around the world (Owusu-Bempah 2010), within the established system of publicly administered child care in the UK, the fostering of children was originally framed in the language of 'family' relationships, with children placed in the care of foster 'parents': a foster 'mother' and a foster 'father'. This choice of vocabulary underlined the surrogate role and official directives emphasised caring for the children 'as if they were foster parents' own' (quoted in Oldfield 1997: 19). Fostering was thus considered an extension of the mothering role requiring those 'natural' female virtues that are characteristic of the familial space. But in order to emphasise that children removed from their families still have birth parents, 'foster parents' are now 'foster carers': terms which encapsulate the two, sometimes divergent, discourses of family and bureaucracy (Schofield *et al.* 2000) that shape the service. Many adults who are thus 'carers' to one child are 'parents' to another and must manage this ambiguity within the same setting.

Generally foster carers described the circumstances and the context of their fostering as fraught with difficulties and lacking official support, in line with the findings of Sinclair *et al.* (2000) and Owusu-Bempah (2010). For some, children's exclusion from school, offending, drug experimentation, graffiti and damage, verbal and physical abuse were everyday experiences. Yet, whilst detailing the incidents very few used descriptions of children that were critical or judgemental. Frequently daily lives were dominated by the needs of troubled children whilst the carers felt unsupported by the social services. Care officials seemed (to the carers) unable or unwilling to provide necessary services (practical, financial, educational, psychological) for the fostered children.

Moral accountability

Laura and Stan, who had fostered over 50 children, had coped with vandalism, violence and behavioural problems innumerable times but were adamant that 'there are no problems with the children. Just huge problems with everything else' (the social services, birth parents and education authorities). Kelly regularly mediated with the school when her foster son sabotaged lessons, entreating for less punishment and more perceptive understanding. It can be argued that all children have agency but the majority of the study carers differentiated this from normal accountability (see also Ribbens McCarthy and Edwards 2000, discussed further below). Cyril summed up current difficulties with, 'I mean you can't blame him 'cos he's a foster child'. These carers found explanations for unacceptable behaviour as they connected lack of moral accountability with children's past experiences.

> Children in care don't show lots of different, well they don't show any more different traits than normal children, except they're far more extreme and now, because you know what they're coming from, you cope with a lot more because you know their problems . . . aren't their own making. (Olivia)

He sort of like moved from place to place bless him . . . you can understand why he's like he is. (Janet considering Craig's oppositional attitudes)

We don't know the *reason*[3] why he was doing it [i.e. violent attacks] . . . a problem because he's away from his mum or what happened to his mum or whatever . . . so that's not really his fault, so you can understand all that. (Gordon)

Foster carers as change agents: saving foster children

Whatever the difficulties with the children, together with their perceived lack of official support, the majority of the study carers seemed to have established their own coping mechanisms. In most of the interviews, foster carers presented themselves as having individually discovered sufficient internal resources in order to confirm commitment. Importantly, they had created their own rewards through the children: they positioned themselves as potentially very powerful in terms of the possibility of modifying children's attitudes and behaviour. They talked of changing young people and thereby 'saving' them for a more positive future. Grace described her own influence upon the children: 'to see a change – them is like magic and they *change*'. Whilst Isambard reflected on making a difference: 'taking a child in who was, who'd been excluded from school and was really, you know – and by the time he left you he was back in mainstream school'. As with other women Hanneke reflected on the long-term meaningfulness of motherhood.

Well I want my [birth] children not to be a burden on anybody, I want them to make sure that they can look after themselves and if you can help another [foster] child do the same it will save all those, I won't say crimes that could have been committed otherwise . . . prevention, trying to do the preventative thing, actually looking ahead.

Many of these foster carers believed that they could save children by giving stability, positive role models, teaching and understanding by means of those notions of home and family which offered a particularistic emotional attachment.

Whilst social workers and teachers, as professional carers, might make some impact, these foster carers believed that they offered something extra. They were more physically and emotionally available to take a personal interest in and concern for the children's performance and well-being. The children's attitudes, activities and psychological states were of concern (Colton 1988, 1989). Their caring was based on a more enduring and committed emotional bond between themselves and each individual young person. Foster children were constructed as dependant and 'in need'; particularly in requiring acceptance and love. Carers, of both genders, depicted their daily lives in terms of emotionality. Keith explained that 'you have got to have feelings' and described how 4-year-old Timmy's initial rejection of him 'brought me to tears once . . . I was really upset, I thought, what am I doing wrong?' Jackie says of the teenagers she prepares for independence:

I do get emotionally involved with them. I cry for them, I'm happy for them ... And it *is emotional.* You know, you want the best for them. You want them to do the best they can do for their selves. So yes, you've *got* to get emotional, if you don't get emotional that means you're cold and if you're very cold then the kids are going to pick up on this.

All the study carers debated the ambiguities of fully, emotionally caring/loving the foster children. Typically, Margaret speaking of the 16/17-year-old young men she fostered opined, 'Well there should be just plenty of love. You want to give those kind of children, 'cos that's what they are.' Hope charted the emotional change that occurred with her care of Lindsey who was placed initially for respite[4] and then became permanent:

I can't just switch off and do things mechanically for her and I, I love this child as my own daughter ... it's been such a gradual thing that before you know when – you're besotted by her ... but I couldn't say to you it happened the second year, third, it was just one of those slow things until now I can feel the warmth in me the same as I think of Arash and Zeeba [her birth children] and the warmth it's that you know, I'm sure there *must* be some difference, but I can't, I don't *feel* any difference.

Hope raised expectations that biology mattered but suggested that caring had inevitably led to an individual bond and to love; she experienced the same warm feelings that she had for her birth children. Others felt that to hold back emotionally would disadvantage the child. Alice said of her toddler foster child how she had determined:

'I'm not going to get involved to the depths that I can't let him go ... I know he's gonna go back. I'm not gonna get that attached that I'm going to get really devastated.' But I can't. You can't *not* get attached ... I can see the difference ... in the way he plays from the first couple of days he was here when I was thinking 'I'm not going to get close' and the way he behaves now, 'cos before he'd do something and he would just look at me across the room and then he'd put it down ... Whereas now, he'll do something and he'll come running up to me with his arms up to show me how clever he is and I think if I tried to keep him at a distance he'd know and that just wouldn't be fair on him.

Whilst acknowledging that he had to go back Alice also stated, elsewhere in the interview, 'he's mine now'; the absence of a genetic tie had been no barrier to an emotional one (Golombok 2000). The social services' training included reference to children leaving so she commenced the placement believing that she should avoid over-emotional involvement. But co-residence had brought a daily, immediate quality into play, a physical quality that sabotaged her intentions. Her construction of their particularistic bond was in terms of the child's needs and she became emotionally tied. Foster-carer training may have taught detachment but carer daily lived experience invoked attachment.

The special relationship

Although generally for foster carers there is no blood relationship,[5] there can grow an affinity, a freely chosen act understood via the needs of the child which may, or may not, be reciprocated. This was demonstrated by the study carers' special relationships with individual foster children. Deconstruction of their narratives suggested that each foster child was seen to be offering the potential to become the all important love object: a caring bond which made life purposeful and provided happiness. In line with Zelizer's (1985) depiction of childhood in contemporary affluent societies, foster children were regarded as priceless in terms of their meaningfulness and emotional value. Yet relationships with fostered children are full of risk. Their tenure and primary alliances are always uncertain and their attitudes and behaviours can, at best, be unpredictable and, at worst, anti-social. Nonetheless these carers appeared to ignore the strong dichotomies presented by childhood – these 'extreme idealizations of child rearing juxtaposed with equally dismaying possibilities' (Walkover 1992: 178). Some of the interviews suggested that the more challenging the children's behaviours then the more the carers would protect and love. Meg, for example, had fostered Wes who was actively criminal:

> I had a lot of feeling for Wes. You know, I really did. I mean I've broken my heart over Wes I've sat [laugh] and cried my eyes out. And I've taken him back no end of times. (And remembering a boy who made an official complaint about her care) Wes would never, have ever, really reported me. I think, I mean, I could hit Wes, Wes wouldn't – he would just accept that as part and parcel.

Meg's care of Wes was 'an expression of moral commitment that requires people to behave towards one another in caring ways' (Brannen *et al.* 2000: 4). Accordingly, she felt it would therefore have been uncaring of Wes if he had invoked foster care regulatory systems and reported her for any breach of foster carer conduct. Furthermore she constructed a true emotional bond as overcoming all obstacles and breaching boundaries including both foster care rules and the rights of looked-after children – 'I could hit Wes.' But it was precisely this emotional, personal bond that she portrayed as providing the quality of care that Wes needed.

Jackie had reported herself to the social worker for breaching these rights with a young man who stayed out until three in the morning:

> I got really angry with him ... When I started telling him off he said to me, 'What do you care?' he says, 'you're only my carer.' With that I just shoved him against the wall and said, 'I bloody *do* care else I wouldn't be in this state.'

By this mechanism of a particularistic tie the foster carers constructed themselves as individually necessary to each child. This raised a notion of self, an ethic of care of a relational self, which was actually enhanced through the foster children.

Foster carers choose to take on the care of extra children. The study carers constructed these young people as victims and exhaustively demanding. Significantly they were also 'bureaucratised', public children whose care was dictated and regulated by the local authority so that foster carers had very circumscribed autonomy. Additionally there was the disadvantage of different time orientations and competing time frames. Understandings of 'family' generally include strong orientations to time past and to a future (Morgan 1996); childhood offers parents both futurity and nostalgia (Jenks 1994). Family is about traditions and a shared history. The foster children brought no shared past and could offer no certain prospects of a future. Biologically related children not only ensure (re)presentation, but signify adults' hope for and meaning in the future; blood children offer ongoing and infinite time. Foster children offer only finite time; these foster carers invested everything into their here-and-now. Thus, even though relationships with children can be precarious, there was an expectation that foster children would give added value to the lives of their carers. The meaning of life was loaded onto them via the significance of a loving particularistic tie.

Ribbens McCarthy *et al.* (2003) identify the significance of dependent children in any claims to moral adequacy on the part of relevant responsible adults. They argue that when adults are positioned as having responsibility for young children, there is a moral imperative that they not only exercise this responsibility for any children in their care, but also accept that children's needs are paramount. In this study, foster carers' moral selves were shaped by their construction of fostered children as vulnerable, innocent and deserving of care via a loving relationship that only they could provide. Their strong ethic of care for others was prominent throughout the study and in the process they constructed themselves as moral beings. Not only did they try to ensure that the children's needs were given priority but their interviews suggested they did so in the face of problems and opposition from the social services department, other agencies such as schools, and the children's birth parents. They presented themselves as giving the children's needs priority before those of themselves and frequently their own families. They regularly chose to change their lives in order to better accommodate the needs of the fostered children.

Meg related how she sat with her fostered sons until the early hours ('because *this* is the time these kids want to talk') and how, although originally house proud, housework and gardening took second place:

> [New foster carers] were asking things about, you know, these kids adjusting to a different – I said, it's not the *kids*. We're the ones that got to adjust. Which it is! I mean OK it's all strange for the kids but we're the ones got to do the adjusting and changing. And we have to do it for every different child we get.

Meg's construction of each young person is that they are individually so precious that she must make personal adaptations to suit their uniqueness. In other interviews each foster carer described personal adaptations to the needs and demands of foster children: Mandy paid for new banisters, Ruth had a wall removed, Janet gave up her evening class and Cyril his sports programmes in favour of the foster child's choice, Gordon altered his work hours whilst Clive and Kelly changed their friendship group for those 'who are sensitive to our boys' feelings'. When asked to consider a theoretical dilemma (posed as a vignette in the research study) of choice between a birth child's school concert or a foster child's court case the majority of carers chose the court case.

An ethic of care

However, in any potential collision of the two ethics – an ethic of care for children and an ethic of self-care – it can be argued that, for these interviewees, these two ethics of care complemented each other. The ethic of self-care for the foster carer was tied in with their self-esteem and self-identity. Looking after the children of others may have been a service but, more importantly, it was also a way of life whereby the carers described their own interests as mutually compatible with the care of these particular others. They did not recognise any division of interests: there was no collision or conflict. Foster care was an essential part of what they were; a sense of self bound up with their love for children and young people, and the motivation for their agency. They considered the challenges and satisfactions provided by foster care: opportunities for education, for occupation, for mental stimulation and for emotional satisfaction. From these they constructed a strong ethic of self-care but one that was constructed in harmony with an ethic of child care. It was not an immoral stance in terms of failing the children since it shored up and complemented the ethic of care that served children's needs. These foster carers constructed fostering as providing a satisfying and personally fulfilling moral career.

Set alongside this are important official reports which have identified the potential for negligent care and actual abuse within foster carer households – for example Waterhouse (2000), Utting (1997) and Berridge and Cleaver (1987). It is not possible to tell whether there were any such carers in my study, only to note that generally in interviews respondents manage self-presentation and parents wish to appear competent and adequate (Baruch 1981). These carers were no different. Parenthood and family life is about being a moral person; Ribbens McCarthy and Edwards (2000) conclude that it is virtually impossible for a responsible adult to produce a viable narrative and thus relate an immoral tale with regard to children. My sample was culled through the carers' own networks and so cannot therefore be fully representative. But if foster care is bound up with notions of being a moral person, could a carer express a negative view of the child as undeserving? Could they admit dislike of a child or experience one as unfulfilling?

Brian and Tricia continued to grieve for a young girl who was removed because her behaviour had threatened their marriage. Independently they described the termination in terms of 'broken hearts' and feeling 'distraught', and retained contact. Celia, Laura, Grace and Stuart had each requested that children be placed elsewhere because of conflict with their birth children, but not one of them criticised the children concerned. Gordon and Emma blamed themselves because their first two boys proved impossible to manage. Jackie maintained supportive contact with a young woman who had stolen and used her cheque book. Georgina intimated that she would request another family for their foster child because hers could not provide the detail of care he required – but insisted that it was the fault of her family and not the boy.

But there were two foster carers who had found fault with the children. Richard had evicted Jake 'on principle'; he had stolen cash when Richard regarded him as of an age to understand theft. Meg insisted upon the removal of a teenager who had ignored her offers of kindness and daily grieved for his mother, refusing to allow Meg to replace her. As a fostered child with his own birth mother he had repudiated his carer's overtures of nurturing and mothering and rejected the special relationship. Upset and frustrated she had verbally scorned his sulking. He had immediately written out a list of what she accepted as valid complaints against her, thereby placing himself as a bureaucratised child and thus outside the framework of personalised care that she believed she could offer. It was thus perhaps only Richard and Meg in this study who had considered that a child could be undeserving of their care; that it was therefore morally acceptable not to continue the responsibility when they were unable to build a particularistic tie.

Beck and Beck-Gernsheim quote Nichteheliche Lebensgemeinschaften that motherhood 'is felt to be a crucial and exceptional test of one's own character' (1995: 110). Foster children can provide the definitive challenge frequently requiring more understanding, patience and unconditional love than other children. In this study, the majority felt it imperative to invoke a special relationship with their foster children in order to cope with any difficulties. The carers expressed personal culpability when they had failed either to access services required by the child or the children left for, what the carers considered to be, unsatisfactory future arrangements. They accepted accountability for the children in their care.

Conclusions

For the study carers the significance and strength of family discourse and family framework was such that they did not view the child as a bureaucratised, public, contractual child with defined rights. Whilst the local authority measures foster children's 'success' in terms of better health, educational achievements and employment, the study foster carers embraced the child as innocent and victimised; as a member of the foster carer family, as 'their' child. From this came the notion of foster children that required the carer to 'save them through love' which frequently worked to the same goals.

Foster children represented the emotional value that made the carers feel not only responsible and important but also emotionally indispensable. Beck and Beck-Gernsheim (1995) posit that parents control their children under a cloak of love: Gillies *et al.* (2001) argue that parental support may carry potential overtones of control and obligation. Certainly, for those foster carers, loving the children provided a route to happiness and thus a meaningful life.

> [Fostering] opened my life . . . when I was at work one day and people are talking about their kids and their grand-kids and I was completely out of it . . . but I'm now part of a wider circle . . . people come up to me and sort of say 'Have you tried this? Have you gone?' . . . and it's a whole different, you know, which I've never been involved in before you know and it's lovely. (Mary)

Likewise Dick reported that neighbours commented 'cor you must be a marvellous person taking on a job with some child like that . . . or you're gonna have nothing but problems'.

By focusing on lived experiences, this qualitative research study examined the carers' own views and experiences and how they constructed their lives. The striking feature was that, although they were a diverse, heterogeneous group, their views, experiences and constructions were consistent across interviews – foster children were their priority. But fostered children can be problematic; they are public children with specified rights. They do not map onto the standard familial notion of dependent children.

Nonetheless these foster carers sought and encouraged a reciprocal emotional bond with their foster children even though this was compromised as they were not 'ordinary' but bureaucratised children. Carers continued to seek to 'save' the children because of their belief in the power of a particularistic loving individual tie. Fostering became a care identity based on love. In different ways the study foster carers constructed the children of others and their care of them as personally worthwhile. Foster care was framed as parenthood by choice. The carers in this study fostered because these children and young people confirmed their moral value, whilst also providing the possibility for emotional connection. Caring reassured the foster carers that they mattered.

Notes

1 With thanks to Jane McCarthy, my doctoral supervisor, for her continued interest and support. Also to Monica Dowling for her contributions to an earlier draft.
2 Throughout this chapter statements are quoted verbatim from the transcripts.
3 Italics indicate original emphasis.
4 Respite care is regular, part-time care of a child, e.g. one weekend each month.
5 There is currently increasing formal emphasis on the provision of 'kinship care' which is authorised foster care of children by relatives. This study did not include kin carers.

11 Intellectual disability and mothering

An engagement with ethics of care and emotional work

Chrissie Rogers, Anglia Ruskin University

Introduction

This chapter is about mothering intellectually disabled[1] children and the broadly defined 'care work' involved that forms a large part of a particular mothering journey. It draws on past PhD research (Rogers 2005) and more recent policy and theoretical discourse and asks, does a nation care for those who are in need of care and support, and how can interdependence be promoted?[2] Conceptually it engages with three spheres of care work. They are the *emotional* – where love and care are psycho-socially questioned; the *practical* – where day-to-day care is carried out; and the *socio-political* – where social intolerance and aversion to difficult differences are played out. Therefore, in this chapter I draw upon an ethics of care (see, for example, Held 2006; Noddings 1995; and Tronto 1993) and love labouring (Lynch 2007; Lynch *et al.* 2009), in attempting to understand what care work and emotional work are for mothers who have an intellectually disabled child or children. In this sense we might consider care and *who cares*?[3] Noddings (1995b) implies that natural caring is something that is maternal but ethical care is outside of this relationship.[4] *Ethical care though is more nuanced than this.*

My PhD research was inspired by my own mothering experience of having an intellectually disabled daughter (Rogers 2003, 2007a) and for this chapter I take an in-depth case whereby one mother's – Tracy's (a pseudonym) – narrative,[5] forms the foundation for discussion. I decided upon Tracy as a case because she has two very different caring narratives around two of her children. Whilst Tracy was not the only participant to have two disabled children (there were 6 in total out of 24) and was not necessarily the most extreme example, her narrative explicitly highlights care work and emotional work within the emotional, practical and socio-political spheres. Thus by drawing on maternal narratives we can move ideas and practices about care work forward in trying to understand the relationships between mothers with disabled children, professionals and everyday life.

Critically, in thinking about mothering and care, it is important to recognise that expectations (particularly in Western cultures) during pregnancy and beyond can be full of hopes and dreams for a child's future. Mothers often see their child(ren) as moving towards independence, autonomy or separateness and often believe them to be extensions of themselves (Smart and Neale 1999: 106).

However a disabled child's position is often in conflict with these maternal expectations and emotions, for example a child with autistic spectrum disorder who is unable to communicate cannot necessarily be an extension of the mother's self without invoking angst about what that self is. Or a child with Down's syndrome may be unable to negotiate full independence, autonomy or separateness and therefore challenge a mother's notion of successfully mothering a fully independent young adult. It has therefore been found that mothers are often left wondering about their own future and how their caring persona (potentially) spills out into their old age as their child becomes a dependent or interdependent adult (Barnes 2006; Bowlby *et al.* 2010). This, indeed, feeds into the notion that disability is a burden to both the individual and society, straddling emotional, practical and socio-political spheres. This has an impact upon policy and practice as well as day-to-day life.

To this end therefore we need to strip back what is considered as care, caring relations and emotional work and understand the *value* of care and emotional support within relationships. Moreover we need to provide a platform for understanding dependence and interdependence and recognise that interdependence will ultimately lead to a great many enabling and socially just practices (McLaughlin *et al.* 2008). Critically the feminist ethics of care literature problematises care in relation to, for example, the capacity to care, caring relations, gendered practice, labour, autonomy and dependence (see, for example, Held 2006; Lynch *et al.* 2009; Tronto 1993). Some disability literature, in a different way, has been very critical of interpretations of care and caring practices (see, for example, Hughes *et al.* 2005; Shakespeare 2006; Thomas 2007). It is these very aspects that are thrashed out here via the narrative of a mother with disabled children.

Extreme care and labour

In attempting to position this chapter I turn to Hooyman and Gonyea's (1999) useful distinction between caring for and caring about and suggest that 'caring about implies affection and perhaps a sense of psychological responsibility, whereas caring for encompasses both the performance or supervision of concrete tasks and a sense of psychological responsibility' (151). Furthermore, research carried out by Lynch (2007) and her colleagues (Lynch *et al.* 2009), provides a comprehensive understanding of care. Lynch (2007) actually suggests that there are three spheres of care: love labouring, general care work and solidarity work. For the purposes of this chapter I particularly (but not exclusively) draw on Lynch's (2007) notion of love labouring, or the care given by the primary carer which is intimate in nature and in this case refers to the mother's emotional work.[6] Critically, practical care work *and* love labouring can cause immense distress for mothers especially those with children who have additional behavioural difficulties such as overt aggression or extreme socially inappropriate behaviour (for example, violence towards family members or criminal damage).

To highlight how *extreme* aspects of caring for, with and about a disabled child can get, at one end of this 'caring' spectrum is murder and suicide. When stories of a mother killing her disabled child hit the media, moral and ethical questions are asked. That might be about the care for the child, the mother's mental health, or the lack of care experienced by such families from external agencies and wider society. In Lynch's (2007) terms this could highlight a lack of both general care work and solidarity work (for example, lack of care from extended family and public services). Cases include: Joanne Hill who was jailed for drowning her 4-year-old daughter who had cerebral palsy (Hornby 2009), Ajit Singh-Mahal admitted killing her 12-year-old autistic son and then attempted to take her own life (BBC 2010) and Fiona Pilkington took her own life and that of her 18-year-old disabled daughter, due to persistent harassment from local young people according to her diaries (Walker 2009). These examples of extreme 'care' are important in attempting to understand the enormity of both practical care work and emotional work that some mothers experience in their mothering journey. What these examples also demonstrate are that in extreme cases the care work and emotional work involved can go against culturally accepted norms – to love and care for your child unconditionally.

Such extreme cases might cause us to question what is 'natural' for example, about killing a child, including whether this can be considered caring, moral or ethical. Here I ask, is it caring and ethical to suggest that the care work carried out with and for a disabled (and/or 'difficult') child is done so out of necessity or obligation rather than love? (See also Nutt, Chapter 10 in this volume, for difficult behaviour and obligation in relation to 'care work', but with foster children.) Tracy, whose narrative this chapter is based upon, said 'only a mother could actually put up with this' and 'there are certain things in life where you haven't got a choice'. Care and ethics in this sense could be about human frailty and vulnerability; as implied by Tracy, who else will do it? Furthermore, intellectually disabled children, one could argue, are at times both vulnerable and frail and therefore unable to care for themselves (see also Nussbaum 2006). Nevertheless, the mother is also frail and vulnerable at times during her maternal journey. Interestingly, Noddings (1995b: 9) talks about the relationship between 'natural' and 'ethical' caring as it is often considered that mothering and a 'mother's love' is 'natural' and caring, but that caring is also moral and ethical and is often fraught with conflict, as identified above (see also Tronto 1993). This chapter draws on a less extreme maternal narrative than those in the media but still one that involves caring for, caring with and caring about disabled children, where care work and emotional work coexist.

Tracy – an introduction

Tracy is a white British working-class mother in her thirties who has four boys aged between 11 and 16. Two of these children, the oldest Dean (a twin) and the youngest Brad, have (unrelated) different types of impairments. Both her disabled children have been assessed for learning difficulties and received a statement of 'special educational needs' (SEN).[7] I spoke to Tracy about her experiences as a mother and how this has impacted upon her day-to-day life over two in-depth interviews a year apart. Interestingly she has two very different stories to tell which seem largely dependent on the fact that even though Dean, her oldest son and a twin, drew on her resources as a carer in practical ways (although there were emotional responses too), Brad had additional behavioural difficulties that meant her care work, emotional work and mothering identity were called into question by herself and those around her.

Dean

Tracy's twins were born 29 weeks into the pregnancy and Dean's lungs collapsed immediately after birth. At five months old Dean left hospital deaf, blind and paralysed. During this period Tracy travelled from East Anglia to London on a daily basis to visit him, even though she had his twin baby brother to care for at home. In the hospital Dean had probes on him which if left too long in one place made small round burn marks due to the low level of heat produced. She knew just this alone must have caused at best discomfort and at worst pain. It also had an impact on her relationships with 'early years' professionals due to the fact that the marks left by the probes looked like old cigarette burns and Tracy was a smoker.

In the early months, seeing Dean lying in the hospital cot, Tracy told me, 'I sometimes looked at him willing him to give up.' On leaving the hospital Dean had his first shunt put in – a piece of medical equipment for draining fluid from the brain for hydrocephalus. Tracy was very able to describe all the medical and technical aspects of caring for her son in a practical way. She told me she had watched the nurses for five months during his hospitalisation and had carried out her own research too (and she was a teenager at the time). This was the beginning of Tracy's caring story.

As we will see unfold in this chapter, living with an intellectually disabled child can push a mother to question her love for her child, which often goes against culturally expected norms – to love your child unconditionally. However, Parker (1997: 17) refers to maternal ambivalence and sees this as a part of ordinary motherhood 'in which loving and hating feelings for children exist side by side'. Moreover in understanding the narratives in this chapter, Moore (1996: 58) suggests, 'Mothering and motherhood are not, contrary to popular belief, the most natural things in the world.' Listening to Tracy's narrative it was clearly emotionally painful to see Dean in hospital with probes and monitors all over his body, not knowing if he would survive. At this point it could be argued that Tracy was experiencing both 'love labouring' (emotional work – feeling and doing) *and* 'solidarity care' (via the public nursing services) (Lynch 2007), as well as carrying out her own practical care work on a daily basis.

Brad

Tracy's experience with her fourth son introduces a different caring story. She spoke to me of Brad's *different* behaviour from birth. She told me that as a baby 'he wouldn't give me eye contact or hold his head up' and 'had a cackle that was quite frightening'. She did go to the health visitors but nothing was indicated as being problematic even though as a toddler Tracy said that 'he was very aggressive'. For example, towards his brothers he would, she told me, 'walk up and kick them for no reason, pull their hair, bite them'. Given the cumulative, disruptive and aggressive nature of Brad's difficulties, she did find her maternal self, emotional responses and caring roles at odds with each other. Tracy emphasised, 'I loved him to bits but there were certain bits that were wrong. I knew there were things wrong . . . But . . . (pause) I could never find the problem that existed.' Later on in the interview she was more graphic in her explanation of this love/hate dualism due to his disruptive and difficult behaviour. Tracy recalled 'there were times when I'd sit there and I'd be like that gritting my teeth, (pause) I hated him, (pause) I loved him, but I hated him. I really detested him, the child he was, and what he did. I was in tears all the time.' This emotional dilemma and emotive language was based on aspects of her life that were dramatically affected, and as his mother she was expected to care for *and* care about Brad – unconditionally.

But what of care when it involves at best disruption to the family as a whole, at worst emotional and physical pain for the mother. Based on this early caring encounter we can begin to see how care could be considered as maternal obligation and emotionally traumatic. Yet, caring for, caring with and caring about, could be considered as quite nebulous terms. But actually how people interpret and experience them is an important issue for the carer, the cared-for, policy makers, caring professionals and wider society.

Where practical care takes over

Research suggests that a disabled child disables a whole family (Runswick-Cole 2007; Rogers 2007b). This is largely based on negative social perceptions of (and sometimes intolerance to) disability (including difficult differences). A social model of disability, whereby barriers to inclusion are considered socially constructed, was a breakthrough in experiences for disabled people, particularly those with a physical impairment. This model translates into family research by suggesting that a disabled child disables the family based on social constructions of difference and disability leaking into and impacting upon family practices. The social model of disability was a reaction to many aspects of disablism, but also in response to the medical model, which pathologised disabled individuals (see Oliver 1996). These socially constructed barriers do have an impact on care work, caring practices and maternal care as this social intolerance leaks into daily life for mothers with disabled children and therefore limits general and solidarity care work. However with regard to the everyday impacts of intellectual disabilities and for those experiencing 'impairment effects' (Thomas 2007) (as experienced by mothers for example), the social model has not moved experience and perception of disability and impairment as far forward as we might have anticipated (Oliver and Barnes 2010; Shakespeare 2006). Moreover, the social model falls short of addressing aspects of *objective difficulties* and emotional responses around impairments and behaviour considered to be outside culturally accepted norms, at a day-to-day level for some families.

Thinking about care work and emotional work (or love labouring) and what this might mean for a mother, especially in the early years, is often about practical necessity and actual dependence. As in Tracy's case, if the shunt for Dean's hydrocephalus was broken and not replaced the side effects could have been life-threatening. Even though Tracy had, as a mother, become a 'researcher' and a 'nurse', she was petrified at the thought of taking Dean home from hospital after watching the nurses for five months. But learning these nursing skills was crucial if she were to care for Dean competently. For example, he would stop breathing while taking his milk from a bottle. She told me 'when I had friends round and we were watching tele[vision] and giving the baby the bottle [we] got wrapped up in conversation . . . and [I'd] look down he'd be blue. . . . he hadn't taken a breath'. She was told by the nurses what to do and pragmatically said that

> what you'd do is pull the bottle out and then we'd have to flick his toes and if that didn't work, pinch his toes and if that didn't work swing him round by his feet. Which sounds really weird [but] it was like second nature. I'd put me coffee down and off we go. Friends were quaking in their boots but it was just second nature coz I'd done it so often.

It is crucial for networks of friends to have some understanding of the care work involved and it is here that the social model is not particularly helpful (especially in the private sphere). For the first 18 months of his life Dean was blind, deaf and paralysed, but Tracy said 'I absolutely adored him, but dreaded the future.'

Tracy emphasised that she was dreading him getting older and bigger and not being able to cope on a practical level. She also thought about how 'he would have no future, nothing to look forward to'. Tracy said she did have lots of family support, 'general care work' (Lynch 2007), but no one took Dean from her to give her a break and said they were 'too frightened'. She went on, 'even though the doctors didn't hold out much hope, by the time he was 2 he could hear, see and sit up'. *Extended* early years care often goes beyond what one would expect as a mother, and as a result can relate to absolute dependence or at best interdependence. (Subsequently Dean went on to develop as a young adult and had some level of interdependence.)

All of this therefore involved extended early years care, practically and emotionally. Dean was nearly 17 at the time of the first interview and Tracy said throughout that she wanted him to become self-sufficient and independent. Care both emotionally and practically that goes beyond expectations of what mothering is on a day-to-day basis needs to be questioned. The narratives show how, sometimes, care work (learning new skills to support a child) and emotional work (thinking and behaving with care) take over other day-to-day activities as the child develops. This day-to-day work is often misunderstood in British policy as partnership discourses suggest that there *is* support 'out there' (DfES 2001a, 2001b, 2005b, 2007b; Rogers 2011) for families with disabled children. Yet the 'war like' experiences between professionals and parents continues (Rogers 2007a, 2011) making care work and emotional work at times unbearable.

For example, significantly on a practical level one of the main challenges facing mothers with an intellectually disabled child is managing or coping with the number of professionals involved in the child's life. As Russell (1997: 79) suggests, 'knowing 17 different professionals isn't partnership. It's a survival exercise with often conflicting advice, everyone with expectations and a bag of homework at the end of the day that makes you feel you should be the real professionals!' This 'homework' could be considered as an aspect of their practical day-to-day care work (Rogers 2011). Tracy was given 'homework' to do with Dean which meant taking on the caring personae of a teacher, nurse, physiotherapist, occupational therapist to name a few. This indicates the mother (in the case of Tracy) might actually be carrying out 'emotional labour', similar to that of paid care professionals (Hochschild 1983; Theodosius 2008). Crucially though this blurs with 'love labouring' (Lynch 2007) due to the intimate relationship and lack of financial exchange. Consequently health, education and social work professionals 'have a piece' of the mother's life and yet the mother continues to learn new skills because she cares for, cares about and indeed cares with her child and desires her child to make progress towards, at least, interdependence. Braun (2001) confirms this idea as she suggests mothers may feel trapped because on one hand they want to *care for* their child without 'public' support and thus conform to dominant norms around being a 'good' mother, and on the other hand they need/want specialist support.

As said, caring professionals such as those in education and health often become involved in the lives of mothers with intellectually disabled children and yet many mothers experience this as interfering rather than caring. Interestingly, drawing on Foucault's notion of the 'medical gaze', Culpitt (1999: 144) introduces the 'welfare gaze', and explains, '[t]he looking was not so much a discovery but a confirmation, an attempt to prove what was already known'. Culpitt suggests that by virtue of claiming welfare, a person is known as dependent, and that 'to seek public support is to define yourself as needy, and by definition dependent' (1999: 144). The same can be said for mothers with intellectually disabled children, who are looking for solutions to problems. Yet the caring professionals are often working within bureaucratic guidelines and state-led agendas, which do not necessarily tap into or draw upon the mother's important and relevant knowledge (Ong-Dean 2009; Tissot 2011). This emotional and practical knowledge may be an important part of the puzzle when attempting to put together a package of care for a child and their mother. I would suggest this is also evident for foster carers too (see Nutt, Chapter 10 in this volume).

Care, resilience, survival and skills development are evident in mothers with disabled children's narratives surrounding extended early years care. However, once thoughts of survival (or not) in any immediate sense wanes an issue of potential lifelong care is considered. This emotional lifelong care however is not always associated with practical care, but 'love labouring' (Lynch 2007). Of course there are indeed practical care issues with lifelong care, but the idea of the future and the emotional responses to 'what next?' are crucial in the caring narrative. Living with their adult child's impairment and what that future holds is critical in ethical care and thinking with care. What is often missing from policy discourse and care professionals' training is the focus on the *family's* lifelong care. Care ought to be privileged and positioned as not simply about the practical day-to-day aspects of care (albeit important) but how practical care work and emotional work coexist. Moreover, in addition to this the mother who is caring for, about and with their 'child' practically and emotionally then faces potential prejudice in addition to self-doubt about their own mothering abilities as can be seen below.

Emotional management and care – caring with difficult behaviour

Mothering a child whose behaviour calls into question her care work and maternal relationship when her child's behaviour is outside socially accepted norms is problematic. The very essence of what it means to be a moral human being can go unnoticed, until the moment a mother's child behaves in a way that is 'immoral', unethical and seemingly without responsibility. Several mothers in my research referred to difficult behaviour that *did* impact upon their caring and emotional responses to aspects of their definitions of moral, ethical and responsible behaviour (Rogers 2007a). This difficult behaviour included public masturbation, self-induced vomiting, boys touching girls inappropriately and criminal damage. Sometimes their care work veered between a duty of care (or obligation) and love/ hate responses that questioned their maternal identity and actual *desire* to care.

Tracy had different experiences with both her sons. She talked about how Dean's behaviour towards girls younger than himself was problematic for her and about Brad's behaviour that was so verbally and physically violent that she feared for his or others' lives. Ultimately she felt responsible for their behaviour. With Dean, Tracy said

> (there were) possible sexual undertones with the younger girls, but I think what his body was saying 'hey I've got lots of hormones' (pause) this was when he was about 14, 15 and 'I've got lots of hormones here I'm a man' but mentally he relates better to smaller children because of his mental age, and he made friends with a little girl . . . and he used to play with her and tickle her and (pause) although nobody ever said that he'd touched her sexually (pause) because of his size, and looking like a full grown man (it was) inappropriate for him to be playing with a 7, 8 year old girl.

This aspect of sexual behaviour too was introduced by other mothers in my research (Rogers 2007a). What Tracy said about Dean's difficult behaviour and his intellectual capacity to understand his actions, did cause her to contemplate her capacity to care; partially based on how *she felt* about this inappropriate behaviour. Critically Tracy's emotional work here goes beyond Dean as it involves the 'care' of others, in this case anyone Dean touched inappropriately.[8]

To then include Brad into this narrative and Tracy's emotional work, she said, 'by the time he went to primary school, parents were complaining about him . . . I was embarrassed because he was totally disrupting a whole class', but this was nothing compared to the disruption on a grander scale as she described here,

> One day when he was 6 I was driving past the school and I saw some guys I knew who were installing windows and I stopped to chat to them and they said 'oh bloody hell, there were some fire engines up here earlier' . . . And they said 'I bet your Brad set fire to the school', and I said 'yeah right' and we were having a right laugh about it (pause) and low and behold when I went to collect him from school that night I got called into the school and he'd burnt down 2 porta cabins [temporary buildings] and their contents! (She exclaimed).

As a result of this behaviour Brad was permanently excluded from school which impacted not only upon Tracy's emotional response to the situation and how she felt, but also on her practical care work as he was not placed in another school immediately. She also told me she was subjected to aggression and hostility from parents who were worried about their own children being around such a 'dangerous and disruptive child'. Consequently due to the nature of Brad's behaviour he was tested and found to have a rare chromosomal syndrome that – according to medical professionals – meant he was more likely to display aggressive behaviour. Tracy at this time said that she felt vindicated as she knew all along that there was 'a problem with Dean' and not with her as a mother.

The incident above was not the only extreme behaviour displayed. Tracy explained Brad had 'lit the gas fire and shoved the newspaper in the grill'; she went on to say that he had 'stolen money from school out of teacher's handbags, police have been involved where he's threatened other children with a knife'. In fact a whole host of events over a period of a few years had happened involving both Tracy's actual day-to-day care work and her emotional work. Graphically Tracy told me 'we've had three portable teles [televisions] thrown from upstairs windows . . . I've had neighbours knocking on my door saying "Brad's hanging out the window" . . . hanging by his fingertips'. Tracy struggled with a lack of support in this case and told me,

> I used to have a really good babysitter for the other three children . . . but once Brad got a little bit older she was sitting in the chair like that and he came up behind her and held a knife at her throat and said 'I'm going to fucking kill you' and she wouldn't step foot inside the house again. Erm (pause) he's thrown knives at me, he's thrown knives at his brothers erm (pause) at this point the social services were a complete waste of space.

Essentially Tracy was not feeling cared for, and it could be suggested that 'general care labour' (Lynch 2007) or extended support networks were not available to her at this time. In addition to the above, before Brad was excluded from school, Tracy had to be present on the school premises at every break time due to his difficult behaviour. This meant that Tracy could never take paid employment during this period.

In thinking about care work and who cares, Tracy said on several occasions about how she phoned up for professional support and told me 'I said (to social services) so basically I've got to kick the shit out of my child before you do anything?' She was refused support at that time, suggesting that there was little 'solidarity work' (Lynch 2007). Eventually Brad was accommodated in a residential school for children with 'challenging behaviour' where he was a weekly boarder. Tracy was desperate for some respite. Even when she did receive some help she said she wanted support and respite not therapy. Tracy simply wanted and needed 'time out' and as a result told me

> a couple of times I thought about taking the lot of them [pills] and a big bottle of booze and just finishing it all . . . I got to the stage where I thought I was a completely lousy mother and they'd be better off without me anyway . . . I was getting to the stage where they would be better off without me.

In getting to this point, that of at the very least considering suicide, we are brought back to the beginning of the chapter where mothers have actually taken their disabled child's life and attempted to take, or actually taken, their own too. These examples above highlight the complexity around dealing with the emotional work and caring for, about and with a child in circumstances that are not easily defined as care work. Critically it is here therefore that social intolerance at its broadest conceptualisation needs recognising as problematic so that emotionally mothers are able to gain day-to-day support when needed.

Crucially in this argument, emotional work was so overwhelming that Tracy told me, 'there comes a time when your energy is so low that it affects your emotional state'. Care work from a political perspective suggests that support can be given (or not), via practical or financial support. However this care and emotional work discussed moves beyond the simple financial and practical into a more ethical debate about *who cares* and what this means for an individual's everyday experience.

Concluding remarks

It is clear that mothering an intellectually disabled child is difficult. Still UK policy directives and guidelines assure us that they promote partnerships between parents and professionals (DfES 2001a, 2001b, 2005b, 2007b). Crucially relationships between parents and professionals must not be about individualistic notions based on particular professionals, but indeed there should be a 'politics of recognition', and moreover that recognition is a 'central component of social justice' (McLaughlin *et al.* 2008: 190). Social justice and care seem tantamount to understanding politically how we can move forward thinking with care and doing care (see also Nussbaum 2006). As seen above, Tracy's narrative suggests there is a significant cost to all these difficulties and that these costs straddle the emotional, practical and socio-political spheres. However none of these 'caring costs' are easily defined due to the messy nature of emotional work, love labouring and care work involved.

In thinking about the policies and directives that influence the issues at stake here – caring through partnership policy and directives for example (DfES 2001b, 2005b, 2007b), even though parents with disabled children have been part of the partnership narrative for nearly three decades, research suggests that this is still benevolent rhetoric (Rogers 2011). For example, why have we got a mother on the edge and even thinking about suicide? Whether this is just a passing thought or a serious consideration we need to think about caring, enabling and just practices for mothers with disabled children and how interdependence might work. This ought to be considered politically as a reaction against social intolerance and toward a more humane and just social position.

In this chapter it seems that sometimes a mother might love and hate her child at the same time, but feels obliged to *care for* them. A mother with a disabled child is obliged to care, one could argue. The constant battle between 'I must do something' (caring for) and 'something must be done' (caring about) is critical in attempting to understand a complicated relationship (Noddings 1995b: 11). 'I must' carries with it obligation (Noddings 1995b: 11). 'I must' is very different to 'I want'. It could be argued that some of the narratives above are driven by 'I must', and others by 'I want'.[9] 'If caring is to be maintained, clearly, *the one – caring must be maintained'* (Noddings 1995b: 26, emphasis added). This is certainly the case for mothers with intellectually disabled children, especially children with challenging behaviours. Critically in the UK the 'Big Society' ideology promoted by the Coalition government of 2010 onwards implies the emphasis in policy will be on families (and the local community) addressing their own local issues (see DfE 2010, for disabled children). This will highlight further the cultural, social and economic divide as those 'with' are able to at best support, at worst manipulate, those 'without'. For example, those with the economic and cultural capital will be able to prescribe what goes on in a 'free school', local club or support network. It is at this point more work on enabling and just practices for families with intellectually disabled children ought to be pursued.

Notes

1 I use the term intellectual disability and intellectually disabled to include a spectrum of children and young people identified in England with additional difficulties in learning, but also as a conceptual term that goes beyond 'learning' in any pedagogical sense. I also, in this chapter, use the term disability for the purposes of brevity but do not mean physical disability although there can be some similar caring stories, that is not for discussion here.

2 Rather than continually talking about dependency that is often associated with disability and care which positions the disabled person as in a powerless position (Hughes *et al.* 2005).

3 I recognise the tension between the Disabled People's Movement (DPM) and feminist understandings of care – that is for the DPM care is often demonised due to the significant oppression that comes with being 'cared for', and yet within feminism care is positioned as problematically oppressive due to the gendered nature of care. These issues cannot be given the necessary airing due to space, but see Hughes *et al.* (2005) and Rogers (forthcoming) for a more nuanced and fuller discussion.

4 This is based on a Kantian interpretation that ethical caring is done out of duty and not out of love, which is an interesting and important point to make, especially as not all maternal caring acts we have seen here are based on what might be described as 'natural caring', but more likely to be interpreted as 'ethical care' (Noddings 1995b).

5 I have chosen a mother rather than a father due to the culturally defined care work that continues to be evident in Western cultures. It is also clear within 'caring' discourses both empirically and theoretically that this work is often carried about by women.

6 'General care work' is associated with secondary care relations, so extended family relations, neighbours and friendship networks could form part of this and 'solidarity work' form part of tertiary care relations or public care work (Lynch 2007: 562).

7 This is based on an assessment in England and Wales carried out by the local education authority so as to identify additional education needs. If a child has a statement of SEN then additional money ought to be allocated to the child (Rogers 2007a).

8 As it happens, inappropriate touching was a period that seemed to subside for Dean as he developed into his later teens and learned that this behaviour was problematic.

9 Some questions the reader might want to think about reading the narratives above are: as a mother she might ask, 'do I love my son who has damaged the rest of our family?' and 'do *I* care for him?' 'Yes I care' she may well say, 'but love? That is more difficult: I both love and hate him.' The love/hate dualism that can come with mothering a child who behaves outside expected norms is apparent in this chapter and needs further exploration. Furthermore, in discussing mothering, whilst I have been unable to go into too much of the gendered role due to the scope of this chapter, in thinking about care and ethics, it is clear that there are gendered issues at work here. Women, for example, who do not express their emotions in response to grief of others or respond tenderly to a crying baby, are considered at best selfish. This is not the case with men (Friedman 1995: 64), but for some of the mothers in my research there are times when practical care takes over from emotional responses in caring for rather than caring about their child.

12 Working at post-divorce family life

The feminist ethics of care as a framework for exploring fathering after divorce or separation

Georgia Philip, University of East Anglia

Introduction

Fathering, particularly in a post-divorce or separation context, remains a complex and contested issue and one which continues to appear high on political and policy agendas (Cameron 2011). Politically, concerns shift from questioning fathers' commitment to their children's lives, to positioning them as an underused or underrated resource; exhorting individuals and institutions alike to 'Think Fathers' (Featherstone 2009). Debates over how separating couples should make provision for and take care of children remain highly pertinent in personal and public contexts, as an ongoing expression of anxiety about 'the state of the family', moral values, and questions of financial liability.

This chapter draws on research exploring fathers' own narratives of fathering after divorce or separation and analyses these in terms of the practical, relational and moral aspects of their caring roles and responsibilities. A central aim of the study was to use a feminist conception of care (Noddings 2003; Ruddick 1995; Tronto 1993) to explore fathering as distinct from, but interconnected with, mothering and attend to the ways in which gender infuses the practices, emotions and moral work involved in caring for children. There remains a need for more 'feminist work on fathering' (Doucet 2006a) which theorises gender relations and the gendered power struggles that shape the personal and social organisation of care for children. However, this has to be done without disregarding the constraints and opportunities these produce for both fathers and mothers, and in particular without ignoring the domestic and caring responsibilities women continue to bear. I am also arguing that the concept of care enables the emotional, practical and moral elements of fathering to be teased out and considered more effectively than other concepts, such as intimacy, allow. Feminist conceptions of care, importantly, incorporate both labour and love, without seeking to either rank these or present them as opposites.

Following this approach my own research revealed the complex and ambivalent responses to gender and caring expressed by divorced or separated fathers. It also demonstrated ways in which gendered patterns of caring for children become fault lines for the renegotiation of parental roles and responsibilities following divorce or separation. My study showed that alongside, or despite, the transformative potential of direct care and caring responsibility, a gendered model of parenting often appears as a default position. This model, which tends to place mothers as primary and fathers as morally equivalent, but secondary, carers, is recognisable in public discourses around not just parenting but also work–life balance (Gatrell 2005) and is not incompatible with promoting father engagement (Featherstone 2009). Within fathers' narratives, this model was also often accompanied by ideas of the 'different but equal' qualities and contributions of fathers and mothers; but here again equality can be presented in terms of moral worth, rather than a division of labour. So, fathers may continue to benefit from the optional, yet morally adequate, aspects of fathering contained within and validated by gendered caring arrangements, in that mothers may continue to carry the bulk of routine care and responsibility for children. However, during the process of separation, fathers (and mothers) may also reassess what such responsibility carries with it, in terms of opportunities for sustaining relationships and retaining parental (and co-parental) authority. My research demonstrated that it is in this kind of difficult rethinking and working out of 'bearable' solutions that possibilities for changing and challenging the gendering of care exist.

This chapter will discuss the value of the feminist ethics of care as a theoretical framework for my analysis of narratives of fathering after divorce or separation. Drawing on data collected during my doctoral research, I will present two case studies, each demonstrating how this body of theory provides an appropriate approach and language for thinking and writing about fathering. The main argument made here is that my application of feminist moral philosophical ideas sheds valuable light on understanding men's experiences of post-divorce fathering. It reveals the complex influence of gendered caring roles and identities, and also a gendered moral space in which such fathering takes place. This kind of nuanced critical analysis is really important for understanding the personal, social and emotional investments involved, and at stake, in caring for children after divorce or separation, and is relevant to researchers, practitioners and policy makers alike.

Researching fathers after divorce or seperation

The broader qualitative study involved 23 previously resident, biological fathers' accounts of fathering after divorce or separation. All the fathers saw themselves as having maintained contact with their children over time and across households.[1] The research consisted of individual interviews with men who were fathering in a range of contexts with a variety of caring arrangements in place. All the fathers had at least one biological child where the relationship with the mother had ended and had been divorced or separated for at least one year.[2] The interviews focused on fathers' caring arrangements for children and how these had developed; on whether/how their working lives had changed with becoming a father and with divorce/separation, and on the emotional and practical aspects of their relationships, and time spent, with children. The volunteer sample of fathers all lived in a comparatively rural region of eastern England, and the majority were of White

British ethnicity. The sample was varied in terms of age, employment, type of contact or caring arrangements in place, and the reported quality of the co-parental relationship with mothers. Overall it constituted a diverse group of fathers who had in common some experience of attempting to sustain contact and relationships with their children, and navigating ongoing co-parental relationships with mothers. The illustrations used in this chapter identify and explore a number of the key themes to emerge from the study with particular reference to the moral aspects of fathers' narratives.

Locating the feminist ethics of care

A central aim of feminist moral philosophical work on the ethics of care has been to expand the concept of care, and critically examine how caring practice becomes gendered. More specifically, the feminist ethics of care seeks to theorise care in a more nuanced way, as a practice, a discipline and a way of thinking, arising out of connection and interconnection with others. To do this, key theorists, such as Ruddick (1995) and Tronto (1993), focus on the mother–child relationship as a significant instance where ethics and everyday life are intertwined. Importantly though, such writers emphasise that they use women's caring experiences as mothers in particular ways. First, in order both to make visible their deeply ethical, deliberative and relational qualities and then to assert the value of such experiences as a model for ethical reasoning in other contexts. Thus theorists of a feminist ethics of care have sought to assert the value and legitimacy of care in moral philosophy and political theory, and to use women's experiences as a lived context from which ethical relationships and moral deliberation can be modelled. The challenge is how to present and make use of women's experiences without further consigning them to be 'natural' or the best carers for evermore, and without idealising or sentimentalising women as mothers.

Alongside this emphasis on the value of care for moral and political theory, the feminist ethics of care also sheds important light on care as a social and relational practice. A number of writers contribute to this (Noddings 2003; Ruddick 1995; Tronto 1993) but in relation to my own research, Ruddick's work on 'maternal practice' and 'maternal thinking' has been particularly helpful. Ruddick produces a rigorous consideration of what constitutes mothering, in terms of a set of *learnt* activities. Ruddick defines 'maternal work' as the commitment to and practice of preservation love, nurturance and training, in response to what she sees as the primary demands of child care: preservation, growth and social acceptability. She then uses this model to develop the concept of maternal thinking, as a distinctive form of reasoning and reflection: 'Maternal work itself demands that mothers think; out of this thoughtfulness, a distinctive discipline emerges' (1989: 24). Having rooted maternal thinking firmly within the experience of mothering, Ruddick's aim is then to demonstrate that it is not limited or tied to women as a group; the challenge is to value women's difference without losing sight of feminist goals of gender equality. Broadly, the position argued is that care as a practice can be understood through mothering, but is not essentially bound to or defined by it.

The feminist ethics of care and fathering

One of the implications arising from Ruddick's work is the question of whether male carers for children could be described as mothering, i.e. whether recognising maternal work as a practice and form of ethics might remove distinctive characteristics between mothering and fathering. In recent years, Doucet (2006a) has engaged directly with Ruddick's ideas, and, most specifically, the question of 'do men mother?' Doucet's response is that they do not. Her work asserts the importance of gender differences in the experience of caring activities and responsibilities, and argues that recognising distinctive qualities to male caring can enrich and expand our empirical and theoretical understanding of care. Doucet emphasises the importance of a nuanced and grounded understanding of male caring and gender difference, but again, from a feminist perspective which can attend to fathering without either simply comparing it to mothering, or disenfranchising mothers in the process (Doucet 2006a).

The conception of care, caring practice and caring responsibility outlined above resonated powerfully with my research interviews and has been the central theoretical framework for my analysis and writing of fathers' stories. In the case studies that follow I aim to show how the feminist ethics of care shed crucial light on the moral and relational aspects of fathers' narratives, and on the importance of gender in shaping the process of caring for children after divorce or separation. My broader argument is that the conceptualisation of care within feminist ethics advances understanding of fathering through its ability to attend to the multifaceted and complex nature of caring practices and relationships. When applied to fathering, this approach draws attention to distinctive perceptions or experiences for men, and to ways in which gendered divisions of caring labour between men and women are reproduced. Through taking this critical approach to exploring how care is gendered, I also suggest that it produces roles, responsibilities and identities of 'fathering', which are relational and morally loaded. So, I now move on to demonstrate male caring as a complex, relational process and as a 'way of thinking' (Ruddick 1995; Doucet 2006a; Lynch *et al.* 2009) by discussing two case studies from my research: Dennis, the 'transformed father', and Micky, the father who 'stayed'.[3] The presentation of each case will enable a more direct exploration of how this moral philosophical perspective can contribute to understanding fathering after divorce or separation. It also illustrates how a feminist conception of care deeply informed my analysis, and my attempts to capture how fathers felt they tried to 'stay close to', 'provide' and 'be there' for their children.[4]

Dennis, the 'transformed father'

Dennis was 45, White British, worked full-time as a family lawyer and was a partner in his firm. He was married to Lynne for 14 years and at the time of interview they had been divorced for 18 months. Dennis has two children: Anna, 14, and Craig, 13. Since their separation the children continued to live with Lynne in the family home, and Dennis had bought a smaller house very close by. Dennis saw his relationships with his children as improving, particularly with his son Craig. Both children regularly spent a weekday evening with Dennis at his new home, and Dennis also described a lot of informal contact, such as phone calls or 'popping in' visits. At the time of interview, he defined his relationship with Lynne as amicable, although there had been a good deal of conflict during the early stages of the separation. They had both used solicitors to manage their divorce, but there were no legal disputes.

The overall narrative that Dennis produced in his interview can be described as one of repentance and transformation. Dennis gave an account of having moved from being a father who had peripheral and highly mediated involvement in his children's lives, to realising the need for, and value of, developing a more direct emotional relationship with them. For him, the ending of his marriage had been a catalyst for thinking and acting differently in terms of caring for his children, and also how he experienced caring responsibility. Here, Dennis is recalling an incident where he removed photographs of his children from his office shortly after separating from his wife. The story illustrates his positioning of himself as a reflective and subsequently transformed father:

> I took the photographs of the children down, cos they actually used to make me incredibly sad, they were maybe two and three, and I thought 'I didn't really know them', y'know, I never spent enough time with them, and, for two years I was working in London and only coming up at weekends (pause) and it was just a time where, I had children but I didn't really know who they were.

Dennis also presents a sense of moral identity through this account of changes to his fathering, both in terms of his caring practice and his experiences of caring. Throughout his interview, Dennis presented himself as a more morally responsible or 'better' father than he had been whilst married. For Dennis, the ability to sustain his fathering role and relationships, or to stay connected to his children, was seen as directly linked to a new or adapted fathering practice. This change primarily involved becoming more attentive and directly available to his children, and to developing what he perceived to be a new kind of relationship with them.

In telling this story, Dennis also provides an example of one of the broader moral themes present across the interviews, that of 'putting children first' (see also Ribbens McCarthy *et al.* 2003). The claim to be putting children first was important, in moral terms, for making non-resident fathering 'legitimate' as long as fathers were seen to be attempting to avoid relational and emotional distance. Fathers presented this primarily in terms of trying to spend consistent, meaningful time with children, taking children's interests or feelings into account and trying to foster a bearable co-parental relationship. For Dennis, his increased availability was linked to spending increased (though limited) time with Anna and Craig. However, it was equally to do with the relational and emotional quality of that time, and the unexpected consequences of directly caring for his children, outside the context of his marriage. Dennis felt that the evenings he spent in sole charge of his children were the key to both his 'realisation' of the value of care and to his changing relationship with them.

you've got to spend time with them, nothing happens without that and even, that small change, and I don't spend as much time with them, as I would like, or I should, but even that small change has made such a difference and I now have my own relationship with them and I really don't think I did before.

Dennis's story also reveals something about the gendering of care for children within heterosexual couple relationships, as well as the experience of parenting beyond divorce or separation, and he was explicit about having actively sought (and been able) to avoid looking after his children whilst he was married. This indicates the more optional nature of certain parenting activities or caring responsibilities for many men, and illustrates how, during the process of separation, the gains attached to this can suddenly be felt as disadvantages as the 'taken-for-granted' nature of relationships with both children and mothers are strongly challenged.

So Dennis constructs an overall narrative about positive changes to his fathering practice and moral identity, and illustrates the moral principle of 'putting children first'. However, the following example presents some of the further complexity of narrating and implementing this apparently powerful idea. For fathers who had older daughters, particularly, an important issue that often arose, was how best to put *girls'* interests first. This demonstrates in another way how ideas about gender and care played out in relation to the one 'cared-for' (Noddings 2003) as well as the one-caring; fathers' comments here are arguably stereotypical in terms of perceptions about girls, but nonetheless they often treated this 'difference' as another aspect of trying to be a 'good father'. Talking about this frequently involved a moral question about whether it should involve fathers doing things they didn't necessarily like. The recurring idea of having to do 'girlie things' and fathers' differing responses to this, revealed the added complexity that gender can add to the general moral principle of putting children first, as it can make the practice of sharing and sustaining common pleasures more of a challenge, or indeed, draw attention to the moral qualities of playing with dolls or going shopping.

Dennis provides a useful illustration of this process, through the contrasting way in which he talks about spending time with his 13-year-old son Craig and his 14-year-old daughter Anna. What is noticeable is the way gender plays a part in shaping Dennis's developing relationships with his children; the easy pleasure he describes in sharing sport with his son, contrasted with the difficulty he has both with finding common ground with Anna, and with talking about this with me. Dennis also makes a statement about the limits of his moral responsibility to put Anna first, considers and then counters this, as if to pre-empt potential moral evaluation and to protect the moral identity he has built up through his narrative.

> sitting there with Craig with, I dunno, him drinking juice, me drinking beer, eating crisps, watching football or rugby or, any other sport that takes our fancy really, I mean it's just blissful, I couldn't be happier doing that.
>
>   I struggle to think of things actually, that we [Anna and I] would both enjoy, because, in some ways, I don't – it sounds a bit selfish maybe, but I don't want to do something, just because she would enjoy it, to have a shared

experience would be nice but equally I do, I do things I don't enjoy, because she enjoys them, but it would be nice to actually have, found some, common interests as well, but we haven't done that, Anna and I.

The case of Dennis, as a father presenting himself as transformed by new contexts and experiences of care and responsibility for his children, reveals some of the moral and relational dimensions of fathering after divorce. Paying attention to these can shed light on both the detail of care as a practice, and the broader ethical questions involved in caring relationships. Focusing on fathers and fathering reveals something of how these processes are perceived and experienced by men, which can increase our understanding of care, and of the complex ways in which gender continues to shape the organisation of caring work and responsibility. Across the interviews, fathers called on, accepted and resisted certain ideas around gender roles and what is expected of men, at different times and for different purposes, as part of the process of accounting for and asserting their responsibilities and relationships with their children.

Micky, the father who 'stayed'

Micky was 27, Black British, and had one daughter, Megan who was nearly 3. He had worked for a number of years as a security guard and also spent a short time in the army. Micky had lived with Megan's mother Laura for about two years, but they were not married. Micky and Laura's relationship broke down after Megan was born, and they split up when she was six months old. For the past two and a half years, Micky and Laura had been in conflict over contact arrangements, which had involved solicitors, mediation and the court system. After the separation, Micky lost his job and had to move out of their flat. He then lived in the YMCA[5] for about nine months, and had at first supervised and then unsupervised contact with Megan via contact centres.[6] During this time, he also attended parenting classes and other courses offered by the YMCA and paid maintenance for Megan through the Child Support Agency. Micky had also received support from a voluntary organisation assisting young adults, and had been a key member of a young fathers group. He had finally got his own flat, and at the time of interview had a job and regular weekend contact with Megan. He had also recently agreed staying over contact with Laura, via the court, and was having Megan to stay every other Saturday night.

Micky's case is significant because he very much presented himself as having 'worked at' being, or becoming, a father. Micky drew on another recurring theme across the interviews, that of 'staying' in order to assert both his commitment to, and enthusiasm for, fathering. Micky used the idea and language of 'staying' as a means of narrating the process of securing contact and 'proving' himself to a range of particular and generalised 'others' (Holdsworth and Morgan 2007). As his interview progressed, he also demonstrated a certain level of reflexivity in considering his own moral orientation to fatherhood and how this was related to the practice of caring for Megan.

In general, one source of claiming a viable moral identity as a divorced or separated father appeared to be the very fact of demonstrating commitment to contact with children. Attempts to sustain contact and relationships with children, and a co-parental relationship with their mother, were often seen to constitute moral acts in themselves. This raises interesting questions in relation both to moral philosophy and to gender. It may be that some acts are considered moral because they are seen as laudable, or deemed to go beyond expectation, whilst others are moral because they simply fulfil an expectation. In the context of post-divorce parenting, fathers and mothers are arguably subject to different moral criteria, in relation to the level or nature of commitment to both children and the co-parental relationship, that they are expected to show.

Whilst all the fathers in the study expressed ideas of a moral commitment to their children, this was not presented straightforwardly in terms of inevitable obligation. The fathers in this study certainly appeared able to lay claim to a moral identity, as men who had not 'walked away' even though it was often seen as an *option* available to them. This optional quality to fatherhood is significant here, because of the way it contributes to making fathering beyond divorce or separation possible to present as a moral act in itself. As part of such moral self-presentation, fathers often contrasted themselves with 'other' fathers, whom they saw to be irresponsible, selfish or indeed amoral.

'Staying', as an aspect of moral identity for fathers, was not only expressed within the context of privately made and 'bearable' contact arrangements, but could also be presented through accounts of engagements with agencies, such as Children's Services, CAFCASS[7] or the Family Court. For a minority of fathers – who had very conflicted relationships with the mothers of their children, had experienced protracted court proceedings and had very limited time with their children – it was very important and potentially difficult to retain a morally adequate father identity. Micky's case is therefore insightful, as he narrated this experience and asserted himself as a committed and capable father, who took both joy and pride in caring for his young daughter.

Micky had experienced a long period of supervised and then unsupervised contact through contact centres, and preserving a sense of moral identity as a father had involved compliance with external agencies. Micky gave an account of his 'journey' through courts, contact centres, the YMCA and parenting classes in terms of being willing and able both to be 'exposed' to professional scrutiny and to 'prove' himself as a responsible father, to his daughter's mother, and to the various agencies involved in their family life.

I actually stayed an extra six months in the YMCA, to guarantee that I was gonna get, a two bedroom flat because me getting a one bedroom flat was a waste of time, because at the end of the day Megan needs to have her own space, yeah, so I stayed, another six months in that flaming place just to guarantee myself to get that sorted, and, once again, I fulfilled everything that the courts wanted me to do.

For Micky, therefore, 'staying' was presented in terms of having shown some moral courage and determination, in the face of obstacles to his fathering which he saw as not always of his own making. His narration of perseverance was a key mechanism through which a sense of moral identity as a father could be sustained. Interestingly, Micky also offered some reflective insight into his motives for 'staying' with his daughter Megan, suggesting that his moral identity had become progressively more bound up with fatherhood, and that his initial reasons for making a legal claim for contact were more to do with a sense of personal grievance.

> At first it was because someone had taken something away from me that belonged to me but then later, I started to feel like I'm doing the right thing, to stand by my kid.

For Micky then, the process of demonstrating commitment to Megan and the practice of caring for her with increasing levels of responsibility or autonomy, have perhaps produced a different 'way of thinking'.

Micky's story was very complex and during the course of his interview he managed to narrate and hold together contrasting aspects of his behaviour, emotions and moral identity. Despite having to account for incidents of anger or aggression, and the need to prove himself, Micky laid claim to a moral identity as a proud and active father, and his interview did resonate with the joy, and surprise, he felt from his experiences of caring directly for Megan.

> I mean, something really simple, and really weird, but crossing the road, yeah, I've actually managed to teach Megan, y'know, 'when you get to the end of the road, you stop, y'know, and you wait for daddy' y'know – and I've instilled that into her, I've done that y'know, that's something I've managed to achieve with Megan.

Conclusion

The cases of both Micky and Dennis have been used to offer some insight into the process of fathering after divorce or separation. Their accounts also reveal something about the provision of care for children, by men, as a lived, relational and moral practice, and a form of moral reasoning. The feminist moral philosophical conception of care offers a framework for interpreting these fathers' experiences and provides unique and important opportunities for analysing family and parental relationships. Care is seen to involve both labour and love; practical and emotional dimensions (Lynch *et al.* 2009), and theorised in this way can contain the complex and ambivalent feelings caring for and caring about can produce. In the wider context, attempts to engage, evaluate or empower fathers can be done with or without an interest in gender equity, and can too easily produce yet another adversarial context for mothers and fathers, or problematise women as a barrier to fully involved fathering (Featherstone 2009). I offer, then, a cautious optimism and a considered warning. Fathering after divorce or separation can produce new contexts of care, which have the potential to change personal, social and political understandings of male caring practice and responsibility. Against this, however, is the pull of a model of parenting that may lay claim to greater gender equality by positioning fathers and mothers as morally equivalent, and yet does not substantially alter expectations of fathers in terms of caring labour and responsibility. The need for a nuanced, careful appreciation of the ongoing gendering of care for children is relevant to a whole range of policy areas. Most specifically, it may be particularly important to policy making in relation to divorcing/separating parents and mediation or support services, in order to be attentive and responsive to the investment and 'work' involved in sustaining family relationships. Utilising the full range of theoretical and empirical literature on care (Ruddick 1995; Sevenhuijsen 1998; Lynch *et al.* 2009; Bowlby *et al.* 2010) can and should be a central resource for this important enterprise.

Notes

1 My focus was clearly on fathers who did have contact arrangements and who spent time with their children with some consistency, but I could not impose quantitative and potentially judgemental limits on what counted as 'regular'. In my recruitment literature I used the phrase 'fathers who see and take care of their children' in order to allow for interpretation and self-selection.
2 This was a decision taken as part of the ethical consideration of the implications of asking fathers to retell painful stories.
3 These terms come from my thematic analysis of the interview narratives.
4 'Staying close', 'Providing' and 'Being there' were all themes that emerged from the interviews.
5 The Young Men's Christian Association is a long-established Christian charity supporting all young people, particularly with issues such as homelessness, education, work and mental health.
6 In the UK contact centres function to facilitate contact between parents and children either where relations between parents are highly conflicted or where a court has made an order that contact be supervised for child-welfare reasons. They are not statutory institutions but are supported through the National Association of Child Contact Centres.
7 The Child and Family Court Advisory and Support Service has existed in the UK since 2001 and is a non-departmental public body which aims to champion the interests of children involved in family proceedings and advise family courts on child-welfare and safeguarding matters.

Part IV

Caring across the life course

Part IV Summary

Caring across the life course

Susie Weller, Elisabetta Zontini and
Jane Ribbens McCarthy

This final part focuses on aspects of the life course often overlooked or taken for granted in debates on care. The term 'life course' has, of late, become the preferred expression to describe the journey from 'cradle to grave', used over and above notions of, for example, life cycle (Bowlby *et al.* 2010). Whilst not unproblematic, the term does take account of the unpredictability and lack of linearity in contemporary life. For authors such as Bowlby *et al.* (2010: 50) 'learning about care is not something we only do at the start of life but takes place continuously'. It is important, then, to be cognisant of the need to avoid any simplistic notions of how dependence, vulnerability and care occur over the life course, avoiding any sense of 'phases' of care, and being aware of how care and dependence are continuous features of human experiences.

The chapters focus primarily on informal care; although each touches upon the intersection and fluid boundaries between informal and formal care contexts. Susie's chapter (13) draws on a UK-based study of young people's sibling relationships to illustrate the shifting nature of caring practices, relations and identities over time and in different spaces. This contribution is followed in Chapter 14 by Elisabetta's work that draws attention to the complex multi-directional caring networks of older Italian migrants in the UK, which span generations as well as countries. Finally, the book draws to a close with Jane's chapter (15) on bereaved family members and the continuation of care after death across a range of cultural contexts, considering how, in this process, variable notions of personhood and relationality are drawn upon and framed.

The first theme uniting our chapters relates to preconceptions about flows of care *within* families and *across* generations. Rather than replicating well-rehearsed discussions about hierarchical flows each chapter challenges dominant ideas about conventional caring relationships. Susie's chapter (13) draws on two illustrative examples that challenge the emphasis in family research on vertical flows of care between, for example, parents and children. Rather, she focuses on the significance of lateral sibling relationships to young people's understandings and experiences of care, highlighting the 'oscillations between caring and power dynamics' (Mauthner 2005: 636). Elisabetta's chapter (14) highlights not only how older migrants continue to be care providers, not merely recipients, but also how lateral care flows occurring in friendship groups and community centres are crucial yet neglected aspects of their caring practices. Furthermore, as Jane's chapter (15) highlights, care after death can involve continuing inter-generational (as well as lateral) flows of care, but reveals the particular dynamics of power that can occur between the living and the dead in variable cultural contexts and belief systems.

The second theme connecting our work centres on the salience of time in shaping caring and power relations. The focus in Susie's chapter (13) on sibling connections raises some interesting issues surrounding timing and norms of reciprocity. For many, siblings are 'always there', even if the relationship is sometimes marked by conflict. The expectation that the relationship will be a long-term, if not lifetime, connection, could mean that care and support is not expected to be reciprocated in the short term. This highlights the importance of thinking about care over the life course, with some young people already considering the sharing of future care for their parents. Similar issues arise in care that continues after death, as highlighted in Jane's chapter (15), with long-term (even unlimited) and reciprocal caring being a feature of continuing bonds after death. At the same time, however, such bonds represent a challenge to ideas of reciprocity, where interests and needs are seen to be attached to particular individuals. This analysis thus unsettles and deepens concerns with how to understand individuality and relationality. The importance of time is also evident in Elisabetta's chapter (14), which argues that the values of older migrants shape their caring practices yet also that values change and get renegotiated through time and in particular contexts.

The chapters also point to the salience of space, highlighting relationality between people, as well as between people and places, thereby demonstrating connections between care of/for self, care of/for others and care of/for the environment (Popke 2006). The examples in Susie's chapter (13) show the significance of micro-spaces (home, school, neighbourhood) to caring and power relations amongst siblings, highlighting the ways in which experiences and understandings of care flow within and between different spaces. Elisabetta's chapter (14) challenges the notion that co-presence is a prerequisite of caring practices as it shows that care can be done from a distance. In relation to care for the dead, while the 'proper' sites for such care may vary across cultural contexts, it is common to find some such sites designated, whether in terms of a family altar in the home or shared burial sites in urban areas, as Jane's chapter (15) demonstrates (Hockey *et al.* 2007).

We also offer some methodological insights for researching caring practices, relations and identities. The studies on which each chapter draws employ different methods. Susie's chapter (13) takes a qualitative longitudinal perspective, which brings to the fore changes and continuities in understandings of key elements of care such as reciprocity, relationality and interdependence that might otherwise be overlooked in a short-term project. Elisabetta's chapter (14) employs an ethnographic approach which allows the author to document the caring practices of a particular group of elders wherever they occur and explore some of their daily practices which may be taken for granted and not mentioned in formal interview settings, such as caring exchanges occurring at community centres or communication and exchanges of information across geographical boundaries. In Jane's chapter (15), autobiographical experiences are used as a starting point for exploring the nuances and subtleties of emotions of caring after death, as well as for pointing to issues that have been neglected in existing debates on selfhood and relationality.

Finally, the chapters also speak to a range of policy and practice debates. Susie's chapter (13) draws attention to the significance of lateral relationships, often neglected by practitioners who either prioritise vertical connections or overemphasise problems such as rivalry, jealousy, conflict, thus neglecting the significance of care and support provided by siblings that often buttress family life, particularly during periods of family crisis. It also speaks to wider policy trends that emphasise independency and personal responsibility as key facets of a 'successful' transition to adulthood, to the detriment of acknowledging the salience of interdependency and relationality in shaping young people's lives – an issue taken up again in Jane's chapter (15). Elisabetta's chapter (14) draws attention to the potential problems for older migrants of policies favouring the mainstreaming of services and general cuts in funding to the non-profit sector. The chapter highlights the importance of community centres as spaces where communal care can be offered and received. It also dispels some of the myths about the caring needs of older migrants both in relation to the belief that they care for their own and/or that they are a drain on the welfare system.

These final chapters provide rich illustrations of care but also point towards further issues for continuing work and debate with regard to the feminist ethics of care, including the notion of embodied relationality, and understandings of selfhood and neediness.

13 Who cares?

Exploring the shifting nature of care and caring practices in sibling relationships

Susie Weller, London South Bank University

Introduction

For many, sibling bonds constitute the most enduring, albeit emotionally ambivalent, relationships in their lives (Cicirelli 1995; Dunn 2004; Edwards *et al.* 2006; Punch 2008). Not only can siblings provide an important range of resources, support and care but also such relationships are instrumental in identity formation (Kosonen 1996; Edwards *et al.* 2005a, 2006; Weller 2007; Edwards and Weller 2010a). As Edwards *et al.* (2006: 68) suggest, 'One way in which children and young people experience their sense of who they are as individuals in a sibling unit is through the way that they care for and about each other.' Yet much of the literature on young people[1] and care focuses on the significance of vertical parent–child connections, or between generations, thus neglecting lateral relations (Mauthner 2005; McIntosh and Punch 2009).

Following Tronto's (1993) assertion that we need to acknowledge 'who cares', along with articulations between caring and social identities, and the ways in which care is indicative of societal power relations, this chapter draws on a UK-based longitudinal study to explore the shifting nature of care as a practice and as a way of relating as siblings (McEwan and Goodman 2010). I begin by framing the discussion within two key debates that point to the salience of time and space in caring practices and relations (see also McKie *et al.* 2004): young people, care and lateral relationships; and geographies of care. I then outline the study on which the chapter draws before presenting two examples that illustrate some of the ways in which over time and in different spaces sibling caring and power relations shape and are shaped by aspects of identity (age, class, culture, gender), values (familial and education-oriented) and challenging events (episodes of crisis). In doing so, I seek to offer insights into the shifting nature of informal caring practices, relations and identities within one life-course phase (Cicirelli 1995; Bowlby *et al.* 2010).

Young people, care and lateral relationships

Within families, care is often posited as a vertical relationship; something bestowed on children by their parent(s) or grandparent(s). There exists a substantial body of literature on care-giving by parents (e.g. McKie *et al.* 2004; Doucet 2006a; Thomson *et al.* 2011; and Philip, Chapter 12 and Rogers, Chapter 11 in this volume), and those 'in loco parentis' (e.g. Mullender 1999; Broad and Skinner 2006). Reflecting dominant understandings of adult–child power relations, children in post-industrial societies are predominantly positioned as net receivers of care. Perhaps one of the most significant areas of literature that challenges this one-directional flow is the work on child carers (e.g. Aldridge and Becker 1993, 2003; Evans 2010). Nonetheless, this example is often portrayed as extraordinary; a challenge to contemporary conceptualisations of childhood as a phase of the life course marked by dependency. Indeed, children are expected to learn to care and to acquire caring responsibilities (including care for self) as part of a 'successful' trajectory to independent adulthood (Bowlby *et al.* 2010; Edwards and Weller 2010a). Furthermore, changes over the past 40 years in post-industrial societies, not least the decline of the youth labour market, shifting gender expectations, and new policies on social security and housing, have seen the prolonging of the period of dependence, thus reshaping caring relationships in families and altering understandings of care over time (Irwin 1995, 2005; Edwards 2002; France 2007; Bowlby *et al.* 2010). The primacy given to vertical flows of care along with changing social and political contexts of care, point to the salience of time in understanding caring relations and identities.

Despite the lack of attention given to care in lateral relationships, the early 1980s to mid-1990s witnessed a growth in interest in childhood sibling support. Yet, in line with much youth research of the time, little emphasis was placed on children's perspectives (Kosonen 1996). More recently work has begun to explore the support provided by siblings during different phases of the life course, for instance, to tackle childhood bullying or provide care for elderly parents (Cicirelli 1995; Kosonen 1996, 1999; Sanders 2004; Edwards *et al.* 2006; Weller 2007). An emphasis on power relations has accompanied this interest in sibling support (McNamee 1997; Mauthner 2002, 2005; Edwards *et al.* 2005a; Punch 2005; McIntosh and Punch 2009). For example, research conducted in both the global 'North' and 'South' has pointed to hierarchical flows of care amongst sisters and brothers, with older siblings tending to look after and protect their younger counterparts (Edwards *et al.* 2006). An articulation between age status and gender is also evident. Evan's (2010) work with sibling-headed households in HIV/AIDS-stricken areas of Africa details how children act as parents/guardians for their younger siblings, with female 'heads of household' more likely to do domestic care work, whilst male 'heads of household' earn money and delegate domestic care to a younger sister(s) (see also Edwards *et al.* 2006; Bowlby *et al.* 2010). The ways in which caring identities and relations evolve over time remains less apparent.

Geographies of care

In considering the shifting nature of care in sibling relationships this chapter is not only concerned with the significance of time but also the salience of space. It draws on, and contributes to, the growing literature on geographies of care, which stemmed from wider drives towards more ethical geographies (Raghuram *et al.* 2009) and a greater consideration of the significance of space (and indeed time) with respect to care from the early 1990s onwards (McKie *et al.* 2004). Much work in this vein draws on, and contributes to, the feminist ethics of care literature with concerns including: the spatiality of everyday practices of care; moral landscapes; ethical spatial relations; shifts in and the distending of care over different spaces, including ethical responsibilities; the spatial organisation of care-giving/receiving; shifts in the location of care; the creation of caring spaces; and ethical consumption (e.g. Philo 1997; Milligan 2000; Smith 2000; Conradson 2003; Parr 2003; Massey 2004; Silk 2004; Popke 2006; Barnett and Land 2007; Lawson 2007; Milligan *et al.* 2007; Raghuram *et al.* 2009; McEwan and Goodman 2010).

Tapping into feminist perspectives, many geographers have viewed care in terms of relationality and interdependency, moving the emphasis away from researching the autonomous individual (Conradson 2003; Popke 2006; Lawson 2007; Raghuram *et al.* 2009). A geographical perspective not only emphasises relationality between people, but also between people and places, thereby recognising the relationships between care of/for self, care of/for others and care of/for the environment (Bondi 2003; Popke 2006; Bowlby *et al.* 2010). Despite the growth in interest in geographies of care little is understood about how sibling caring practices and relations shift within and across different spaces. For siblings, and indeed families more broadly, home is often presented as the primary site of care in which such practices are performed and identities fostered (Punch 2008). The emphasis on home neglects the significance of other spatial contexts important to young people, such as neighbourhoods or schools, and the micro-spaces within them, the macro-level contexts that shape them, and the interconnected nature of such spaces (Edwards *et al.* 2006, Bowlby *et al.* 2010). This chapter seeks to take a nuanced approach exploring change and continuity in sibling caring practices, relations and identities over time and in different spaces.

Researching sibling relationships over time

This chapter draws on an eight-year project that forms part of Timescapes; the first major qualitative longitudinal programme to be funded in the UK.[2] Project one of Timescapes – 'Your Space! Siblings & Friends'[3] – documents the meanings, experiences and flows of young people's prescribed (sibling) and chosen (friendship) relationships, exploring how such relationships relate to their sense of self as their individual and family biographies unfold. It follows in-depth the lives of over 50 young people born between 1989 and 1996 and from a diverse range of backgrounds. Data have been gathered in three Waves (2002, 2007, 2009) using in-depth interviews and a flexible range of tools including games, vignettes and photography (see Weller 2010). Whilst care did not feature as an explicit element of the study it undoubtedly flowed through many of the narratives and participants' continued involvement also inferred a sense of care towards the project. Furthermore, our approach was guided by an ethic of care, and the longitudinal nature of the project amplified caring elements of the research relationship not least the (generally) growing emotional connection and sense of responsibility felt towards participants.

Shifting caring practices, identities and relations amongst siblings

Across all three Waves we asked participants to discuss instances of support provided to and by their siblings. Examples also emerged in more general dialogue. This chapter draws on two illustrative examples – Alisha and DJ Kizzel[4] – that are, by no means, intended to be representative. Rather, their narratives highlight the diversity of experience and are illustrative of some of the broader trends relating to the ways in which identities, values and challenging episodes shape, and are shaped by, shifting caring practices, relations and identities.

Alisha's story

The first example focuses on Alisha; a middle-class, British Pakistani young woman who lives with her mother, a self-employed business woman, in an affluent area in South-East England. She has one sister, Malika, five years older than herself. She first took part in 'Your Space!' in 2002 when she was 11 years old. Across her three interviews Alisha described sharing a relatively close, albeit quarrelsome, relationship with Malika. The amount of time they spent together altered a little, particularly when Malika moved away to university during Wave 2. For Alisha, home, and to a lesser extent school, represented key sites in her sibling geographies of care. Salient to her understandings were the values of her immediate family (mother, sister), which were shaped, in part, by her cultural background, gender and class, and encompassed moral expectations about altruism, honesty, kindness, love, politeness and respect. Throughout, Alisha presented the uncaring practices of her extended family, such as the lack of help they gave her mother, in juxtaposition to this ethos of care. Moreover, the importance of two interrelated episodes of family crisis – her father's alcoholism and intermittent presence, and Malika's mental health issues – became apparent. On synthesising all three interviews the intersection between the ethos of care instilled in Alisha by her mother, and her lived experience of family crisis became evident. Over time and in different spaces (namely home[5] and school) this ethos of care was not only reshaped by but also implicated in the sisters' shifting caring identities.

It was during Wave 1 that Alisha first suggested that care formed an inherent part of being/having a sibling. She said 'A brother or sister can be anybody, any type of person at all who is caring . . .' She spent much time at home with Malika and, whilst they argued, she spoke of the protection her sister provided. Home represented the epicentre of the familial ethos of care. It was, however, scarred by what she regarded as her father's uncaring practices, not least the ill-treatment of her mother and sister. The space was successively constructed as caring and uncaring depending on his absence/presence (see also Conradson 2003; Bowlby *et al.* 2010). Her emphasis on his untidiness spoke volumes about the lack of care he brought to the home. She imagined what the space might be like without him and her desires were fulfilled when he left the family home between Waves 1 and 2. Highlighting her quest to forge caring spaces there, Alisha described how she, Malika and their mother redecorated, symbolically remaking the home and illustrating the connection between care for self, others and environment (Popke 2006).

Primarily couched in terms of the presence/absence of talking/listening, Alisha presented two key dimensions to her sibling caring practices and relations, shaped by these broader experiences of uncaring. In sister–sister relationships a number of studies have shown that 'talk' is a significant feature (Gordon *et al.* 2000; Edwards *et al.* 2005a, 2006). On the one hand, Alisha discussed how Malika spoke at her in a maternalistic 'mini-mother' manner (see also Mauthner 2002, 2005; Edwards *et al.* 2005a, 2006). For instance, after listing the sanctions placed on her by Malika, she concluded 'She's basically like a mum. Have to get on with my homework, have to do what she says and respect her.' Whilst her sister's actions may have been intended to be caring they were not necessarily perceived to be so (see also Tronto 1993; Raghuram *et al.* 2009). Rather, such 'mini-mothering' often led either to them not talking or to conflict, during which Alisha assumed a subservient role, apologising even if she did not think it was necessary. On the other hand, there were instances where Alisha suggested that she protected her sister. She believed Malika had been treated disproportionately badly by the wider family and sought to protect her by refraining from voicing her own concerns. She said 'I don't really tell her as much as I could do. I don't tell her that much at all ... I don't want to disturb her.' Alisha's narrative surrounding concerns for her sister's, rather than her own, welfare demonstrated the ways in which she cared for and about Malika. Alisha's narrative also pointed to more hidden power relations and her positioning of herself as strong and resilient in comparison to Malika, who had received formal therapeutic care to deal with such traumas. In line with Sharp *et al.*'s (2000) notion of entanglements of power, as comprising dominating and resisting elements, this example demonstrates the 'oscillations between caring and power dynamics' (Mauthner 2005: 636).

The ethos of care so evident in Wave 1 continued to be salient during Wave 2. Whilst research suggests that those from middle-class families are more likely to view themselves as individuals who happen to be siblings (Edwards *et al.* 2006), Alisha's cultural upbringing emphasised a sense of self as an integral part of a family unit with an enduring ethical responsibility to care for one another. For instance, she helped out in her mother's shop and undertook domestic work. Outside the home Alisha also operationalised this ethos by doing voluntary work with children, and adults with disabilities. Her second interview contained less explicit mention of the family's traumatic experiences, although the legacy of these was apparent especially in terms of her appreciation of her sister's protective stance when their parents had argued; 'it was my sister who would cover my ears and take me to my room'. She did, however, also discuss the continuation of her sister's 'mini-mothering' as both positively and negatively received. By now though, she expressed a sense in which her sister's caring practices were not always spatially or temporally appropriate; perhaps even ill-conceived. Encounters at school in the recent past were experienced as surveillance, for instance, 'the teachers would always talk about me to her'. At home, help with homework was sometimes perceived as impatient and uncaring, making her '[feel] insecure or stupid'.

Wave 2 was also marked by a small shift in the flow of caring and power relations, although Alisha's attempts to use her own expertise in drama to help Malika with an acting course were dismissed as she was younger. Other examples of caring practices were more implicit and, akin to Wave 1, one of the most significant ways in which Alisha cared for her sister revolved around gendered practices associated with talk/listening. She cared for Malika by complying with her demands, understanding her personal problems, and forfeiting her own desires to talk intimately. These examples also point to Alisha's perception that Malika saw herself as the elder, authoritative voice, whilst she assumed the position of the younger, subservient listener. In part, power relations centred on what she viewed as a generational gap between herself and Malika, with both sisters reproducing dominant notions of age-based hierarchical sibling relationships, which intersected with cultural-based expectations around respect for elders. Furthermore, Alisha assumed she could/would acquire greater caring responsibilities as part of her trajectory to adulthood (see also Bowlby *et al.* 2010; Edwards and Weller 2010a; Ribbens McCarthy and Edwards 2011).

Examples of the influence of the familial ethos of care persisted in Wave 3. For instance, cultural and gendered expectations surrounding sustained care over the life course were evident in her negotiations with Malika over the short- and long-term care of their mother. By now, however, Alisha had begun to reflect critically on the familial ethos. She spoke of feeling the need to balance the differing demands of her Asian and British backgrounds, including her post-feminist rejection of what she regarded as Asian gendered expectations. She also discussed how her outlook was shaped by the morals of a religion she did not practice. Furthermore, she considered the pitfalls of her mother's fervour for honesty and generosity, including the possible exploitation of the care-giver. She also described her dual duties of care for her sister and her friends as draining, thereby drawing attention to the labour required in caring relations (Ribbens McCarthy and Edwards 2011). By this stage then the ethos of care outlined in earlier interviews had been reconstructed by Alisha's own critical reflection, shifting identity and lived experiences.

Akin to Wave 2, Malika continued to play the protective and, sometimes, controlling 'mini-mother' whilst Alisha still retreated in the face of conflict. Suggesting a greater awareness of the power relations in their relationship Alisha noted 'she's got a very clever way of getting me to do what she wants'. However, a far more influential happening began to shape their caring relationship. Partly as a result of earlier traumas Alisha's sister was diagnosed with mental health issues and was, again, in receipt of formal therapeutic care. The situation had resulted in a more seismic, but complex, shift in caring and power relations between the sisters. Alisha felt a duty and responsibility to help Malika and, believing that her mother was unable to cope with the enormity of the situation, she stepped in to source information and provide support, 'my Mum doesn't really understand eating disorders ... so I've spent a LOT of time trying to explain it ... I've offered to take her [sister] to appointments'. Furthermore, echoing previous accounts, Alisha continued to assume the position of the dutiful listener having little opportunity to discuss aspects of her own life, thus mirroring a one-way therapeutic-type relationship. Although at times Malika remained domineering Alisha's caring practices speak to Mauthner's (2002) notion of 'shifting positions' in caring and power relations, which often occur in the face of illness or challenging circumstances (Edwards *et al.* 2005b). Concurrently, as the younger sister Alisha found her new caring identity challenging, again reflecting hierarchical-based understandings of care in sibling relationships.

Echoing Bowlby *et al.*'s (2010) argument that 'The ways in which we experience care reflects our age, gender, ethnicity, health and social status, and will be influenced by our beliefs and values about families and relationships' (15), Alisha's story points to the intersection between age-based and gendered identities and flows of care in sibling relationships (Edwards *et al.* 2006), along with a cultural–familial emphasis on an enduring ethical responsibility to care for one another. It also highlights the complexity and oscillating nature of caring and power relations, particularly in the context of challenging events (see also Mauthner 2005). Space and time – particularly shifting home spaces in Alisha's example – are undoubtedly salient in shaping such practices, relations and identities.

DJ Kizzel's story

The second example focuses on DJ Kizzel; a working-class White British young man who lives with his parents, both employed in the service industry, in social housing in a disadvantaged area of South-West England. He also lives with his younger brother, John, and sister, Ella (two and four years younger, respectively). He was 8 years old when he first took part in 2002. Over the course of the research, and akin to many other working-class participants, DJ Kizzel viewed his sense of self as an integral part of a sibling group (see also Edwards *et al.* 2006). Across all three interviews he described spending much time with his siblings at home and in the local park. Coupled with his school these sites formed the locus of his main geographies of care. It is important to note that whilst he spent much time with his siblings, and alluded to their collective sibling identity, like Alisha his relationships with them were marked by regular conflict and entangled power relations, akin to those outlined by Sharp *et al.* (2000). A further salient element to his narrative was the sustained bullying he experienced at school and in his local area. On bringing together all three interviews, the relationship between different aspects of identity (age, class, gender), and critical episodes of bullying at school and in the local area to his caring practices and relations as a sibling became apparent.

During Wave 1 he perpetually presented himself as a victim of uncaring practices across a range of geographies. For example, he described instances of torment perpetrated by his younger siblings at home 'cos [John] made a dent there [points to forehead] because he threw one of those metal trains at me'. He also spoke of bullying at school and in the local area and it was often difficult to disentangle his narratives of 'uncaring' in these different spaces. The prevalence of victimisation in his narrative appeared heavily implicated in his understandings of care, which focused on protection (or a lack of). Whilst he desired to be protected, his father's interjections[6] during this first interview highlighted a paternalistic discourse of care within the family, which as the eldest male sibling meant he was expected to be able to care for and protect himself (see also Edwards *et al.* 2006). His father said: 'you are a big lad you can sort yourself out'. Other research suggests that sibling relationships are gendered, with brothers prioritising 'activities' over 'talk' (Gordon *et al.* 2000; Edwards *et al.* 2005a, 2006). DJ Kizzel's father reinforced this notion suggesting that he ought to be 'doing care' by protecting himself and his siblings.

DJ Kizzel's emphasis on bullying overshadowed the few examples he gave of sibling caring practices. For example, whilst they argued at home, the neighbourhood and the park represented spaces in which they protected one another (see also Edwards *et al.* 2006). He did suggest that he looked after John at school, and there were also glimpses of reciprocity when DJ Kizzel himself noted 'sometimes he [brother] gives me some of his dinner [at school]'. Whilst Bowlby *et al.* (2010: 93) argue that 'care between older and younger children is also an important form of caring behaviour in which divisions of gender and age are expressed, learned and reinforced', DJ Kizzel's lived experiences of sustained bullying appear to have disrupted dominant hierarchical, age-based, notions of flows of care (see also Edwards *et al.* 2005b; McIntosh and Punch 2009). He did not appear to wish to relate to his siblings as a paternalistic protector, in part due to his desire to be protected, and because he believed he would take care of, or assume responsibility for, his siblings when he was older.

Four years later Wave 2 was marked by a more overt discussion of caring practices, particularly the ways in which his siblings cared about him at home and when out in the local area. For instance, John helped him with his homework and both siblings spontaneously organised a party for him. In this respect care was again discussed in gendered terms as actions (kind gestures) and non-actions (a lack of conflict) afforded to him by his siblings. He also expressed a greater sense of care for self, and interdependence and reciprocity, particularly with John. Again, much of this discussion focused on protection as the main caring practice, and whilst gendered in nature, again, did not conform to more hierarchical, aged-based notions of flows of care. The brothers stuck up for one another in the park and both anticipated future caring relations: 'If anyone bullies him [at school] then I'll stick up for him' to which John interjected 'If anyone bullies you then I will stick up for you'. Akin to Wave 1 DJ Kizzel continued to view caring responsibilities as integral to his future trajectory to adulthood (see also Bowlby *et al.* 2010; Edwards and Weller 2010a; Evans 2010; Ribbens McCarthy and Edwards 2011).

Importantly, DJ Kizzel believed his sibling relationships had improved over time and his more positive experiences of care, as opposed to conflict, at home had wider implications for his ability to deal with the challenges he continued to face at school. He said 'my brother and sister have stopped arguing with me and that

... we're friends now and that has helped me better in school'. Akin to Wave 1, he seemed to downplay his own agency, suggesting that it was the caring practices of his siblings within the protective space of his home that now provided him with the resources to cope with bullying at school and in the local area (Weller 2007). Such changes in his home-based experiences of care led him to question the efficacy of more formal care arrangements in his school. For example, he criticised his teachers' lack of engagement with the school bullying policy and felt disappointed that they indicated it was his responsibility to prove there was a problem, thereby pointing to, what authors such as Lawson (2007) describe as, an individualised notion of responsibility to care for self. This example shows how experiences of care in one particular arena can spill over into how care is understood, expected and received in other spaces (Bowlby *et al.* 2010).

Wave 3 was marked by a new-found self-assurance and he immediately started talking about positive changes in his life. There was still a sense of ambivalence in his sibling relationships and although they appeared to argue at times (particularly the brothers) they shared close relationships. He enjoyed their trips to the park; a space once characterised by bullying/protection illustrating, as Conradson (2003) suggests, that the same spaces may enable caring at certain times and not at others. This space was particularly significant in that due to his diagnosis of dyspraxia and Attention Deficit Hyperactivity Disorder[7] he did not feel confident to go far from home on his own. Again, disrupting conventional age-based sibling hierarchies it was John who enabled him to visit the park. The giving of care by DJ Kizzel was perhaps more evident than in his previous accounts. He recounted home-based practices such as helping Ella tidy her room, and following his parents' requests had to 'look after 'em [siblings] sometimes when they go out'. Whilst on the face of it such examples might signal a small shift towards more hierarchical flows of care, DJ Kizzel felt his siblings challenged his authority, thereby discrediting the responsibility of care he had been given by his parents. Perhaps Ella and John had never viewed their sibling identities in this manner before. Concurrently, he seemed to be a somewhat reluctant care-giver, wishing to continue to defer such responsibilities until a future time.

Nonetheless, much of his Wave 3 narrative pointed to a growing sense of interdependency, not least the siblings' shared responsibility for caring for the home and for one another, thus reflecting McIntosh and Punch's (2009) argument that responsibilities are not static but negotiated in sibling relationships. Importantly this, arguably class-based, sense of collective identity emphasised the protection of the sibling unit as a key caring practice (see also Edwards *et al.* 2006).

To illuminate how DJ Kizzel's caring practices and relations were shaped by his lived experiences in different arenas it is fruitful to look to Bowlby *et al.*'s (2010: 94) idea that 'What is learned and practiced by way of caring can be contingent on the nature of the spaces in which we have access.' His encounters of conflict and care in different spaces were intrinsically interlinked; his sense of (un)caring at home by his siblings was not separated out from, but rather shaped by, the (un)caring he faced at school and in the local area. Caring practices and relations continually ebbed and flowed through and between spaces and comprised entangled power relations that were, by no means, clear-cut (Sharp *et al.* 2000). Much of his story did challenge notions of hierarchical, and at times gendered (paternalistic notions of 'doing care'), flows of care in sibling relationships (Edwards *et al.* 2006). Nonetheless, such practices, relations and identities were consistently shaped by class (collectivity and interdependence).

Conclusions

Siblings are said to constitute amongst the longest relationships in life (Punch 2008). Yet, the significance of sisters and brothers as a source of care and support is often taken for granted. This chapter has sought to go some way to remedy this oversight by focusing on two illustrative examples that demonstrate how over time and in different spaces sibling caring and power relations shape and are shaped by aspects of identity (age, class, culture, gender), values (familial and education-oriented) and challenging events (episodes of crisis). In doing so, I have aimed to offer insights into the shifting nature of informal caring practices, relations and identities within one life-course phase (Cicirelli 1995; Bowlby *et al.* 2010).

By taking a spatial–temporal perspective I have sought to challenge preconceptions about flows and spaces of care, highlighting shifts as well as factors that remain consistently salient. A longitudinal perspective is well placed to examine such changes and continuities, arguably providing a new methodological dimension to literatures concerning both geographies of care and feminist ethics of care. For instance, exploring such relationships over the long term can illuminate change and continuity in understandings of key elements of care such as reciprocity, relationality and interdependence.

Whilst this chapter is concerned with informal care amongst siblings the two examples raise some important issues for practice and policy. The credence afforded to vertical connections over lateral relationships, coupled with an overemphasis on the mitigation of sibling relations deemed problematic (rivalry, jealousy, conflict) by practitioners has led to the neglect of care amongst siblings (Edwards *et al.* 2005a; Mauthner 2005). Yet, the examples provided by Alisha and DJ Kizzel highlight the ways in which every day practices of care scaffold family life, often playing a crucial role during episodes of family crisis. Indeed, as Kosonen's (1996) research reinforces, children are more likely to turn to their siblings than their fathers for support. Accordingly, schools ought to be encouraged to recognise the significance of siblings in providing support with school work, friendships and family life, and services need to ensure that in practice siblings are placed together at times of family change/crisis (Tickle 2008; NSPCC 2010). Moreover, for policy and practice to be effective the way in which care flows within and between different spaces needs to be recognised (see also Gillies and Robinson, Chapter 4 and Laurent, Chapter 3 in this volume). Tangentially, this chapter speaks to wider policy trends that emphasise independency and personal responsibility as key facets of a 'successful' transition to adulthood, arguably to the detriment of acknowledging the salience of interdependency and relationality in shaping young people's pathways.

Notes

1 In this context young people is used to denote children and teenagers under the age of 18.
2 Funded by the Economic and Social Research Council, please see: www.timescapes. leeds.ac.uk
3 Conducted with Professor Rosalind Edwards.
4 Participants chose their own pseudonyms.
5 The family moved on several occasions during the study, so home is used in a relatively generic sense here, as a place of significance, rather than a specific building.
6 For all three interviews DJ Kizzel's parents and/or siblings were present at various times, often contributing to the discussion.
7 We became aware of this diagnosis during Wave 2.

14 Care arrangements of transnational migrant elders

Between family, community and the state

Elisabetta Zontini, University of Nottingham

Introduction: the ageing of labour migrants

According to the 2001 census, ageing labour migrants are a growing group in the UK, yet their experiences have until recently largely been ignored in academic literature (Burholt 2004; King *et al.* 2005; for exceptions see Gardner 2002 and Ramji 2006). This lack of attention is surprising given the growing concern and recognition of ageing across Europe and the economic and social contribution that this group of migrant workers had for both their countries of origin and settlement (White 2006).

Drawing on the experiences of Italians in the UK, this chapter will explore the caring arrangements of this group of transnational elders, focusing in particular on the role that families, community and the state have on their everyday life. Looking at feminist ethics of care as well as the transnational care literature, this chapter sees the elderly not just as care receivers and 'needy' dependants, but as individuals interconnected to others who are involved in complex multidirectional caring networks that span generations as well as countries (Reynolds and Zontini 2006). Thus, this research considers care as occurring not just in the sphere of private and intimate relationships but as encompassing wider relations at the community level and beyond (Hill Collins 1995; Tronto 1995a). It explores how these different spheres are negotiated, drawing attention to the role of gender, identity, values and to the elders' particular transnational experiences. It does so through the use of two case studies, that of Mrs Moretti and Mr Gallo who well illustrate the kind of gendered experiences common to other Italians of their class and generation living in the UK.

Transnationalism and caring

Care has started to receive a growing attention in the transnational literature. One important area of enquiry has been the focus on 'global care chains' which has centred on the effects of globalisation on the distribution of care worldwide (Ehrenreich and Hochschild 2002; Hochschild *et al.* 2000; Yeates 2009). This literature focuses on the care drain affecting countries in the global South as a result of the increase in female migration and growing demand in care-related jobs in the global North. It highlights how affluent women of the global North offload their devalued caring tasks to poorer women in the South who migrate to take up such tasks, while simultaneously devolving their own caring duties to even less fortunate women in their country of origin. This literature is important because it highlights the public and global nature of seemingly private and local arrangements, such as the hiring of foreign domestic workers and also the low status and devalued nature of care work worldwide. However, this literature also seems to imply that co-presence is a prerequisite of caring practices and that increased globalisation and transnationalism undermine families and the ability of their members to care for each other. Recent feminist literature on transnationalism rejects this position, arguing that care can be done from a distance and that a family's geographical separation does not mean the demise of care. This has been observed in the literature on transnational motherhood (Hondagneu-Sotelo and Avila 1997; Erel 2002; Parreñas 2001) as well as in the emerging literature on transnational care-giving which has started to explore the consequences of geographical distance in affecting caring practices towards the elderly and the ways in which different migrant groups are addressing this problem (Baldassar and Baldock 2000; Goulbourne and Chamberlain 2001; Burholt 2004; Evergeti and Zontini 2006; Reynolds and Zontini 2006; Zontini 2006; Wilding 2006). Drawing on the feminist ethics of care, these studies have shown that elder care is multidirectional, can be done from a distance and that older migrants are both providers and receivers of care in their transnational families.

As I argue elsewhere, the example of elderly migrants is good for refining theories of transnationalism (Zontini under review). Equally, however, a transnational lens is increasingly important to interpret current experiences of ageing. In multicultural societies like Britain, large numbers of elders have connections elsewhere (Goulbourne *et al.* 2010). Yet, outside the transnational care-giving literature, their experiences are usually only looked at in relation to their situation in the country of settlement (Afshar *et al.* 2008). The few studies available on migrant elders focus on their exclusions and marginalisation (Nazroo *et al.* 2004). A policy agenda shapes studies concerned with their experiences, the main focus being an exploration of their access (or lack of it) to mainstream resources (Walker *et al.* 2001). Their experiences, however, are wider than that and include their relationships not just with local services and institutions but also with family members, communities and places both locally and elsewhere. In public discourse, they are usually seen from two contrasting positions, either as simply needing care and thus as a drain on state resources or as belonging to families that 'look after their own', where children will automatically take up the task of looking after their elders (Mand 2008). As Mand (2008) has argued in relation to South Asians, the caring needs and resources of migrant elders are more complex than that and require further detailed analysis.

The division made in the feminist literature between 'caring for' and 'caring about' is particularly useful for understanding the experiences of older migrants (see Reynolds and Zontini 2006). They, in fact, do not only receive and provide what can be described as practical, day-to-day hands-on support but also the less tangible care that includes 'contact and emotional support and refers to emotional functions connected with sociability, advice, comfort and self-validation' (Reynolds and Zontini 2006: 5). As Reynolds and Zontini (2006) have highlighted, for migrants *caring about* activities include communication by telephone, letters, emails, visits, participation in family decision-making and financing the purchase of care. Also, caring about might mean managing access to services and institutions or even preventing access if it is deemed to be impacting on other issues (as I will show later). Sevenhuijsen's (2002: 131) definition of the moral subject as a person who 'lives in a network of relations and (inter)dependence, in which he/she has to balance different forms of care: for the self, for others and for the relations between these' chimes with the experiences of the older migrants (especially women) at the heart of this study. In line with the feminist ethics of care these older people do not necessarily see autonomy and independence as values and consider themselves as part of families that are heavily interconnected. Authors such as Sevenhuijsen (1998, 2002) have developed the idea of relational autonomy whereby they stress the 'always, already connected' nature of people and agency. This framework is useful for interpreting the experiences of older people, especially in relation to gender. Both men and women in my study saw themselves in relational terms, as Hill Collins (1995) has also found in relation to African American communities in the United States. However, as we know, men and women care differently (Arber *et al.* 2003; Doucet 2006a; Afshar *et al.* 2008). The feminist ethics of care literature sees care as potentially feminist not feminine, as a practice of human activity that can be learned, improved and carried out by everyone. Yet most of the attention in the literature is on the experiences of women. Tronto (1995) explicitly calls for extending the ethics of care beyond the experiences of women and the realm of the family.

I start from this premise and look at gender differences in caring, and at care in other arenas. In much of the care literature families are seen as the main source of care for older people (Phillips 2007). In this chapter, however, I do not want to take the role of families for granted and explore instead the wider caring networks that these older migrants may or may not have access to. Also, because of their experiences as migrants who have lived in two or more countries, I want to see how their 'bifocality' (Vertovec 2009) has shaped their values as well as their commitments and the networks they can access. Vertovec (2009) defines bifocality as the ways in which the outlook and daily experiences of migrants are shaped by communication, frequent travel and other transnational practices. Guarnizo (1997) has described this particular outlook as 'transnational habitus' to denote how certain migrants maintain a dual frame of reference derived from values and practices of two different geographical contexts – in this case the UK and Italy – but also from a lifetime as mobile subjects constantly travelling and exchanging information between the two locations. This chapter is concerned with how ageing migrants – both male and female – give and receive care irrespective of where it occurs.

The study

This chapter is based on a research project recently completed in the British city of Nottingham as well as on insights from a previous ESRC-funded project on Italian

Families and Social Capital (see Goulbourne *et al.* 2010). Methodologically, the Nottingham project involved participant observation in two community centres, at community and family events such as special dinners, religious celebrations, day trips as well as in-depth interviews with older Italian migrants, their family members and community and social workers. A total of ten more formal interviews were conducted with members attending the two centres or drawn from networks originating there. We interviewed both men and women ranging in age from early sixties to mid-eighties, with the majority of them being 70 or above. All had migrated in the 1950s and 1960s at the apex of Italian emigration, initially in response to British employers recruiting labour in Southern Italy for their factories and subsequently as a result of chain migration. As a consequence of the latter, the majority of those attending the two community centres studied came from a single village in Southern Italy. I will call this village Montegiuliano. This is an isolated rural village on the top of a hill in a Southern Italian region. People there were mainly involved in agriculture but since the first villagers gained employment in the factories of Nottingham, emigration has become the main source of income for the village and its inhabitants. Although very few went back to live there, most maintain strong links and continue to visit and invest in properties there. All interviewees, both men and women, had been factory workers in and around Nottingham before retiring.

Getting old: giving and receiving care

When participants left Italy they had planned to return. As Baldassar (2001, 2007) wrote in relation to Italians migrating to Australia, they too had licence to leave from their families but also the obligation to return. Baldassar (2007: 287) describes Italian migrants of the same cohort in Australia as 'heavily homeland-focused', not intending to settle abroad but hoping to save enough money for an eventual return. Because of that they kept close contacts with their families and friends back home. Contrary to their plans, however, the migrants at the heart of this study are ageing in the UK where the majority of their immediate families now reside. For the most part they are resigned to the idea of not returning to Italy and to die in the UK (see also Ganga 2006).

In what follows I briefly present the stories of two Italian elders, one man and one woman, to show how care is given and received by this group, focusing in particular on the role of gender and on families, community and the state. What will become apparent is how the values of this particular group shape their caring practices but also how values change and get renegotiated in particular contexts. These two stories were selected because they are typical of the gendered experiences of care of this particular group of migrants.

Mrs Moretti

Mrs Moretti, aged 70, has four children and has been living in the UK since 1962. She had been a factory worker since her children started school until she had to take early retirement due to health reasons. She was the main carer for her husband until he died a year after we met her and looks after her granddaughter when her children work. She is also at the heart of her family in the UK and abroad. Mrs Moretti clearly draws pride and satisfaction from her caring roles, enjoying the time she is now spending with her youngest granddaughter and Sundays when her house is full with her adult children and grandchildren.

> Every Sunday this house is always full with me and the kids. Every day on Sunday I get up early and I cook and then we have lunch and they are here all day. I love it when, you know, when I see everybody at the table, you feel really full and proud.

Drawing on the feminist ethics of care, we could argue that her sense of self is tied up with those she cares for and that she is involved in reciprocal caring practices where she both gives help and receives emotional rewards from others. Mrs Moretti, however, clearly also resents her role, reminding us that care should not be romanticised as it is also – and at the same time – labour, as many feminist writers have long pointed out (Held 2006; Noddings 2003; Ruddick 1998; Sevenhuijsen 2000). In her own words 'I'm 70 and haven't seen anything, nothing. I remember my life as washing, cooking, cleaning and looking after everybody.' Mrs Moretti feels she hasn't had a fair deal. 'I've been working inside and outside [the home] when I finish work I start again.' She adds:

> I spent my life working, not just one or two years. I would like to get up in the morning and even go to Bramcote on the bus just to be free . . . My husband he goes out to Victoria Centre [shopping mall] and at 12 o'clock he wants the dinner on the table, he goes out in the morning and come back at 12 o'clock and wants the dinner, I can't go far because I got to come back for him.

Interestingly, her resentment involves also her transnational 'duties'. As Vertovec (1999), has written all migrants spend their lives assessing the relative advantages of at least two locations (their place of origin and of settlement), often being torn between which one to choose (Gardner 2002).

Mrs Moretti, however, is very clear that she is better off in the UK than she would be in her village of origin and now finds even visiting difficult.

> Well, my husband he wants to go back . . . a couple of years ago we was fighting and I say 'well look if you want to go back you go back and I stay here' . . . It's alright in Italy, you know, nice air but I think about my family, I can't stay without my family without my grandchildren. You think I got all the children here . . . I say 'look if you want to go you go but I come every 6 months or every year' but he can't go cos he can't do nothing. . . . [there] I still got to wash cos I haven't got a washing machine there I have to wash by hand, I have to cook everyday and I'm not going anywhere . . . There he's on holiday . . . I am worse than here and then all his family come to see you . . . and you make coffee and you make coffee and you make coffee all day long . . . it's no

good for me. I'm not on holiday I work double the time there . . . And me I have to go back to Montegiuliano to have that life for good? No chance! At least here I go to town, I got my bus pass . . . my grandchildren are here . . . I can have a meal, have a laugh, I got my group, it's a different life, no chance!!

Here we see how Mrs Moretti views caring as crucial for her identity and sense of self when she talks about not being able to live without her children and grandchildren but also as work and an unwanted burden, especially in relation to the kind of 'kin work' (Di Leonardo 1992) she would be expected to do in Italy.

Sadly, over the course of fieldwork it became apparent that Mrs Moretti is increasingly struggling with her caring roles also in Nottingham due to her deteriorating health. However, she finds it difficult to seek help both within and outside the family. At present she is still coping although with increasing difficulty. She is not sure who will help her when she becomes too frail. She does not seem to think that her family would provide care for her. She believes that families are changing in the UK and that labour market demands are different from those in Southern Italy where a lot of people are either out of work or work short hours. She thinks that in the UK it is harder for the younger generations to look after their elders. Asked who will look after her if her knee gets worse she replied:

Well I don't know, up to now I don't get help from nobody, not even my husband. Well if I need help I don't know, I don't know will they gonna repay you what I do for everybody? I'll have to wait and see . . .

Mrs Moretti is not alone in her concerns. There seems to be growing academic attention to the enduring capacity of families to care for their members as a result of modernisation and globalisation (Phillips 2007). Also this was a topic openly discussed by the women at the community centre. On one occasion, they reflected on their prospects of ending up in a care home. All but one discussed the possibility in positive terms and saw it as better than moving in with their own children.

My research suggests this is unusual given that this goes against the Italian family ideal (see Zontini 2010). On the one hand it seemed that they were preparing themselves for what they saw as inevitable; on the other hand they appeared to dread the idea of losing control and the leading role at the heart of the families' networks they now seem to enjoy. They were saying that once you go and live with your children, power shifts towards them and you'll have to live by their rules which they would find quite difficult to accept. Others, such as Mrs Moretti, did not want to interfere with their children's lives and felt they didn't want to become a burden. Only one woman saw going into a care home as a terrible thing, she hoped she will be looked after by her son who, in his mid-forties, still lived with her.

Mr Gallo

Mr Gallo, aged 77, and his wife, aged 82, live in what could be called an extended family with their son (who is divorced) and his teenage children and his wife's widowed brother. Rather than them being looked after by the younger generation (Mr Gallo had recently had a stroke) the opposite seems to be the case. Mr Gallo and his wife moved to a bungalow built in the garden of their very large house in order to allow their son and children to move in. Mrs Gallo said that she is the only one trying to clean and look after the house but now she finds it too difficult to do which means that the house looks quite dirty and in disrepair.

Mr Gallo's health deteriorated over the course of the project. As a result of his stroke, he told us that he had lost 100 per cent of his hearing in one ear and 75 per cent of sight in one eye, but what seemed to upset him the most was the prohibition to drive further than two miles from his home. This might be so for two reasons. One could be similar to what Gardner (2002) has found in relation to her Bangladeshi informants – the importance for men to be independently mobile which is linked to their identity. Not being able to drive and go where he wants is a clear sign that he is now an old person. In his interview he spent a lot of time narrating how he used to drive to Italy by car when he was younger (he told us he did it 22 times). The second reason revolves around the real consequences that this might have for him and his family. Mr Gallo thinks that things might 'get difficult' now he can't drive as far, especially for his wife and her brother, as it was Mr Gallo who drove them places for shopping and other needs, such as doctors appointments.

Mr Gallo's migratory project had always been to return to Italy. As he explained:

> Well you see it don't matter how long you been in England when you born in Italy not only for me if you are born in a different country you always think you want to go back, that was my feeling and if I not try one day I might cry and say oh I wish I had gone to Italy but I try and I been to Italy and I realise it's not for me anymore. I try two weeks there and oh no not the way they living there oh my God no.

He tried to return when he was in his early forties. However, things did not work out for him. Life in Turin, where he had found a factory job, was expensive and he did not manage to find a suitable accommodation for reuniting with his family. Missing his wife and children he returned to Nottingham. In addition to economic difficulties, he also had discovered that his values had changed and found it difficult to 'integrate' back in Italy. Italy though remained important for him and his wife and, until his health allowed it, they went back for a long summer holiday every year.

Now that he cannot travel anymore Mr Gallo's main activity and source of pride and self-esteem is his role as chairperson of the Southill community centre which Mrs Moretti also attends. This is one of the two community centres where once a week Italian elders can spend an afternoon playing cards (men) and bingo (women), drinking coffee and chatting with each other. Once a month they have a special meal when more people attend than at the weekly meetings. The older Italians treat the meal as a very special occasion. Men attend in suits and women dress up and wear their best jewellery. Mr Gallo's role involves collecting and administering the money from the other members, negotiating the rent of the room from the council and organising the monthly meal and other activities.

Neither Mrs Moretti nor Mr Gallo get any help from the council or other state institutions even though Mr Gallo has recently had a stroke and Mrs Moretti looked after her husband full-time until he eventually died. I would now like to draw out some points in relation to the caring needs and resources of older migrants such as Mrs Moretti and Mr Gallo, considering in turn family, community and the state as the key sites where care is offered and received.

Role of the family

Contrary to what is argued by proponents of the individualisation thesis (Beck and Beck-Gernsheim 2002; Bauman 2003; Giddens 1992), what emerges from the study is that families are still strong. Much care work continues to be done in the family, for instance a lot of intergenerational care work. However, care is gendered (Arber *et al.* 2003; Doucet 2006a; Afshar *et al.* 2008). Women and men provide and receive care differently. Mr Gallo helps his family financially. He gave his big house to his son and grandchildren allowing them to live in it for free while he and his wife occupy the small bungalow at the back of the garden. He is also the link between the family and other institutions. He drives his wife and brother-in-law where they need to go and negotiates on their behalf with health and other authorities by making appointments, filling in forms and – given his better English – talking to doctors for them. He does not receive much care from the male members of his family such as his son and grandchildren in spite of his recent stroke. Mrs Moretti looked after her husband as well as her grandchildren. She is also the centre of her (transnational) family networks which include both Nottingham and Montegiuliano.

As Mrs Moretti's and other stories show, ageing women continue to be at the centre of these families' networks of care. They are, however, increasingly frail and struggle to maintain this role. This role is both valued by them as they derive pride, a sense of identity and self-esteem from it but it was also resisted. As we can infer from Mrs Moretti's interview this role is problematic for them and they strive for a certain degree of autonomy (at least in old age). If we look at Mrs Moretti's interview there is much resistance talk (very similar narratives were given by other women). This is very different from the narratives of the Bangladeshi women studied by Gardner (2002: 131) who tended to give accounts that depicted them as 'good women', unquestioning providers of care for their husbands, children and elderly relatives. Those who have studied Diasporic Italian women elsewhere describe them in terms of selflessness and sacrifice with a communal and family-oriented notion of self pushing them towards 'compulsory altruism'. However, the older women in this study were not just self-sacrificing subjects, passively resigned to their gender and cultural role as care providers. They were also actively renegotiating their role.

The Italian women had no reservations in talking about care in ambivalent terms, seen both as labour and love (Held 2006; Noddings 2003; Ruddick 1998; Sevenhuijsen 2000). There is much resistance talk also in relation to transnationalism. These women described how they are cutting down on visits because of the work it involves (see Alicea 1997; Zontini 2004). Perhaps this could be linked to the fact that these Italian women had also been paid workers. They seem to differentiate themselves from women of their generation who had not migrated (and perhaps also from other migrant women who had never worked outside the home) for whom their caring role remained unquestioned. Their values have changed but it seems not those of their husbands, and this often results in conflicts, the most common ones being around the issue of return.

Women, however, continue to be reluctant to seek support from the younger generations in their families, being aware of changes that are occurring in families in Britain such as long working hours (also for women), job instability and family break-up (Williams 2004). Interestingly, they are wary of shifting their roles from the 'one-caring' to the 'cared-for' (Noddings 2003). As Noddings recognises, these relationships are reciprocal but asymmetrical and often unequal, something my interviewees seemed to be aware of. The women in the study wanted the prominent role in the families' networks that their caring role gave them and were reluctant to relinquish it by going to live with their children. Afshar *et al.* (2008) defines this as 'power to' as it is derived from the central role that older women have in what she termed 'the moral economy of kin'.

Men seem to be in charge of organising trips back home and driving there, providing financial assistance especially to the younger generations and liaising between the family and outside organisations. For men the ideal scenario would be to return to Italy as a successful migrant thus completing their migratory project. They would like to go back to their village owning a property there and living on their pensions. However, since their wives often refuse to go, they have to come to terms with continuing to live in the UK. For them, contrary to white British elders, successful ageing is also linked to relational autonomy as it is for their wives (see Afshar *et al.* 2008). Being surrounded by family and friends is a sign of success and gives them a sense of well-being.

Role of the community

The two community centres that these older Italians attend offer an important socialising role. Older Italians meet there as a specific group: as Italians of a particular generation and class and as former immigrant factory workers. These are places where commonalities and shared experiences bring people together and where their ethnic identity is reproduced. They are good for their socialisation, the development of self-help networks and for the generation and maintenance of their social capital. Both Mrs Moretti and Mr Gallo like 'having their group'. The importance of community centres for older migrants has been highlighted by other studies (Cook 2010; Afshar *et al.* 2008). The older African Caribbean women interviewed by Afshar *et al.* (2008) reported that they had to 'stick together' in order to survive and because of that they had strong friendship and community bonds that lasted a lifetime. They also emphasised the importance of 'shared identities, language, culture and tradition in their lives' (2008: 8). The social support provided in such centres was crucial and provided them with a sense of belonging.

However, these are also places where subtle exclusions operate based on hierarchies of gender, status and respectability. The space there is very gendered and also hierarchical. Men and women sit at different tables. Men play cards and the women are divided into those who play bingo and those who sit at the periphery of the group and chat. There is a separate table where the male committee members and the chairperson sit talking about 'important' issues to do with the running of the group. Women do not know anything about what the committee discusses and decides as there are no women on it. Some elders whose stories I have not reported here felt excluded from the 'inner circles' of the group and stopped attending. They also resented the gossip and the social control. On the whole, however, they are viewed as positive places giving the elders a sense of purpose and of community (see Cook 2010; Afshar *et al.* 2008).

From my research and that of others it emerged that such community centres are important spaces of intra-generational care and solidarity. They empower older people through what Afshar *et al.* (2008) have termed 'power with', i.e. power derived from participation in collective activities. However, their future seems precarious (Cook 2010). During fieldwork we witnessed the elderly gradually losing their autonomy. At one point the council stopped allowing them to cook their monthly meal for themselves because they were deemed too old by health and safety regulations. This was a big disappointment for them. At first they hired external caterers but they were not happy with them and then they said they could not afford them anymore. They started to pay the council to bring 'meals on wheels', but this was problematic. The committee started to be quite worried about the meal because the members were not enjoying the food and thought that 'meals on wheels' were 'making them feel old'. Subsequently they resisted the authorities and started cooking again even though they knew they were not supposed to do so.

As we have seen from the examples above, care is offered and received not just in families and across the generations but also in community groups and among peers. Friendship and co-ethnic networks seem to be as important for the elders I worked with as their immediate and distant families. At these centres they keep an eye on each other, they exchange information, they comfort each other and provide an opportunity for leisure and entertaining that enriches their quality of life.

Role of state institutions

The last area I want to explore is the interviewees' relationship with the state and other institutions which, as the above examples have shown, is characterised by mistrust. They had developed such mistrust through their pre-migration experiences in Italy and although less pronounced than towards Italian institutions, it extended to British ones as well. One example of this was provided by Maria. She is in her eighties and has problems with one of her arms. She did have a local authority home help which she did not pay for, but she said she was 'nosy' and spent time 'looking in the drawers' rather than cleaning. In the end Maria said 'no more the woman was coming round to find out about us not to clean'. After that

Maria and her husband started to pay the neighbour to do the cleaning instead of having what they saw as state officials looking into their life.

All the elders we interviewed were reluctant to seek support from the state and other institutions. Rather than seeking help they were increasingly relying on special aids which helped them cope with their everyday life. Mr Gallo explained that he sees a lot of people who are really struggling but they do not access formal support. He said:

> I know and you know that you got so many things in this country you can have but the Italian people they are proud, there is no way they go begging, to me it's not begging, if it's the law you are not going begging, but that's how they see it.

Their mistrust of institutions resulted in some resistance strategies such as their refusal to cooperate with officials including health workers. We witnessed an episode at the community centre where a health worker came in to advise them on swine flu. The elders were not listening to her presentation, chatting loudly and even laughing while she talked. Again this can be seen as resistance strategies as explained by Gardner (2002). They seemed to resent the health worker intruding in their space and life trying to tell them what to do. Their sense of identity is also tied up with their ability to care for each other and their community without such formal/external help.

For this group of elders caring about included also negotiating the most appropriate forms of care inside and outside the family. This includes not only accessing services but also preventing access to services that are deemed unsuitable. Akin to Buckman's (2010) work with Muslim carers, Italians do not have problems in accessing health services. The same cannot be said for social care services which, as we have seen, are often viewed with great suspicion.

Conclusions

This chapter has explored how ageing migrants access and provide care. Due to their migration experience, the family has become at once more and less significant for these migrants. The immediate family has become more important as they are now removed from their extended family. The extended family has lost some of its significance (though not completely through transnational connections) and friends and community organisations have gained an enhanced role in the lives of these elders. The state and its services play a limited role. This is interesting because it contradicts the current public rhetoric on immigration which is increasingly depicting migrants as a burden for the state and the welfare system (Pero 2008).

Being connected to others and involved in strong and dense networks of support is surely positive for the elders. However, as I have argued elsewhere, there are also problems with that, especially for the younger generations who feel the pressure of both their family's values and those of the more individualistic mainstream society (Zontini 2010; see also Shah 2007) and for women more generally. Women enjoy the power that their central role in caring networks gives them while at the same time they also strive for some degree of autonomy which will mean more control over their time and resources. Men too are active members of these networks of care, albeit in different ways, through community activities, negotiating with external agencies and driving, as we have seen.

Reaching 'relational autonomy' seems difficult, especially for women. As Gilligan (1995) has highlighted, women judge themselves in terms of their ability to care. Being a good carer seems very important to the Italian women considered here, yet it seems difficult to balance this with the caring for self, as many of them are doing more than their body/health allows them. For Gilligan care is different from self-sacrifice but for many of the elderly women I worked with it is not. Self-sacrifice was a feature of much of their lives and, as Hill Collins (1995) has highlighted, is a feature of poor minority women's lives elsewhere. This does not mean to say that they have no agency, as we have seen for instance when they refuse to return to Italy or decide to curb their transnational activities.

Globalisation does not affect care just in relation to care chains and care deficits in the global South. It also impacts on the day-to-day caring practices of an increasing number of people who have migrated and maintain connections with elsewhere. Interestingly migrants such as those considered in this study have values and are involved in practices that differ from those of the white British elders around them (Afshar *et al.* 2008). Such values are quite in tune with what is proposed by proponents of the feminist ethics of care. In fact, for both men and women their sense of self is relational and communal rather than autonomous and individualistic. Their goal for successful ageing is not to prolong independence but achieving interdependence with kin, friends and co-ethnic groups across the transnational social field. Yet, the case studies also highlight some of the problems with the feminist ethics of care, i.e. how to disentangle in practice care from feminine practices and how to guarantee that care for others does not happen at the expense of self. Identity and self-interest were closely linked to care for others, yet the older women in this study found it hard to break away from these caring arrangements. Feminist ethics of care authors would need to pay more attention to the degrees of choice some individuals have in relation to their role and position in caring networks and to the cultural and class specificity of certain arrangements.

Both the feminist ethics of care as well as the transnational caring literature have tended to focus on the family and more specifically on the mother–child relationship when looking at care. My chapter shows the importance of extending the attention to care beyond the family and the experiences of women, as men, friends and co-ethnics can become active members of networks of care. Community centres have emerged as spaces where communal care can be offered and provided and where transnational links can be maintained and reinvigorated when travelling becomes difficult. Their future, however, due to current policies favouring the mainstreaming of services and general cuts to funding in the non-for-profit sector, remains uncertain (Cook 2010).

15 Caring after death

Issues of embodiment and relationality

Jane Ribbens McCarthy, The Open University

> Death isn't romantic . . . death is not anything . . . death is . . . not. It's the absence of presence, nothing more . . . the endless time of never coming back . . . a gap you can't see, and when the wind blows through it, it makes no sound.
>
> (Stoppard 1973, *Rosencrantz and Guildenstern are Dead*)

Introduction

Death most fundamentally would seem to concern the absence of presence, and the loss of the living embodied other is the apparently hard inescapable truth to be faced. This brings sharply into relief the part that bodies play in our relationships and in caring for others. While the significance of bodies and embodied experience has been discussed in general terms with regard to the development of caring capacities (Hamington 2004), in this chapter I will consider the particular significance of embodied relationality in the contexts of caring after death.

One form of care that has been established and institutionalised in many contemporary Western societies since the later decades of the twentieth century is care of the seriously and terminally ill through what is termed 'palliative care', both as part of the hospice movement and as part of general medicine (National Council for Palliative Care 2012), and closely following on, bereavement care (e.g. see Cruse Bereavement Care 2011). What is less apparent in the cultural contexts of many European and New World societies is the notion that care may continue past death, despite the apparent 'loss' of the 'other'. The idea of caring for the other as an embodied practice after death may thus seem like a contradiction in terms: a hollow, even macabre, mockery of what is no longer possible. Rituals certainly exist to 'honour the dead' and show respect to their memories, especially if they are deemed to have died heroically (Hallam and Hockey 2001). More everyday memorialisation is also apparent in specific locations such as cemeteries – although the meanings of such activities may be contested (Woodthorpe 2011). But the notion of 'caring-for-the-other after death' may at first glance appear to be anomalous, except in some amorphous sense of remembered affection or nostalgia with respect of 'caring-about-the-other'. Surely when the other is removed from the neediness of corporeal being, does this not render the notion of 'caring after death' meaningless at best and pathological at worst?

The opening quote from Stoppard suggesting that death is 'the absence of presence' may at one level be seen to encapsulate a profound truth. I want to argue that this is also simplistic and fails to capture the complexities of relationality after death. Beyond remembrance of the dead, for example, Meyer and Woodthorpe (2008) suggest the importance of 'the material presence of absence' that may be signified through memorialisation, including the possibility that such absence may be agentic. In my discussion here I will explore the significance of the absence and presence of material bodies for care practices and for the understandings of relationality that may underpin caring after death.

At the same time I also want to consider the bodies of the living and the ways in which grief and loss may be experienced as physical pain in one's own body, suggesting that the relationality of caring – even in contemporary US and European societies – may incorporate an embodied relational self in which threats to the physical well-being of another may be experienced directly as implicating one's own physical well-being. Such embodied relationality highlights one of the deep paradoxes in the costs and benefits of care that arise when we recognise how individual well-being and flourishing may be bound up with that of others (Sayer 2011). I am thus focusing on the experience and phenomenology of grief in the context of the death of someone who is personally significant in order to consider the theoretical implications for understandings of relationality which underpin much feminist discussion of care more generally (e.g. Sevenhuijsen 1998). As Lofland points out, grief is an emotion 'which touches directly on the mutual interdependence of selves and societies, of actors and others, of me and you' (1985: 181).

In what follows I start with a brief review of some relevant threads and concepts from the rather disconnected literatures of care, bereavement and family studies. I then explain my personal interest in the topic as a result of being widowed ten years ago and consider whether and how published accounts of personal grief may be sociologically useful. Drawing on such sources, I explore experiences of the absence of the embodied other and of embodied relationality alongside a wider consideration of the social and cultural contexts of care after death.

Theoretical themes and debates

As Philip *et al.* (Chapter 1 in this volume) discuss, feminist theorising of care has pointed to fundamental human issues of dependency, vulnerability and the potential for suffering. At the same time the feminist ethics of care has foregrounded personal and specific relational connections rather than abstract principles (Tronto 1993). Care is theorised to encompass labour and love, caring for and about, and also care receiving. Here I want to consider all these themes – and the paradoxes that accompany them – in regard to the specifics of a relationship with someone who has died and the suffering that may result. In the process we may see how feminist concerns with the moral theorising of care are inseparable from affective relational processes which yet also potentially point to broad political issues of human belonging.

As a concept, 'relationality' has been core to much feminist theorising of care and feminist challenges to the unreconstructed rights-bearing autonomous individual of conventional moral and philosophical theorising (e.g. Donchin 2000, 2001; Sevenhuijsen 1998). Yet the concept remains complex, elusive and difficult to grasp, potentially encompassing a range of connections of varying types (Mason 2004). While it has thus become relatively well established for feminist work to centre on the notion of the relational individual rather than the autonomous individual, I suggest that the discussion needs to go further to recognise the depth and complexity of notions of personhood that are fundamentally bound up with interpersonal connections (Ribbens McCarthy 2012). At the same time the cross-cultural psychologist Kağitçibaşi (2005) argues that even feminist work that explores the notion of 'relational autonomy' is in danger of reproducing the Western view of relatedness and autonomy as antagonistic, and instead uses the term 'close-knit selves' to describe forms of connection that may be hard to see within the cultures of European and New World societies. Nevertheless it is important not to romanticise the relationality of connections, nor to subsume the needs of the individual into the needs of the group (Smart 2007). In my discussion here I will endeavour not to lose sight of the (bereaved) individual, even as I seek to explore how far suffering in relation to death can highlight how far individual needs and vulnerability may be bound up with the relational connection to the dying and deceased.

In terms of work on bereavement, theories in New World and European societies were for many years dominated by the idea that it is important to 'let go' of the deceased in order to reconnect with the living, but in more recent times this view has been significantly challenged (Howarth 2000). Theories of continuing bonds after death developed from the 1990s, were stimulated particularly by the edited collection published by Klass and colleagues in 1996, which led to further theoretical and empirical work to consider the forms and implications of relationships between the living and the dead. This work may be seen to raise parallel issues of the blurring of boundaries and the (culturally shaped) experience of deeply close-knit selves that may be found in relationships between living individuals, with the potential to deepen our understandings of relationality.

Empirical studies in Western cultures have found continuing bonds to be significant after death through activities, thoughts and conversations, with the deceased person her/himself experienced as either passive or active in the relationship (Bennett and Bennett 2000; Foster *et al.* 2011; Howarth 2007). In Japan the dead person is seen to have considerable continuing agency with important repercussions for the living (Klass 2001). At the same time, for both the Japanese and the bereaved in Western societies, such continuing bonds may comprise a *felt* experience as much as an active or cognitive one, of just 'being with' deceased family members and ancestors – 'like waving to a friend across the street' (Klass 2001: 748).

Some recent contributions to the literature on families and relationships also provide some relevant themes for consideration here, most notably Mason's (2008) treatment of 'tangible affinities' which provides useful conceptual thinking.

Affinity in Mason's discussion refers to being 'bound by some tie' (2008: 42) and she describes such ties as 'tangible' even though they may also be 'ethereal', by which she means that they may refer to 'matters that are considered beyond (rational) explanation' (2008: 37). She suggests that even these ethereal affinities can be described as tangible 'because they feel vivid, real, palpable (or almost) and resonant in lived experience' (2008: 42). Mason's account also draws attention to the part played by 'sensory affinities', which she uses to consider and develop anthropological discussion of kinship and materiality and the connections between bodies themselves.

The embodied nature of 'family practices' is also explicit in Morgan's discussion in which he suggests that 'the body is necessarily a relational body' (2011: 90). In close family relationships, Morgan argues, the sense of belonging that is encapsulated by the 'we' refers to an embodied relationality. His discussion includes a brief mention of the significance of family members who have died who may be 'relatively disembodied' (2011: 91). To know who 'belongs' to a family thus requires attention to 'embodied traces which provide reminders of others who have been there' (2011: 98). Yet Morgan also suggests that the giving and receiving of care generally involves a strong sense of embodiment, thus implicitly raising the conundrum of whether it is possible to care after death.

Between them, these literatures draw our attention to forms of care and embodied relationality beyond the boundaries of life and death, the tangible and intangible, the material and the supernatural; themes which I pursue next through personal accounts of bereavement.

Introducing autobiographical experiences

My concerns in pursuing these questions have developed from my own experiences of the terminal illness and death of my second husband Peter in January 2000, leaving me as a single parent to our 5-year-old daughter. This experience led me into academic work on bereavement, and particularly the bereavement experiences of young people (Ribbens McCarthy 2006, 2007) – a personal motivation that has been common among members of the Women's Workshop (Philip *et al.*, Chapter 1 in this volume; Ribbens 1998), as well as others interested in the sociological usefulness of autobiographical writing (e.g. Ellis 1993, 1995; Ribbens 1993; Rogers 2009). Indeed, autoethnography has now become recognised as a legitimate sociological enterprise for the interpretation of cultural understandings (e.g. Ellis 2009; Chang 2008). Unlike some autobiographical sociology, however, I am not offering here an extended story of my experience with Peter, but use certain specific features of my (remembered and retold) experience to ask questions of other published autobiographies of bereavement – most particularly how my experiences drew my attention forcefully to the significance of what might be termed corporeal relationality along with the absence of the embodied other who had been my husband/partner and father to our daughter.

Historians have long used personal diaries and published autobiographies as sources for their analyses, alongside attention to the circumstances of the production of such materials (e.g. Loftus 2006). Autobiographical accounts of death, dying and bereavement were just beginning to be published at the time of Peter's terminal illness and seeming to break the 'taboo' of going public with experiences of dying and bereavement. Such publications have since expanded and might now be seen to constitute a particular autobiographical genre. Even though it is a decade since Peter's death I have still found them to make compelling reading as I continue to explore and seek to understand personal meanings and emotions of grief and whether or not my own experiences resonate with others'.

The titles I have obtained and quote below (although I have read several more that I do not use here), are the result of serendipitous word of mouth and searching on booksellers' databases. Drawing on these powerful personal writings enables a particular consideration of how to understand care and relationality after death. Such autobiographical accounts are of course embedded in cultural contexts as well as the personal biographies of the authors, being written from the affluent circumstances of contemporary New World and European societies. At the same time, in what follows I will explore them alongside published research evidence of experiences of death in various cultures. I turn next to consider the absence of the embodied or enfleshed other, before considering the significance of the experiences of the embodied living.

Caring for and about the dead – the loss of the enfleshed other

In contemporary New World and European societies, people now predominantly die in hospitals with undertakers taking 'care of' the body and the funeral arrangements. This entails a loss of the body itself from the care of those who 'care(d) about' the person. My husband Peter died in a hospice and I found the moment when the undertakers came to remove his body quite excruciatingly painful, as it felt they were taking away what was mine. It was MY right and responsibility to care for and about this body and I so wanted to keep him with me as an integral part of me. Such strong emotions about the possession of the deceased remains are not unique to my experience (Hockey *et al.* 2007).

Yet after death 'the enfleshed self' (which is the term Woodward suggests to 'foreground the living, breathing body' – 2009: 23) becomes unsustainable (Hockey *et al.* 2007), such that the continuing corporeal presence becomes de-personalised – it is 'the' body, 'the' remains – the person to whom we are related is somehow no longer 'there' and what is left is no longer seen to constitute them. At the same time, as Klass observes (2006: 850), 'Survivors' physical relationship with remains can be very complex'. Some may want to encounter the corpse in order to confront the reality of its lifelessness, while in other cultures or historical periods, physical proximity and care of the remains may constitute a sense of continuing closeness. People may thus keep and care for deceased remains close-by as when Klass refers to 'Greek village women who cradle the skulls of their dead' (Holst-Warhaft 2000, quoted in Klass 2006: 850), or when Victorian women had jewellery made from their deceased husbands' hair (Hallam and Hockey 2001). Such evidence resonates with my own anecdotal knowledge of an English widow who kept the ashes of her husband with her for many months, taking them with her in a shopping trolley wherever she went.

There are issues then of a continuing relationality through the lifeless remains which may also constitute a focus for continuing care for the dead. Francis *et al.* (2001) describe cemeteries as 'a public theatre for the creation and continued expression of relationships with the deceased' (2001: 227). This work highlighted the continuing care that was apparent in the physical tending of the graves in London cemeteries, and the implications for the relational identities of such carers, e.g. a parent of a stillborn child. A continuing physical connection could be seen to be consequential for some, e.g. a Cypriot widower who would not return to live in Cyprus because his wife was buried in London (Francis *et al.* 2005, discussed by Klass 2006). Indeed Klass points out the importance of the physical care of the dead in many cultures – providing food and care of (and sometimes close contact with) the remains.

Care of the dead may also occur through the medium of other material objects than the corporeal remains or the site where they are deposited. This is most apparent in cultures other than those of contemporary European and New World societies. Thus a study of widows and widowers in Japan includes the following comment, revealing elements of the benefits as well as the routine obligations of caring:

> A man in his 60s who had lost his wife one year earlier ... said, 'Every morning I offer an orange at the family altar in my house because it was my wife's favorite fruit. I can glance at her pictures on the altar and it comforts me very much.'
>
> (Asai *et al.* 2010: 43)

Continuing care for the dead might be expressed in other ways too such as, 'Wishing to put the deceased at rest by bringing up children/grandchildren proudly' and 'Being eager to pray that the soul of the deceased will rest in peace' (Asai *et al.* 2010: 44).

Rather more menacingly, traditional Chinese beliefs point to the need for the living to continue to care ritually for the dead through the making of offerings which may then help to ransom the deceased from hell (Chan *et al.* 2005). Spiritual beliefs concerning the afterlife are also apparent in Japanese culture where, Klass (2001) suggests, grieving may include a focus on whether or not the living have been able to fulfil their obligations to the dead, both when they were alive and since their death. But the bereaved also have an obligation to let go of such regrets in order to enable the deceased to go on to become a Buddha. At the same time there may also be elements of fear in these obligations since dead spirits may become dangerous if the appropriate rituals are not performed for them.

In autobiographical accounts in contemporary secularised Western cultures, the living are less likely to feel a sense of responsibility for the care of the departed soul. Comfort in continuing to care directly for the remains is also less obvious once the funeral or cremation and distribution of ashes has been completed. Although care of cemeteries remains of core concern for many, it is the materiality above rather than below ground that is the focus of the care. Thus it is the separation from the embodied, enfleshed other – alive and dead – that is railed against. Certainly I knew what it was to want to jump into the grave with Peter – again being parted from his corporeal presence felt unbearable. The profound sense of relationality bound up with the physical body is expressed here by Wolterstorff on the burial of his son:

> I buried myself that warm June day. It was me those gardeners lowered on squeaking straps into that hot dry hole . . . It was me over whom we slid that heavy slab more than I can lift. It was me on whom we shovelled dirt. It was me we left behind after reading psalms.
>
> (Wolterstorff 1987: 42)

Bereavement researchers discuss one aspect of grieving as a 'yearning' for the other that is gone and it is apparent from Western autobiographical accounts that yearning for the dead may be strongly focused on the desire for their physical presence, as powerfully expressed by Hancock after the death of her husband:

> I wanted him in the present, in the flesh. Especially the flesh, as it happens. To caress and cling to.
>
> (Hancock 2008: 8)

> That night I had a vivid dream that John was there with me. I reached out and touched him. I felt the roughness of his bristles. Saw the cleft in his chin and the scar. The silky receding hair, and his blue, blue, wryly smiling eyes. I went to hold him, but he turned deliberately and drifted away. I tried to call out to him but my voice wouldn't work. I woke weeping, hideously alone. Knowing he had really gone. Finally. For ever.
>
> (Hancock 2008: 24)

Such sensory affinities of voice, touch and smell (Bennett and Bennett 2000; Mason 2008) are key aspects of relationality to include here – as for example with the reminders bereaved parents and children might purposefully or unintentionally encounter after the death of a child:

> I see her and I can also, you know, smell her. She smells like clean-ness. I can also . . . just taste . . . cause she liked cheese and I can just taste it. Whenever I eat something that's cheesy I remember her. It makes me feel closer to her.
>
> (Sibling quoted in Foster *et al.* 2011: 433)

The longing for the physical living presence of the deceased is thus central to these accounts of personal grief, with the desire to care for the dead sometimes going a small way towards mitigating the loss of the living. Solace may also sometimes be found through a linking object such as a favourite item of clothing (which may provide sensory reminders of comfort as well as loss) or a strong continuing attachment that transcends the physical world (Bennett and Bennett 2000), perhaps an indication of Mason's (2008) ethereal affinities. However, both the attachment to linking objects and the transcendence of the physical world may be more approved and supported in some cultural contexts than others (Hallam and Hockey 2001). Creating or finding a presence despite absence of the enfleshed other may thus be a socially unsupported struggle for bereaved individuals in contemporary Western contexts.

The bodies of the living

While a focus on the bodies of the dead may thus reveal important aspects of the experiences, forms and emotions of continuing bonds involved with caring for and about deceased loved ones, there is much also to be learned about relationality by focusing on the impact of profound grief on the bodies of the living. Loss may thus be *felt* and experienced as a threat, damage or trauma to the physical body of the living, with some sense of emerging from this physical trauma over time. Such personal accounts of physical pain and (some) recovery speak powerfully to the experiential strength of the connections – for good or ill – we may forge with those we care about and the ways in which such connections are physically as well as emotionally embedded to constitute a deeply relational – perhaps close-knit – embodied self.

Indeed such embodied connections may also be attested to by research showing the extent of raised mortality rates and somatic disorders among the bereaved. There is thus strong evidence suggesting that the experience of widowhood may be associated with significantly raised mortality levels even over many years (Boyle *et al.* 2011), and similar patterns have been found with other forms of bereavement such as loss of a child (Foster *et al.* 2011; Parkes and Prigerson 2010). Such evidence points to the potentially mortal outcome of loss through death, most particularly through heart disease – perhaps evoking the image of the broken heart.

What is particularly striking about the experience of such embodied relationality is that the pain may be felt in quite specific parts of the body. Sometimes this may seem to be underpinned by the circumstances of the death, as with a woman who experienced great pain in her chest after her son was killed in a car crash when the steering wheel impacted into his chest (Parkes 2011, personal communication). Similarly, Ellis writes after the death of her brother in an air crash: 'I swallow and it is MY head hitting the front seat as we crash' (Ellis 1993: 720).

This physical trauma of the embodied relational self was most apparent to me when I was first given the news – when Peter was just coming round from brain surgery – that his brain tumour was a secondary cancer and he would certainly die. At this point I felt as if someone had lobbed an axe into my chest and that I was then expected to carry on walking around in the world with an axe in my chest and tears pouring down my face. This extreme physical trauma did not lessen for several days after I was given the news, making care of our young daughter almost impossibly difficult to manage. And in reading others' autobiographical accounts I have found that I am not alone in such graphic and specific sensations:

The horror of that moment was physical [when her husband told her that his cancer was terminal]. A bullet of ice seemed to penetrate my body and shoot through my heart, my limbs, every nerve, every finger and every toe.

(Want 2010: 160)

As with many another woman, the sense of loss sometimes manifested itself in a searing physical pain, somewhere in the guts.

(Stott quoted in Whitaker 1984: 32)

Hunniford (2008) repeats what a woman said to her about the death of her own mother when she was a teenager:

It's like your arm has been chopped off. It's like something physical has happened to you but nobody can see it. Sometimes you want to scream, 'Don't you realise that half my body is missing?'

Hunniford goes on to discuss this in relation to her own experiences after the death of her adult daughter:

She's right. I felt it too: the early stage of grief is really physical. It's like being hit in the stomach with a bat, it's like being winded, but of course that doesn't come close . . . The pain is very real.

(Hunniford 2008: 87)

Want also discusses the physicality of early grieving:

It was unlike anything I had ever known. It was inhuman, bestial. Gritting my teeth, clenching the muscles of my mouth and neck and locking my hands and arms in a fierce grip, I tried to brace myself against the waves of what I knew to be the worst emotional pain that I, or any human being ever could have felt. It was piercing, searing, stifling. Instead of offering me some sort of release it seemed to tighten its hold on me. I thought it was going to destroy me and was genuinely surprised when I survived each successive onslaught.

(Want 2010: 202–3)

Walterstorff discusses the expectation placed on men to be 'strong' in this regard:

And why is it so important to act strong? I have been graced with the strength to endure. But I have been assaulted and in the assault wounded, grievously wounded. Am I to pretend otherwise? Wounds are ugly, I know. They repel. But must they always be swathed?

(Wolterstorff 1987: 27)

Such physical pain can recur and take one unawares even years after the death, as I have found myself, and as Hunniford here describes:

I have moments of pure joy . . . but then suddenly a wave hits and that joy is savagely interrupted by a searing, shocking stab through my heart. It all becomes too much and I realise I've learnt nothing at all. My heart is broken.

(Hunniford 2008: 301)

Conclusions – culture, materiality and the boundaries of self

Writing from a European perspective in the seventeenth century, Donne famously expressed a sense of universal connection through the Catholic notion that each death diminishes everyone (in Whitaker 1984: 110–11), so 'never send to know for whom the bell tolls, it tolls for thee'. Such an idea is marginalised in contemporary Western secularised cultures and it is apparent that care after death is closely interlinked with key historically and culturally variable understandings of the nature of the individual or person and of transformations after death. Japanese beliefs in continuing bonds, for example, are embedded in an understanding of individual identity by reference to social harmony with 'dependence or interdependence, not autonomy, [as] the core social value' (Klass 2001: 743), and a different understanding of dependency as a positive part of relationships.

Even so, as I have discussed, while death in contemporary Western societies is understood to mean the 'loss' and absence of the embodied significant other this does not necessarily mean the loss of a relational connection to them – and its continued embodiment through that relationality. At the same time such experiences may challenge accepted Western understandings of 'matter', the divisions between life and death and the boundaries between self and other, with the associated notions of 'internal' and 'external' realities (Howarth 2000). In his classic account of personal grief after the death of his wife, C.S. Lewis challenges conventional Western notions of the significance of 'matter' when he writes about his detailed remembrance of their 'carnal love':

'But this', you protest, 'is no resurrection of the *body*. You have given the dead a sort of dream world and dream bodies. They are not real.' Surely neither less nor more real than those you have always known.

(quoted in Whitaker 1984: 76)

Bringing together some of the themes of feminist work on care, and aspects of contemporary theorising on continuing bonds, I would argue is mutually enriching. At the same time as the focus on care and the relational self may thus shed light on continuing bonds after death, the focus on the embodied nature of the bonds that are mourned and yet also continued may shed light on a particular aspect of how relationality is manifested in lived experience. The depth and extent of the embodied nature of grieving and loss points to the extent and depth of our 'close-knit selves' – a depth that is certainly marginalised, even rendered invisible, by the pervasive Western notion of the autonomous self who must 'let go' of their deceased loved ones.

Even in the absence of the enfleshed other, relationality can mean that – at least in some cultural understandings – the well-being of related individuals is perceived to be intrinsically and explicitly bound up together, 'the well-being of the living and the dead are mutually dependent' (Klass 2001: 749) as in this detailed example from Japan:

> when the adult daughter is depressed, her deceased mother is feeling lonely and neglected. The cure for both their negative feelings is for the adult daughter to go to the shrine where she does the simple rituals that re-establish her bond with her mother. At the end of the ritual the deceased mother is satisfied and the young woman's mother is less depressed. The relation between the living daughter and her ancestor/mother is thus symmetrical; *the well being of each depends on the other.*
>
> (Klass and Goss 1999: 551, emphasis added)

> care for the dead is including the dead within the family remembering them and acting in ways they approve. In return, the dead provide comfort and guidance.
>
> (Klass and Goss 1999: 553)

Furthermore, Klass (2006) argues for the broader political significance of such understandings of connection and their mediation through continuing bonds with the dead since these affinities occur within the contexts of family, community and ethnic identities, which also extend to political identities and narratives (and see also Klass and Goss 1999, on the significance of relationships with the dead for national and religious affiliations). This points to the political significance of continuing bonds as well as of care (Lynch *et al.* 2009; Barnes 2006). On the basis of these aspects of care for and about the dead and the nature of grieving, which have been largely absent from Western work on death and bereavement, Klass calls for an extension to attachment theory to cover 'each level of social membership or identity' (2006: 854).

The emphasis on attachment from which loss has been theorised (Silverman and Nickman 1996), involves the giving and receiving of (at least some forms of) care. Such care emanates from the bond with the attachment figure, a bond which is not clearly severed by death but may involve a continuing *inter*active relationship. It may be however that 'relationality' might be a (more) useful framework here rather than (or alongside) 'attachment', which is so heavily steeped in ideas of child development and dyadic bonds. The notion of the 'relational self', which is at the heart of feminist theories of care, can provide for a sense of connection and close-knit selves that may encompass intimate, family, community and ethnic ties and sense of belonging – albeit that these ties may be of varying intensities and carry varying degrees of ambivalence. But in the process we may also see how deeply – and sometimes irrevocably – the well-being of the individual may be inseparable from the well-being of the other.

Some of the parallels with theorising about care are apparent from the early days of debates on continuing bonds. Thus Silverman and Nickman conclude the 1996 collection by suggesting that mourning may involve learning to live with paradoxes in terms of presence/absence of presence, the feeling of being bereft/ not being bereft, and continuity/disruption. One of the most significant contributions of the literature on care, in my view, is that it seeks to recognise similar deep paradoxes concerning human connections and to encompass and keep in view the gains and the losses, the labour and the love, which are at stake in caring for our most significant others. Such tensions are also certainly present in the continuing bonds that may be apparent after death, while the autobiographical accounts discussed here provide powerful testimony that challenges even the embodied boundaries of the self, an embodiment which is revealed to be deeply relational. But perhaps the deepest paradox here is that while on the one hand what emerges from this discussion is the potentially deeply embodied nature of relationality – to the extent of creating a real threat to the physical well-being of the living – there is also evidence of the potential for overcoming the boundaries of the flesh in such a way that a profound sense of relationality may continue in the absence of material embodiment.

References

Abu-Lughod, L. (2002) 'Do Muslim women really need saving? Anthropological reflections on Cultural Relativism and its others', *American Anthropologist,* 104(3): 783–90.

Afshar, H., Franks, M., Maynard, M. and Wray, S. (2008) *Women in Later Life: Exploring race and ethnicity*, Maidenhead: Open University Press.

Agar, M.H. (1996) *The Professional Stranger: An informal introduction to ethnography*, Bingley: Emerald Group Publishing.

Ahmad Nia, S. (2002) 'Women's work and health in Iran: A comparison of working and non-working mothers', *Social Science & Medicine*, 54(5): 753–66.

Aldridge, J. and Becker, S. (1993) 'Punishing children for caring: The hidden costs of young carers', *Children & Society*, 7(4): 376–87.

Aldridge, J. and Becker, S. (2003) *Children Caring for Parents with Mental Illness: Perspectives of young carers, parents and professionals*, Bristol: Policy Press.

Alicea, M. (1997) '"A chambered Nautilus": The contradictory nature of Puerto Rican women's role in the social construction of a transnational community', *Gender and Society*, 11(5): 597–626.

Anning, A. and Edwards, A. (2006) *Promoting Children's Learning from Birth to Five: Developing the New Early Years Professional* (2nd edn), Maidenhead: Open University Press.

Anning, A., Cullen, J. and Fleer, M. (2004) *Early Childhood Education, Society and Culture*, London: Sage.

Appleton, J., Christenson, S. and Furlong, M. (2008) 'Student engagement with school: Critical conceptual and methodological issues of the construct', *Psychology in the Schools*, 45(5): 369–86.

Apthekar, B. (1989) *Tapestries of Life: Women's work, women's consciousness and the meaning of daily experience,* Amherst: University of Massachusetts Press.

Arber, S., Davidson, K. and Ginn, J. (2003) *Gender and Ageing: Changing roles and relationships*, Maidenhead: Open University Press.

Armstrong, H. (2009) 'Foreword', in W. Piersall and H. Armstrong (eds) *Mom Blogging for Dummies*, Hoboken, NJ: Wiley.

Asai, M., Fujimori, M., Akizuki, N., Inagaki, M., Matsui, Y. and Uchitomi, Y. (2010) 'Psychological states and coping strategies after bereavement among the spouses of cancer patients: A qualitative study', *Psycho-Oncology,* 19: 38–45.

Bahramitash, R. (2003) 'Islamic fundamentalism and women's economic role: The case of Iran', *International Journal of Politics, Culture and Society*, 16(4): 551–68.

Bahramitash, R. and Esfahani, H.S. (2009) 'Nimble fingers no longer! Women's employment, in Iran', in A. Gheissari (ed.) *Contemporary Iran: Economy, society, politics*, Oxford: Oxford University Press.

Baldassar, L. (2001) *Visits Home: Migration experiences between Italy and Australia,* Melbourne: Melbourne University Press.

Baldassar, L. (2007) 'Transnational families and aged care: The mobility of care and the migrancy of ageing', *Journal of Ethnic and Migration Studies,* 33(2): 275–97.

Baldassar, L. and Baldock, C. (2000) 'Linking migration and family studies: Transnational migrants and the care of ageing parents', in B. Agozino (ed.) *Theoretical and Methodological Issues in Migration Research. Interdisciplinary and international perspectives,* Aldershot: Ashgate.

Bamberger, J. (2011) *Mothers of Intention: How women and social media are revolutionizing politics in America,* Houston, TX: Bright Sky Press.

Barber, T. (2002) 'A special duty of care: Exploring the narration and experience of teacher caring', *British Journal of Sociology of Education,* 23(3): 383–95.

Barnes, M. (2006) *Caring and Social Justice,* Basingstoke: Palgrave Macmillan.

Barnett, C. and Land, D. (2007) 'Geographies of generosity: Beyond the "moral turn"', *Geoforum,* 38(6): 1065–75.

Baruch, G. (1981) 'Moral tales: Parents' stories of encounters with the health professions', *Sociology of Health and Illness,* 3(3): 275–95.

Bauman, Z. (2003) *Liquid Love,* Cambridge: Polity.

BBC One (2004) *Real Story: Nurseries undercover.* 10 August. Online. Available HTTP: < http://news.bbc.co.uk/1/hi/programmes/real_story/3552332.stm> (accessed 6 December 2011).

BBC News (2010) *Woman Admits Killing Autistic Son, 12, with Bleach.* Online. Available HTTP: <http://www.bbc.co.uk/news/uk-england-london-12933888> (accessed 6 December 2011).

Beaulieu, A. (2010) 'Research note: From co-location to co-presence: Shifts in the use of ethnography for the study of knowledge', *Social Studies of Science,* 40(3): 453–70.

Beck, U. and Beck-Gernsheim, E. (1995) *The Normal Chaos of Love,* Cambridge: Polity.

Beck, U. and Beck-Gernsheim, E. (2002) *Individualization,* London: Sage.

Beck-Gernsheim, E. (2002) 'From "Living for Others" to "A Life of One's Own"', in U. Beck and E. Beck-Gernsheim, *Individualization,* London: Sage.

Belenky, M.F., Clinchy, B.M., Goldberger, N.R. and Tarule, J.M. (1997) *Women's Ways of Knowing* (10th anniversary edn), New York: Basic Books.

Belkin, L. (2011) 'Queen of the Mommy Bloggers', *New York Times Magazine.* Online. Available HTTP: <http://www.nytimes.com/2011/02/27/magazine/27armstrong-t. html?pagewanted=all> (accessed 1 November 2011).

Bell, L. (1995) 'Just a token commitment? Women's involvement in a local babysitting circle', *Women's Studies International Forum,* 18(3): 325–36.

Bell, L. (1998) 'Public and private meanings in diaries: Researching family and childcare', in J. Ribbens and R. Edwards (eds) *Feminist Dilemmas in Qualitative Research: Public knowledge and private lives,* London: Sage.

Bell, L. and Ribbens, J. (1994) 'Isolated housewives and complex maternal worlds: The significance of social contacts between women with young children in industrial societies', *Sociological Review,* 42: 227–62.

Bennett, G. and Bennett, K.M. (2000) 'The presence of the dead: An empirical study', *Mortality,* 5: 139–57.

Berridge, D. and Cleaver, H. (1987) *Foster Home Breakdown,* Oxford: Blackwell.

Birch, M. (1996) 'The Goddess/God within: The construction of self-identity through alternative health practices', in K. Flanagan and P.C. Jupp (eds) *Postmodernity, Sociology and Religion,* Basingstoke: Macmillan.

Birch, M. (1997) 'The quest for self discovery: The reconstruction of self-identity stories in alternative therapy groups', unpublished PhD thesis, Oxford Brookes University.

Bishop, S.L., Yardley, L. and Lewith, G.T. (2007) 'A systematic review of beliefs involved in the use of complementary and alternative medicine', *Journal of Health Psychology*, 12(6): 851–66.

Bloome, D., Power Carter, S., Morton Christian, B., Otto, S. and Shuart-Faris, N. (2005) *Discourse Analysis and the Study of Classroom Language and Literacy Events: A microethnographic perspective*, Mahwah, NJ: Lawrence Erlbaum.

Bondi, L. (2003) 'A situated practice for (re)situating selves: Trainee counsellors and the promise of counselling', *Environment and Planning A*, 35: 853–70.

Bourdieu, P. and Passeron, J.C. (1994) 'Language and relationship to language in the teaching situation', in P. Bourdieu, J.C. Passeron and M.S. Martin (eds) *Academic Discourse: Linguistic misunderstanding and professorial power*, The Hague: Polity.

Bowlby, S., McKie, L., Gregory, S. and Macpherson, I. (2010) *Interdependency and Care over the Lifecourse*, London: Routledge.

Boyle, P.J., Feng, Z. and Raab, G.M. (2011) 'Does widowhood increase mortality risk? Testing for selection effects by comparing causes of spousal death', *Epidemiology*, 22: 1–5.

Braedley, S. and Luxton, M. (eds) (2010) *Neoliberalism and Everyday Life*, Montreal: McGill-Queen's University Press.

Brannen, J., Hepinstall, E. and Bhopal, K. (2000) *Connecting Children: Care and family life in later childhood*, London: Routledge Falmer.

Braun, D. (2001) 'Perspectives on parenting', in P. Foley, J. Roche and S. Tucker (eds) *Children in Society: Contemporary theory, policy and practice*, Basingstoke: Palgrave.

Broad, B. and Skinner, A. (2006) *Relative Benefits: Placing children in kinship care*, London: BAAF.

Broadhurst, K., Paton, H. and May-Chahal, C. (2005) 'Children missing from school systems: Exploring divergent patterns of disengagement in the narrative accounts of parents, carers, children and young people', *British Journal of Sociology of Education*, 26(1): 105–19.

Brown, P. and Levinson, S.C. (1987) *Politeness: Some universals in language usage*, Cambridge: Cambridge University Press.

Bryk, A. (1988) 'Musings on the moral life of schools', *American Journal of Education*, 96(2): 256–90.

Buckman, S. (2010) 'Performing Allah's work: Experiences of Muslim family carers in Britain', unpublished PhD thesis, University of Nottingham.

Burholt, V. (2004) 'Transnationalism, economic transfers and families' ties: Intercontinental contacts of older Gujuratis, Punjabis and Sylhetis in Birmingham with families abroad', *Ethnic and Racial Studies*, 27(5): 800–29.

Caldwell, B. (1991) 'Educare: New product, new future', *Developmental and Behavioural Paediatrics*, 12(3): 199–204.

Caldwell, B. (2002) 'The Educare of children in the twenty-first century', in J. Gomes-Pedro, J.K. Nugent, J.G. Young and T.B. Brazleton (eds) *The Infant and Family in the Twenty-First Century*, New York: Routledge.

Calixte, S. and Johnson, J. (2009) 'Marginality in the mamasphere: Queers racializing the family tree', in M. Friedman and S.L. Calixte (eds) *Mothering and Blogging: The radical art of the MommyBlog*, Bradford, ON: Demeter Press.

Cameron, D. (2011) 'David Cameron: Dad's gift to me was his optimism', *Daily Telegraph*. Online. Available HTTP: <http://www.telegraph.co.uk/news/politics/david-cameron/8584238/David-Cameron-Dads-gift-to-me-was-his-optimism.html> (accessed 6 December 2011).

Campbell, C. and McLean, C. (2002) 'Social capital and social exclusion in England: African-Caribbean participation in local community networks', in C. Swann and A. Morgan (eds) *Social Capital for Health: Insights from qualitative research,* London: Health Development Agency.

Card, C. (1990) 'Caring and evil', *Hypatia,* 5(1): 101–8.

Carter, D. (2005) 'Living in virtual communities: An ethnography of human relationships in cyberspace', *Information, Communication & Society,* 8(2): 148–67.

Carter, H. (2011) 'Birmingham Nursery Worker Arrested on Suspicion of Child Abuse', *The Guardian.* Online. Available HTTP: <http://www.guardian.co.uk/society/2011/jan/06/nursery-worker-arrested-suspicion-child-abuse> (accessed 6 January 2011).

Casey, E. and Martens, L. (2007) *Gender and Consumption: Domestic cultures and the commercialisation of everyday life,* London: Ashgate.

Chan, C., Chow, A., Ho, S., Tsui, Y., Tin, A., Koo, B. and Koo, E. (2005) 'The experience of Chinese bereaved persons: A preliminary study of meaning making and continuing bonds', *Death Studies,* 29: 923–47.

Chang, H. (2008) *Autoethnography as Method,* Walnut Creek, CA: Left Coast Press.

Charles, M. and Charles, D. (1999) 'Sales negotiations: Bargaining through tactical summaries', in M. Hewings and C. Nickerson (eds) *Business English: Research into practice,* Harlow, Essex: Pearson Education.

Cicirelli, V.G. (1995) *Sibling Relationships across the Life Span,* New York: Plenum.

Clarke, A.J. (2004) 'Maternity and materiality: Becoming a mother in consumer culture', in J. Taylor, L. Layne and D. Wozniak (eds) *Consuming Motherhood,* New Brunswick, NJ: Rutgers University Press.

Clarke, A.J. (2007) 'Consuming children and making mothers: Birthday parties, gifts and the pursuit of sameness', *Horizontes Antropológicos,* 13(28): 263–87.

Clarke, E. (1957) *My Mother Who Fathered Me,* London: George Allen Unwin.

Clarke, L. and Roberts, C. (2002) 'Policy and rhetoric: The growing interest in fathers and grandparents in Britain', in A. Carling, S. Duncan and R. Edwards (eds) *Analysing Families: Morality and rationality in policy and practice,* London: Routledge.

Clegg, S. and Rowland, S. (2010) 'Kindness in pedagogical practice and academic life', *British Journal of Sociology of Education,* 31(6): 719–35.

Collins, P.H. (1994) 'Shifting the center: Race, class and feminist theorizing about motherhood', in E.N. Glenn, G. Chang and L.R. Forcey (eds) *Mothering: Ideology, experience and agency,* London: Routledge.

Colton, M. (1988) *Dimensions of Substitute Child Care: A comparative study of foster and residential care practice,* Aldershot: Avebury.

Colton, M. (1989) 'Attitudes of special foster parents and residential staff towards children', *Children and Society,* 3(1): 3–18.

Coltrane, S. (1996) *Family Man: Fatherhood, housework and gender equity,* Oxford: Oxford University Press.

Connell, R. (2005) *Masculinities,* London: Polity.

Connell, R. (2010) 'Understanding neoliberalism', in S. Braedley and M. Luxton (eds) *Neoliberalism and Everyday Life,* Montreal: McGill-Queens University Press.

Conners, C. (2009) 'Meter Politikon: On the "politics" of mommyblogging', in M. Friedman and S.L. Calixte (eds) *Mothering and Blogging: The radical art of the MommyBlog,* Bradford, ON: Demeter Press.

Connor, M. and White, J. (2011) *Black Fathers: An invisible presence in America* (2nd edn), London: Routledge.

Conradson, D. (2003) 'Geographies of care: Spaces, practices, experiences', *Social & Cultural Geography*, 4(4): 451–4.

Cook, J. (2010) 'Exploring older women's citizenship: Understanding the impact of migration in later life', *Ageing and Society*, 30: 253–73.

Craig, C. (2007) *The Potential Dangers of a Systematic Explicit Approach to Teaching Social and Emotional Skills (SEAL): An overview and summary of the arguments*, Centre for Confidence and Well-being, Online. Available HTTP <http://www.centreforconfidence. co.uk/docs/SEAL summary.pdf> (accessed 17 January 2011).

Crawford, R. (2006) 'Health as a meaningful social practice', *Health,* 10(4): 401–20.

Cruse Bereavement Care (2011) *Cruse Bereavement Care*. Online. Available HTTP: <http://www.crusebereavementcare.org.uk/> (accessed 10 October 2011).

Cuffaro, H.K. (1995) *Experimenting with the World. John Dewey and the early childhood classroom,* New York: Teachers College Press.

Culpitt, I. (1999) *Social Policy and Risk,* London: Sage.

Daly, M. (2002) 'Care as a good for Social Policy', *Journal of Social Policy,* 31: 251–70.

De Tona, C. (2011) 'Mothering contradictory diasporas: Negotiation of traditional motherhood roles among Italian migrant women in Ireland', in L. Baldassar and Gabaccia, D. (eds) *Intimacy and Italian Migration. Gender and domestic lives in a mobile world*, New York: Fordham University Press.

Department for Children, Schools and Families (DCSF) (2008) *Statutory Framework for the Early Years Foundation Stage*. Online. Available HTTP <http://nationalstrategies. standards.dcsf.gov.uk/node/151379> (accessed 18 November 2010).

Department for Children, Schools and Families (DCFS) (2009) *Lamb Inquiry: Special educational needs and parental confidence,* Nottingham: Department for Children, Schools and Families.

Department for Education (DfE) (2010) *Every Disabled Child Matters: Spending Review 2010,* Runcorn, Chesire: Department for Education.

Department for Education and Employment (DfEE) (1998) *Meeting the Childcare Challenge,* London: HMSO.

Department for Education and Skills (DfES) (2001a) *Code of Practice on the Identification and Assessment of Special Educational Needs,* London: Department for Education and Skills.

Department for Education and Skills (DfES) (2001b) *Special Educational Needs and Disability Act,* London: Department for Education and Skills.

Department for Education and Skills (DfES) (2002) *Birth to Three Matters*, London: Department for Education and Skills.

Department for Education and Skills (DfES) (2003) *Every Child Matters. Green Paper,* Norwich: The Stationery Office.

Department for Education and Skills (DfES) (2004a) *Choice for Parents, the Best Start for Children: A ten year childcare strategy,* London: Department for Education and Skills.

Department for Education and Skills (DfES) (2004b) *Every Child Matters: Change for children*, London: Department for Education and Skills.

Department for Education and Skills (DfES) (2004c) *Children Act,* London: HMSO.

Department for Education and Skills (DfES) (2005a) *Primary National Strategy: Excellence and enjoyment, social and emotional aspects of learning guidance booklet,* Nottingham: Department for Education and Skills.

Department for Education and Skills (DfES) (2005b) *Higher Standards, Better Schools For All: More choice for parents and pupils,* London: Department for Education and Skills.

Department for Education and Skills (DfES) (2007a) *Secondary National Strategy: Social and emotional aspects of learning for secondary schools guidance booklet,* Nottingham: Department for Education and Skills.

Department for Education and Skills (DfES) (2007b) *Every Parent Matters,* London: Department for Education and Skills.

Dermott, E. (2008) *Intimate Fatherhood: A sociological analysis,* London: Routledge.

Dewey, J. (1929/1987) *The Later Works, 1925–1953,* in J.A. Boydston (ed.) *Volume 4 1929: The Quest for Certainty,* Carbondale: Southern Illinois University Press.

Dewey, J. (1933/1998) *How We Think,* Boston, MA: Houghton Mifflin.

Di Leonardo, M. (1987) 'The female world of cards and holidays: Women, families and the world of kinship', *Signs,* 12(3): 440–53.

Di Leonardo, M. (1992) 'The female world of cards and holidays: Women, families and the work of kinship', in B. Thorne with M. Yalom (eds) *Rethinking the Family: Some feminist questions,* Boston, MA: Northern University Press.

Domínguez, D., Beaulieu, A., Estalella, A., Gómez, E., Schnettler, B. and Read, R. (2007) 'Virtual ethnography', *Forum Qualitative Sozialforschung / Forum: Qualitative Social Research,* 8(3). Online. Available HTTP: <http://nbn-resolving.de/urn:nbn:de:0114-fqs0703E19> (accessed 7 December 2011).

Donchin, A. (2000) 'Autonomy and interdependence: Quandaries in genetic decision-making', in C. Mackenzie and N. Stoljar (eds) *Relational Autonomy: Feminist perspectives on autonomy, agency and the social self,* Oxford: Oxford University Press.

Donchin, A. (2001) 'Understanding autonomy relationally: Toward a reconfiguration of bioethical principles', *Journal of Medicine & Philosophy,* 26: 365–87.

Doucet, A. (2000) '"There's a huge difference between me as a male carer and women": Gender, domestic responsibility, and the community as an institutional arena', *Community, Work and Family,* 3(2): 163–84.

Doucet, A. (2001) '"You've seen the need perhaps more clearly than I have": Exploring gendered processes of domestic responsibility', *Journal of Family Issues,* 22(3): 328–57.

Doucet, A. (2006a) *Do Men Mother? Fathering, care, and domestic responsibility,* Toronto: University of Toronto Press.

Doucet, A. (2006b) '"Estrogen-filled worlds": Fathers as primary caregivers and embodiment', *Sociological Review,* 54(4): 696–716.

Doucet, A. (2009) 'Gender equality and gender differences: Parenting, habitus, and embodiment (The 2008 Porter Lecture)', *Canadian Review of Sociology/Revue Canadienne de Sociologie,* 46(2): 103–21.

Doucet, A. (2011) '"It's not good for a man to be interested in other people's children": Fathers and public displays of care', in E. Dermott and J. Seymour (eds) *Displaying Families: New theoretical directions in family and intimate life,* London: Palgrave Macmillan.

Doucet, A. McKay, L. and Tremblay, D-G. (2009) 'Parental leave policy in Canada', in S. Kammerman and P. Moss (eds) *The Politics of Parental Leave Policies: Children, parenting, gender and the labour market,* Bristol: Policy Press.

Douglas, A. (2009) 'Web 2.0, Meet the mommyblogger', in S.L. Calixte and M. Friedman (eds) *Mothering and Blogging: The radical art of the MommyBlog,* Bradford, ON: Demeter Press.

Dowling, M. (1996) *Children and Young People's Experiences of Care,* Surrey Social Services and Royal Holloway, University of London.

Drew, P. (ed.) (2005) *Conversation Analysis,* Mahwah, NJ: Lawrence Erlbaum.

Driscoll, C. and Gregg, M. (2010) 'My profile: The ethics of virtual ethnography', *Emotion, Society and Space,* 3(1): 15–20.

Duncan, S. and Edwards, R. (1999) *Lone Mothers, Paid Work and Gendered Moral Rationalities,* London: Macmillan.

Dunn, J. (2004) *Children's Friendships: The beginning of intimacy,* Oxford: Blackwell.

Ecclestone, K. and Hayes, D. (2008) *Affect: Knowledge, Communication, Creativity and Emotions-Review, Beyond Current Horizons,* Online. Available HTTP <http://www.beyondcurrenthorizons.org.uk/affect-knowledge-communication-creativity-and-emotion/> (accessed 17 January 2011).

Edwards, R. (ed.) (2002) *Children, Home and School: Regulation, autonomy or connection?* London: RoutledgeFalmer.

Edwards, R. and Gillies, V. (2005) *Resources in Parenting: Access to capitals project report,* Families & Social Capital ESRC Research Group Working Article, No. 14, London South Bank University.

Edwards, R. and Weller, S. (2010a) 'A sideways look at gender and sibling relationships', in J. Caspi (ed.) *Sibling Development: Implications for mental health practitioners,* New York: Springer.

Edwards, R and Weller, S. (2010b) 'Trajectories from youth to adulthood: Choice and structure for young people before and during recession', *21st Century Society,* 5(2): 125–36.

Edwards, R., Mauthner, M. and Hadfield, L. (2005a) 'Children's sibling relationships and gendered practices: Talk, activity and dealing with change', *Gender and Education,* 17(5): 499–513.

Edwards, R., Hadfield, L. and Mauthner, M. (2005b) *Findings: Children's understanding of their sibling relationships,* York: Joseph Rowntree Foundation.

Edwards, R., Hadfield, L., Lucey, H. and Mauthner, M. (2006) *Sibling Identity and Relationships: Sisters and brothers,* London: Routledge.

Eelen, G. (2001) *A Critique of Politeness Theories,* Manchester: St Jerome Publishing.

Eggins, S. and Slade, D. (1997) *Analysing Casual Conversation,* London: Cassel.

Ehrenreich, B. and Hochschild, A. (2002) 'Introduction', in B. Ehrenreich and A. Hochschild (eds) *Global Woman: Nannies, maids and sex workers in the new economy,* London: Granta Books.

Eide, B.J. and Winger, N. (2005) 'From the children's point of view: Methodological and ethical challenges', in A. Clark, A.T. Kjørholt and Moss, P. (eds) *Beyond Listening,* Bristol: Policy Press.

Elfer, P. (2007) 'Babies and young children in nurseries: Using psychoanalytic ideas to explore tasks and interactions', *Children & Society,* 21(2): 111–22.

Ellen, R.F. (1984) *Ethnographic Research: A guide to general conduct,* London: Academic Press.

Ellis, C. (1993) '"There are survivors": Telling a story of sudden death', *Sociological Quarterly,* 34: 711–30.

Ellis, C. (1995) *Final Negotiations: A story of love, loss and chronic illness,* Philadelphia, PA: Temple University Press.

Ellis, C. (2009) *Revision: Autoethnographic reflections on life and work,* Walnut Creek, CA: Left Coast Press.

Ellyatt, W. (2009) 'Learning and development: Outcomes – own goals', *Nursery World,* Online. Available HTTP: <http://www.nurseryworld.co.uk/inDepth/920092/Learning---Development-Outcomes---Own-goals/> (accessed 30 December 2010).

e-Marketer (2011) *Report Roundup: Demographics.* Online. Available HTTP: <http://www.emarketer.com/blog/index.php/report-roundup-demographics/> (accessed 1 November 2011).

Erel, U. (2002) 'Reconceptualizing motherhood: Experiences of migrant women from Turkey living in Germany', in D. Bryceson and U. Vuorela (eds) *The Transnational Family. New European frontiers and global networks*, Oxford: Berg.

Evans, R. (2010) *The Experiences and Priorities of Young People who Care for their Siblings in Tanzania and Uganda.* Online. Available HTTP: <http://www.reading.ac.uk/ges/Aboutus/Staff/r-evans.aspx> (accessed 10 January 2011).

Evergeti, V. and Zontini, E. (2006) 'Introduction: Some critical reflections on social capital, migration and transnational families', *Ethnic and Racial Studies*, 29(6): 1025–39.

Fatherhood Institute (2010) *Fatherhood Institute Research Summary: African Caribbean Fathers*. Online. Available HTTP: <http://www.fatherhoodinstitute.org/2010/fatherhood-institute-research-summary-african-caribbean-fathers/> (accessed 7 December 2011).

Fawcett, M. (2009) *Learning through Child Observation* (2nd edn), London: Jessica Kingsley.

Featherstone, B. (2009) *Contemporary Fathering, Theory, Policy and Practice,* Bristol: Policy Press.

Ferreira, M. and Bosworth, K. (2000) 'Context as a critical factor in young adolescents' concepts of caring', *Journal of Research in Childhood Education*, 15(1): 117–28.

Finch, J. (1989) 'Kinship and friendship', in J. Witherspoon and L. Brook (eds) *British Social Attitude. Special International Report*, Aldershot: Gower.

Finch, J. (2007) 'Displaying families' in *Sociology*, 41(1): 65–81.

Finch, J. and Mason, J. (1993) *Negotiating Family Responsibilities*, London: Routledge.

Fine, M.D. (2007) *A Caring Society*, Basingstoke: Palgrave Macmillan.

Flesch, H. (2010) 'Balancing act: Women and the study of complementary and alternative medicine', *Complementary Therapies in Clinical Practice,* 16: 20–5.

Florian, L. and Black-Hawkins, K. (2011) 'Exploring inclusive pedagogy', *British Educational Research Journal*, 37(5): 813–28.

Foner, N. (2009) 'Gender and migration: West Indians in comparative perspectives', *International Migration*, 47: 3–29.

Foster, T.L., Jo, G.M., Davies, B., Dietrich, M.S., Barrera, M., Fairclogh, D.L., Vannatta, K. and Gerhardt, C.A. (2011) 'Comparison of continuing bonds reported by parents and siblings after a child's death from cancer', *Death Studies,* 35: 420–40.

Foucault, M. (1984) *The Care of the Self. The history of sexuality Vol 3,* London: Penguin.

France, A. (2007) *Understanding Youth in Late Modernity*, Maidenhead: Open University Press.

Francis, D., Kellaher, L. and Neophytou, G. (2001) 'The cemetery: The evidence of continuing bonds', in J. Hockey, J. Katz and N. Small (eds) *Grief, Mourning and Death Ritual*, Buckingham: Open University Press.

Fredricks, J.A., Blumenfeld, P.C. and Alison, H.P. (2004) 'School engagement: Potential of the concept, state of the evidence', *Review of Educational Research,* 74(1): 59–109.

Friedman, M. (1995) 'Beyond caring: The de-moralization of gender', in V. Held (ed.) *Justice and Care: Essential readings in feminist ethics,* Boulder, CO: Westview Press.

Friedman, M. and Calixte, S.L. (2009) *Mothering and Blogging: The radical art of the MommyBlog*, Bradford, ON: Demeter Press.

Frydenberg, E., Ainley, M. and Russell, V.J. (2005) *Student Motivation and Engagement,* Schooling Issues Digest: Australian Department of Education, Science and Training, Online. Available HTTP <http://www.dest.gov.au/sectors/school_education/publications_resources/schooling_issues_digest/schooling_issues_digest_motivation_engagement.htm> (accessed 17 January 2011).

Furedi, F. (2004) *Therapy Culture: Cultivating vulnerability in an anxious age*, London: Routledge.

Ganga, D. (2006) 'From potential returnees into settlers: Nottingham's older Italians', *Journal of Ethnic and Migration Studies*, 32(8): 1395–1413.

Gardner, K. (2002) *Age, Narrative and Migration: The life course and life histories of Bengali elders in London*, Oxford: Berg.

Gatrell, C. (2005) *Hard Labour: The Sociology of Parenthood*, Milton Keynes: Open University Press.

Gaunt, C. (2008) 'Nursery deputy manager guilty of force-feeding children', *Nursery World*. Online. Available HTTP <http://www.nurseryworld.co.uk/news/832560/Nursery-deputy-manager-guilty-force-feeding-children/> (accessed 10 January 2010).

Gee, J.P. (2005) *An Introduction to Discourse Analysis: Theory and method* (2nd edn), New York: Routledge.

Gerber, M. (2002) *Caring for Infants with Respect* (expanded edn), Los Angeles, CA: Resources for Infant Educarers (RIE).

Gerber, M. (2005) 'RIE principles and practices', in S. Petrie and S. Owen (eds) *Authentic Relationships in Group Care for Infants and Toddlers – Resources for Infant Educators: Principles into practice*, London: Jessica Kingsley.

Ghorayshi, P. (1996) 'Women, paid-work and the family in the Islamic Republic of Iran', *Journal of Comparative Family Studies*, 27(3): 453–66.

Gibson, L. (2004) 'The mountain behind the clouds: The professionalisation and integration of CAM in the UK', unpublished PhD thesis, Lancaster University.

Giddens, A. (1991) *Modernity and Self-identity: Self and society in late modern age*, Cambridge: Polity.

Giddens, A. (1992) *The Transformation of Intimacy: Sexuality, love and eroticism in modern societies*, Cambridge: Polity.

Gillard, D. (2011) *Education in England: A brief history*, Online. Available HTTP <http://www.educationengland.org.uk/history/> (accessed 17 January 2011).

Gillies, V. (2008) 'Childrearing, class and the new politics of parenting', *Sociology Compass*, 2(3): 1079–95.

Gillies, V. (2010) 'Is poor parenting a class issue? Contextualising anti-social behaviour and family life', in M. Klett-Davies (ed.) *Is Parenting a Class Issue*, London: Family and Parenting Institute.

Gillies, V. (2011) 'Social and emotional pedagogies: Critiquing the new orthodoxy of emotion in classroom behaviour management', *British Journal of Sociology of Education*, 32(2): 185–202.

Gillies, V. and Lucey, H. (2007) *Power, Knowledge and the Academy*, Basingstoke: Palgrave Macmillan.

Gillies, V. and Robinson, Y. (2010a) 'Managing emotions in research with challenging pupils', *Ethnography and Education*, 5(1): 97–110.

Gillies, V. and Robinson, Y. (2010b) 'Shifting the goalposts: Researching pupils at risk of school exclusion', in M. Rob and R. Thomson (eds) *Critical Practice with Children and Young People*, Bristol: Policy Press.

Gillies, V., Ribbens McCarthy, J. and Holland, J. (2001) '*Pulling Together, Pulling Apart*': *The Family Lives of Young People*, London: Joseph Rowntree Foundation/Family Policy Studies Centre.

Gilligan, C. (1982) *In a Different Voice: Psychological theory and women's development*, Cambridge, MA: Harvard University Press.

Gilligan, C. (1995) 'Moral orientation and moral development', in V. Held (ed.) *Justice and Care: Essential readings in feminist ethics*, Boulder, CO: Westview Press.

Gilligan, C. (2011) *Joining the Resistance*, Cambridge: Polity.

Goffman, E. (1967) *Interaction Ritual: Essays on face-to-face behaviour*, New York: Doubleday.

Goleman, D. (1997) *Emotional Intelligence: Why it can matter more than IQ*, New York: Bantum.

Goleman, D. (1999) *Working with Emotional Intelligence*, London: Bloomsbury.

Goleman, D. (2006) 'Emotional Intelligence: What does the research really indicate?' *Educational Psychologist*, 41(4): 239–45.

Golombok, S. (2000) *Parenting: What really counts?* London: Routledge.

Goodfellow, J. (2001) 'Wise practice: The need to move beyond best practice in early childhood education', *Australian Journal of Early Childhood*, 26(3): 1–6.

Goodfellow, J. (2008) 'Presence as a dimension of early childhood practice', *Australian Journal of Early Childhood*, 33(1): 17–22.

Gordon, T., Holland, J. and Lahelma, E. (2000) *Making Spaces: Citizenship and difference in schools*, Basingstoke: Macmillan.

Goulbourne, H. (1989) 'The contribution of West Indian groups to British politics', in H. Goulbourne (ed.) *Black Politics in Britain*, London: Avebury.

Goulbourne, H. and Chamberlain, M. (eds) (2001) *Caribbean Families in Britain and the Trans-Atlantic World*, Basingstoke: Macmillan Caribbean.

Goulbourne, H., Reynolds, T., Solomos, J. and Zontini, E. (2010) *Transnational Families, Ethnicities, Identities and Social Capital*, London: Routledge.

Graham, H. (1983) 'Caring: A labour of love', in J. Finch and D. Groves (eds) *A Labour of Love*, London: Routledge & Kegan Paul.

Gu, Y. (1990) 'Politeness phenomena in modern Chinese', *Journal of Pragmatics*, 14: 237–57.

Guarnizo, L.E. (1997) 'The emergence of a transnational social formation and the mirage of return migration among Dominican transmigrants', *Identities*, 4(2): 281–322.

Gumperz, J.J. (1992) 'Contextualization and understanding', in A. Duranti and C. Goodwin (eds) *Rethinking Context: Language as an interactive phenomenon*, Cambridge: Cambridge University Press.

Gumperz, J. J. (1999) 'On interactional sociolinguistic method', in S. Sarangi and C. Roberts (eds) *Talk, work and institutional order*, Berlin: Mouton de Gruyter.

Gumperz, J.J. (2001) 'Interactional Sociolinguistics: A personal perspective', in D. Schiffrin, D. Tannen and H. Hamilton (eds) *The Handbook of Discourse Analysis*, Oxford: Blackwell.

Hallam, E. and Hockey, J. (2001) *Death, Memory and Material Culture*, Oxford: Berg.

Hamington, M. (2004) *Embodied Care: Jane Addams, Maurice Merleau-Ponty, and Feminist Ethics*, Champaign: University of Illinois Press.

Hancock, S. (2008) *Just Me*, London: Bloomsbury.

Hansen, K.V. (2005) *Not-So-Nuclear Families: Class, gender, and networks of care*, Piscataway, NJ: Rutgers University Press.

Hattar-Pollara, M., Meleis, A.I. and Nagib, F.H. (2003) 'Multiple role stress and patterns of coping of Egyptian women in clerical jobs', *Journal of Transcultural Nursing*, 14(2): 125–33.

Heidegger, M. (1962) *Being and Time*, New York: Harper and Row.

Held, V. (1983) 'The obligations of mothers and fathers', in J. Trebilcot (ed.) *Mothering: Essays in feminist theory*, Savage, MD: Rowman and Littlefield.

Held, V. (2006) *The Ethics of Care: Personal, political, and global*, Oxford: Oxford University Press.

Heshusius, L. (1995) 'Listening to children: "What could we possibly have in common?" From concerns with self to participatory consciousness', *Theory into Practice*, 34(2): 117–23.

Hill Collins, P. (1990) *Black Feminist Thought*, London: Routledge.

Hill Collins, P. (1995) 'Black women and motherhood', in V. Held (ed.) *Justice and Care: Essential readings in feminist ethics*, Boulder, CO: Westview Press.

Hill Collins, P. (2004) *Black Sexual Politics: African-Americans, gender and the new racism*, London: Routledge.

Hine, C. (2000) *Virtual Ethnography*, London: Sage.

Hine, C. (2008) 'Virtual ethnography: Modes, varieties, affordances', in N.G. Fielding, R.M. Lee and G. Blank (eds) *Handbook of Online Research Methods*, London: Sage.

HM Government (2004) *The Children Act 2004*, London: HMSO.

HMSO (1967) *Children and their Primary Schools: A report of the Central Advisory Council for Education (England) (The Plowden Report)*, London: HMSO.

Hoagland, S. (1990) 'Some concerns about Nel Noddings' caring', *Hypatia*, 5(1): 109–14.

Hochschild, A. (1983) *The Managed Heart: Commercialization of human feeling*, Berkeley: University of California Press.

Hochschild, A. (2002) 'Love and gold', in B. Ehrenreich and A. Hochschild (eds) *Global Woman: Nannies, maids and sex workers in the new economy*, London: Granta Books.

Hochschild, A. (2003) *The Commercialization of Intimate Life*, Berkeley: University of California Press.

Hochschild, A.R., Hutton, W. and Giddens, A. (2000) 'Global care chains and emotional surplus value', in A. Giddens and W. Hutton (eds) *On the Edge Living with Global Capitalism*, London: Jonathan Cape.

Hockey, J., Kellaher, L. and Prendergast, D. (2007) 'Sustaining kinship: Ritualization and the disposal of human ashes in the United Kingdom', in Mitchell, M. (ed.) *Remember Me: Constructing Immortality: Beliefs on immortality, life, and death*, London: Routledge.

Hohmann, U. (2007) 'Rights, expertise and negotiations in care and education', *Early Years*, 27(1): 33–46.

Holdsworth, C. and Morgan, D. (2007) 'Revisiting the generalised other: An exploration', *Sociology*, 41(3): 401–17.

Holland, J. (2004) '"Lost for Words" in Hull', *Pastoral Care*, 22: 22–6.

Hollway, W. (2006) *The Capacity to Care: Gender and ethical subjectivity*, London: Routledge.

Holmes, J. (1995) *Women, Men and Politeness*, Harlow, Essex: Addison Wesley Longman.

Hondagneu-Sotelo, P. and Avila, E. (1997) '"I'm here, but I'm there". The meanings of Latina transnational motherhood', *Gender and Society*, 11(5): 548–71.

Hooyman, N. and Gonyea, J. (1999) 'A feminist model of family care: Practice and policy directions', *Journal of Women and Ageing*, 11(2/3): 149–69.

Hornby, M. (2009) 'Review Reports Back on Murder of Disabled Girl', *The Independent*. Online. Available HTTP: <http://www.independent.co.uk/news/uk/crime/review-reports-back-on-murder-of-disabled-girl-1783563.html> (accessed 13 December 2011).

Houston, B. (1990) 'Caring and exploitation', *Hypatia*, 5(1): 115–19.

Howarth, G. (2000) '"Dismantling the boundaries between life and death', *Mortality*, 5: 127–38.

Howarth, G. (2007) 'The rebirth of death: Continuing relationships with the dead', in M. Mitchell (ed.) *Remember Me: Constructing immortality. Beliefs on immortality, life, and death*, London: Routledge,

Hoyle, D. (2008) 'Problematizing Every Child Matters', *Encyclopaedia of Informal Education*. Online. Available HTTP: <www.infed.org/socialwork/every_child_matters_a_critique.htm> (accessed 7 December 2011).

Hughes, K. (2004) 'Health as individual responsibility, possibilities and personal struggle', in P. Tovey, G. Eastwood and J. Adams (eds) *Mainstreaming of Complementary and Alternative Medicine*, London: Routledge.

Hughes, B., McKie, L., Hopkins, D. and Watson, N. (2005) 'Love's labour's lost? Feminism, the disabled people's movement and an ethic of care', *Sociology*, 39(2): 259–75.

Hunniford, G. (2008) *Always With You*, London: Hodder.

Irwin, S. (1995) *Rights of Passage: Social change and the transition from youth to adulthood*, London: UCL Press.

Irwin, S. (2005) *Reshaping Social Life*, Abingdon: Routledge.

Jackson, S. (1992) 'Towards a historical sociology of housework: A materialist feminist analysis', *Women's Studies International Forum*, 15(2): 153–72.

Jenks, C. (1994) 'Child abuse in the postmodern context: An issue of social identity', *Childhood*, 2: 111–21.

Jenks, C. (1996) *Childhood*, London: Routledge.

Johnstone, B. (2002) *Discourse Analysis*, Oxford: Blackwell.

Kağitçibaşi, Ç. (2005) 'Autonomy and relatedness in cultural context: Implications for self and family', *Journal of Cross-Cultural Psychology*, 36: 403–22.

Kahn, T. (2011) *The XY Factor: Addressing gender issues in the early years*, London: Pre-school Learning Alliance.

Kamali, A. (2004) 'Women: Double poverty', *Social Welfare Quarterly* [Iran], 3(12): 181–201.

Kamerman, S.B. and Moss, P. (eds) (2009) *The Politics of Parental Leave Policies: Children, parenting, gender and the labour market*, Bristol: Policy Press.

Kendall, S. and Kinder, K. (2005) *Reclaiming Those Disengaged from Education and Learning: A European perspective*, Slough: NFER.

King, R., Thomson, M., Fielding T. and Warnes, T. (2005) *Gender, Age and Generations*, State-of-the-art-report- IMISCOE Network of Excellence on Immigration, Integration and Social Cohesion in Europe. Amsterdam: IMISCOE.

Kittay, E.F. (1999) *Love's Labor: Essays on women, equality, and dependency*, New York: Routledge.

Kittay, E.F. (2005) 'Dependency, difference and the global ethic of care', *Journal of Political Philosophy*, 13(4): 443–69.

Klass, D. (2001) 'Continuing bonds in the resolution of grief in Japan and North America', *American Behavioral Scientist*, 44: 742–63.

Klass, D. (2006) 'Continuing conversations about continuing bonds', *Death Studies*, 30: 843–58.

Klass, D. and Goss, R. (1999) 'Spiritual bonds to the dead in cross-cultural and historical perspective: Comparative religion and modern grief', *Death Studies*, 23: 547–67.

Klass, D., Silverman, P.R. and Nickman, S.L. (1996) *Continuing Bonds: New understandings of grief*, London: Taylor & Francis.

Koehn, D. (1998) *Rethinking Feminist Ethics*, London: Routledge.

Kosonen, M. (1996) 'Siblings as providers of support and care during middle childhood: Children's perceptions', *Children & Society*, 10: 267–79.

Kosonen, M. (1999) '"Core" and "kin" siblings', in A. Mullender (ed.) *We are Family: Sibling relationships in placement and beyond*, London: British Agencies of Adoption and Fostering.

Kozinets, R.V. (2010) *Netnography: Doing ethnographic research online*, London: Sage.

Kuhse, H., Singer, P. and Rickard, M. (1998) 'Reconciling impartial morality and feminist ethic of care', *Journal of Value Inquiry*, 32: 451–63.

Lakoff, R. and Ide, S. (eds) (2005) *Broadening the Horizon of Linguistic Politeness*, Philadelphia, PA: John Benjamins.

Laming, Lord (2003) *The Victoria Climbié Inquiry Report*. Online. Available HTTP: <http://publications.everychildmatters.gov.uk/eOrderingDownload/CM-5730PDF.pdf> (accessed 25 November 2010).

Larrabee, M.J. (ed.) (1993) *An Ethic of Care: Feminist and interdisciplinary perspectives*, London: Routledge.

Lawrence, J. (2009) 'Blog for rent: How marketing is changing our mothering conversations', in M. Friedman and S.L. Calixte (eds) *Mothering and Blogging: The radical act of the MommyBlog*, Bradford, ON: Demeter Press.

Lawson, V. (2007) 'Geographies of care and responsibility', *Annals of the Association of American Geographers*, 97(1): 1–11.

Lee-Treweek, G. (2010) 'Born to it and then pushed out of it: Folk healing in the new complementary and alternative medicine marketplace', in R. Moore and S. McClean (eds) *Folk Healing and Health Care Practices in Britain and Ireland*, Oxford: Berghahn.

Leffers, M.R. (1993) 'Pragmatists Jane Addams and John Dewey inform the ethic of care', *Hypatia*, 8(2): 64–78.

Lenz Taguchi, H. (2010) *Going Beyond the Theory/Practice Divide in Early Childhood Education*, Abingdon, Oxon: Routledge.

Lewis, C.S. (1961) *A Grief Observed*, London: Faber and Faber.

Libbey, H.P. (2004) 'Measuring student relationships to school: Attachment, bonding, connectedness, and engagement', *Journal of School Health*, 74(7): 274–83.

Licuanan, P. (1994) 'A moral recovery program: Building a people – building a nation', in M.B. Dy Jr. (ed.) *Values in Philippine Culture and Education: Philippine philosophical studies 1*, Washington, DC: Council of Research in Values and Philosophy.

Lievesley, N. (2010) *The Future Ageing of the Ethnic Minority Population of England and Wales: Older BME people and financial inclusion report*, London: Runnymede.

Lister, R. (2002) 'Sexual citizenship', in E.F. Isin and B.S. Turner (eds) (2002) *Handbook of Citizenship Studies*, Thousand Oaks, CA: Sage.

Locher, M.A. (2004) *Power and Politeness in Action: Disagreements in oral communication*, Berlin: Mouton de Gruyter.

Lofland, L.H. (1985) 'The social shaping of emotion: The case of grief', *Symbolic Interaction*, 8: 171–90.

Loftus, D. (2006) 'The self in society: Middle class men and autobiography', in D. Amigoni (ed.) *Life Writing and Victorian Culture*, Aldershot: Ashgate.

Long, A.F., Mercer, G. and Hughes, K. (2000) 'Developing a tool to measure holistic practice: A missing dimension in outcomes measurement within complementary therapies', *Complementary Therapies in Medicine*, 8: 26–31.

Lopez, L.K. (2009) 'The radical act of "mommy blogging": Redefining motherhood through the blogosphere', *New Media & Society*, 11(5): 729–47.

Lovat, T. (2010) 'Synergies and balance between values education and quality teaching', *Educational Philosophy and Theory*, 42(4): 489–500.

Lowdell, C., Evandrou, M. and Bardsley, M. (2000) *Health of Minority Ethnic Elders in London: Respecting diversity*, London: The Health of Londoners Project.

Luff, P. (2012) 'Challenging assessment', in T. Papatheodorou and J. Moyles (eds) *Cross-Cultural Perspectives on Early Childhood*, London: Sage.

Luxton, M. and Vosko, L.F. (1998) 'The Census and women's work', *Studies in Political Economy*, 56(Summer): 49–82.

Lynch, K. (2007) 'Love labour as a distinct and non-commodifiable form of care labour', *Sociological Review*, 55(3): 550–70.

Lynch, K. (2010) 'Carelessness: A hidden doxa of higher education', *Arts and Humanities in Higher Education*, 9(1): 54–67.

Lynch, K., Lyons, M. and Cantillon, S. (2007) 'Breaking silence: Educating citizens for love, care and solidarity', *International Studies in the Sociology of Education*, 17(1): 1–19.

Lynch, K., Baker, J. and Lyons, M. (eds) (2009) *Affective Equality: Love, care and injustice,* Houndsmill: Palgrave Macmillan.

McCarthy, J. and Edwards, R. (2011) *Key Concepts in Family Studies*, London: Sage.

McClean, S. (2005) '"The illness is part of the person": Discourses of blame, individual responsibility and individuation at a centre for healing in the North of England', *Sociology of Health and Illness,* 27(5): 628–48.

McEwan, C. and Goodman, M.K. (2010) 'Place geography and the ethics of care: Introductory remarks on the geographies of ethics, responsibility and care', *Ethics, Place and Environment,* 13(2): 103–12.

McGuire, M.B. (1995) 'Alternative therapies: The meaning of bodies in knowledge and practice', in H. Johannessen, S.G. Olesen and J.Ø. Andersen (eds) *Studies in Alternative Therapy 2. Body and nature,* 15–32, Odense: INRAT/Odense University Press.

McGuire, M.B. (2008) *Lived Religion. Faith and practice in everyday Life,* New York: Oxford University Press.

McIntosh, I. and Punch, S. (2009) '"Barter", "deals", "bribes" and "threats": Exploring sibling interactions', *Childhood,* 16(1): 49–65.

McIntosh, S. and Houghton, N. (2005) *Disengagement from Secondary Education: A story retold,* London: Learning and Skills Development Agency.

McKie, L., Gregory, S. and Bowlby, S. (2004) *Caringscapes: Experiences of caring and working,* Centre for Research on Families and Relationships Research Briefing, No. 13, Edinburgh: CRFR.

McLaughlin, J., Goodley, D., Clavering, E. and Fisher, P. (2008) *Families Raising Disabled Children: Enabling care and social justice,* Basingstoke: Palgrave Macmillan.

McMillan, M. (1919) *The Nursery School,* London: Dent.

McNamee, S. (1997) '"I won't let her in my room": Sibling strategies of power and resistance around computer and video games', in. J. Seymour and P. Bagguley (eds) *Relating Intimacies: Power and resistance,* Basingstoke: Macmillan.

Magnuson, E. (2008) 'Rejecting the American dream. Men creating alternative life goals', *Journal of Contemporary Ethnography,* 37(3): 255–90.

Malaguzzi, L. (1998) 'History, ideas and basic philosophy. An interview with Lella Gandini', in C.P. Edwards, L. Gandini and G.E. Forman (eds) *The Hundred Languages of Children. The Reggio Emilia approach – Advanced Reflections* (2nd edn), Westport, CT: Ablex Publishing.

Mand, K. (2008) 'Who cares? "external", "internal" and "mediator" debates about South Asian elders' needs', in R. Grillo (ed.) *The Family in Question: Immigrant and ethnic minorities in multicultural Europe,* Amsterdam: Amsterdam University Press.

Mann, C. and Stewart, F. (2000) *Internet Communication and Qualitative Research: A handbook for researching online.* London: Sage.

Manning, S. (2011) 'Move Over, Mumsnet! Meet the New Breed of Cyber Mothers', *The Independent.* Online. Available HTTP: <http://www.independent.co.uk/life-style/health-and-families/health-news/move-over-mumsnet-meet-the-new-breed-of-cyber-mothers-2302856.html> (accessed 1 November 2011).

Manning-Morton, J. and Thorp, M. (2006) *Key Times: A framework for developing high quality provision for children from birth to three,* Maidenhead: Open University Press.

Marcus, L. (2008) 'Compensation sought for children abused at nursery', *Nursery World.* Online. Available HTTP: <http://www.nurseryworld.co.uk/news/809087/Compensation-sought-children-abused-nursery/> (accessed 10 November 2010).

Markham, A. and Baym, N. (eds) (2009) *Internet Inquiry: Conversations about method,* Thousand Oaks, CA: Sage.

Marsiglio, W. (2008) *Men on a Mission: Valuing youth work in our communities*, Baltimore, MD: Johns Hopkins University Press.

Martin, J. (2010) 'The making of a good teacher in the 20th Century', in M. Rob and R. Thomson (eds) *Critical Practice with Children and Young People*, Bristol: Policy Press.

Mason, J. (2004) 'Personal narratives, relational selves: Residential histories in the living and telling', *Sociological Review*, 52: 162–79.

Mason, J. (2008) 'Tangible affinities and the real life fascination of kinship', *Sociology*, 42: 29–46.

Massey, D. (2004) 'Geographies of responsibility', *Geografiska Annaler*, 86B: 5–18.

Mauthner, M. (2002) *Sistering: Power and change in female relationships*, Basingstoke: Palgrave Macmillan.

Mauthner, M. (2005) 'Distant lives, still voices: Sistering in family sociology', *Sociology*, 39(4): 623–42.

Mauthner, N.S. (1995) 'Postnatal depression: The significance of social contacts between mothers', *Women's Studies International Forum*, 18(3): 311–23.

Mauthner, N.S. (2002). *The Darkest Days of My Life: Stories of postpartum depression*, Cambridge, MA: Harvard University Press.

Mauthner, N.S. (2010) '"I wasn't being true to myself": Women's narratives of postpartum depression', in D.C. Jack and A. Ali (eds) *Cultural Perspectives on Women's Depression: Self-silencing, psychological distress and recovery,* Oxford: Oxford University Press.

Mauthner, N.S. (2012) 'Accounting for our part of the entangled webs we weave: Ethical and moral issues in digital data sharing', in T. Miller, M. Mauthner, M. Birch and J. Jessop (eds) *Ethics in Qualitative Research* (2nd edn), London: Sage.

Mauthner, N.S. and Doucet, A. (2003) 'Reflexive accounts and accounts of reflexivity in qualitative data analysis', *Sociology,* 37(3): 413–31.

Mauthner, N.S. and Parry, O. (2009) 'Qualitative data preservation and sharing in the social sciences: On whose philosophical terms?' *Australian Journal of Social Issues,* 44(3): 289–305.

Mauthner, N.S. and Doucet, A. (forthcoming) *Narrative Analysis: The Listening Guide Approach*, London: Sage.

Mauthner, N.S., Parry, O. and Backett-Milburn, K. (1998) 'The data are out there, or are they? Implications for archiving and revisiting qualitative data', *Sociology,* 32(4): 733–45.

Mauthner, M., Birch, M., Jessop, J. and Miller, T. (2002) *Ethics in Qualitative Research,* London: Sage.

Memel, E. and Fernandez, L. (2005) 'RIE Parent – Infant Guidance Classes', in S. Petrie and S. Owen (eds) *Authentic Relationships in Group Care for Infants and Toddlers – Resources for Infant Educators: Principles into practice*, London: Jessica Kingsley.

Mendelsohn, J. (2010) 'Honey, don't bother Mommy. I'm too busy building my brand', *New York Times*. Online. Available HTTP: <http://www.nytimes.com/2010/03/14/fashion/14moms.html?pagewanted=all> (accessed 1 November 2011).

Merwin, M. (2002) 'Let sleeping students lie? Using interpersonal activities to engage disengaged students', *College Student Journal*, 36(1). Online. Available HTTP < http://findarticles.com/p/articles/mi_m0FCR/is_1_36/ai_85007772/pg_4/> (accessed 14 December 2010).

Meyer, M. and Woodthorpe, K. (2008) 'The material presence of absence: A dialogue between museums and cemeteries', *Sociological Research Online*, 13(5): 13.

Miller, C.R. and Shepherd, D. (2004) 'Blogging as social action: A genre analysis of the weblog', in L.J. Gurak, S. Antonijevic, L. Johnson, C. Ratliff and J. Reyman (eds) *Into the Blogosphere: Rhetoric, community, and culture of weblogs*. Online. Available HTTP: <http://blog.lib.umn.edu/blogosphere/ blogging_as_social_action...> (accessed 1 November 2011).

Miller, T. (2011) *Making Sense of Fatherhood. Gender, caring and work,* Cambridge: Cambridge University Press.

Milligan, C. (2000) 'Bearing the burden: Towards a restructured geography of care', *Area,* 32: 49–58.

Milligan, C., Atkinson, S., Skinner, M. and Wiles, J. (2007) 'Geographies of care: A commentary', *New Zealand Geographer,* 63:135–40.

Moghadam, F.E. (2009) 'Undercounting women's work in Iran', *Iranian Studies,* 42(1): 81–95.

Mohseni Tabrizi A.R. and Seyedan, F. (2004) 'Social origins of women's depression', *Woman in Development and Politics (Women's Research),* 2(2): 89–102.

Money, R. (2005) 'The RIE Early Years "Curriculum"', in S. Petrie and S. Owen (eds) *Authentic Relationships in Group Care for Infants and Toddlers – Resources for Infant Educators: Principles into practice,* London: Jessica Kingsley.

Moore, H.L. (1996) 'Mothering and social responsibilities in a cross-cultural perspective', in E. Bortolaia Silva (ed.) *Good Enough Mothering: Feminist perspectives on lone motherhood,* London: Routledge.

Morand, D.A. (1996) 'Dominance, deference, and egalitarianism in organizational interaction: A sociolinguistic analysis of power and politeness', *Organization Science,* 7(5), 544–56.

Morgan, D.H.J. (1996) *Family Connections: An introduction to family studies,* Cambridge: Polity.

Morgan, D.H.J. (2011) *Rethinking Family Practices,* Basingstoke: Palgrave Macmillan.

Morris, S. and Gabbatt, A. (2009) 'Nursery worker Vanessa George pleads guilty to sexually abusing children', *The Guardian.* Online. Available HTTP: <http://www.guardian.co.uk/society/2009/oct/01/vanessa-george-sex-abuse> (accessed 10th January 2010).

Morrison, A. (2010) 'Autobiography in real time: A genre analysis of personal mommy blogging', *Cyberpsychology: Journal of Psychosocial Research on Cyberspace,* 4(2): article 5.

Morrison, A. (2011) 'Suffused by feeling and affect: The intimate public of personal mommy blogging', *Biography,* 34 (1): 37–55.

Morton, F. (2009) 'Developing an appreciation of babies and young children's behaviour – why do they do what they do?', in H. Fabian and C. Mould (eds) *Development and Learning for Very Young Children,* London: Sage.

Moyles, J. (2001) 'Passion, paradox and professionalism in early years education', *Early Years,* 21(2): 81–95.

Mullender, A. (ed.) (1999) *We are Family: Sibling relations in placement and beyond,* London: BAAF.

National Council for Palliative Care (2012) *National Council for Palliative Care.* Online. Available HTTP: <http://www.ncpc.org.uk/> (accessed 28 February 2012).

National Council for Voluntary Organisations (2009) *An Overview of Charitable Caregiving in the UK,* London: NCVO.

National Strategies (2009) *Early Years Foundation Stage.* Online. Available HTTP: <http://nationalstrategies.standards.dcsf.gov.uk/earlyyears> (accessed 18 November 2010).

Nazroo J. (1997) *The Health of Britain's Ethnic Minorities,* London: Policy Studies Institute.

Nazroo, J., Bajekarl, M., Blane, D. and Grewal, I. (2004) 'Ethnic inequalities at older ages', in A. Walker and C. Hagan Hennessy (eds) *Growing Older: Quality of life in old age,* Buckingham: Open University Press.

Nguyen, H. (2007) 'Rapport building in language instruction: A microanalysis of the multiple resources in teacher talk', *Language & Education,* 21(4): 284–303.

Niikko, A. (2004) 'Education – a joint task for parents, kindergarten teachers and kindergarten student teachers', *International Journal of Early Years Education,* 12(3): 259–74.

Nissen, N. (2008) 'Herbal healthcare and processes of change: An ethnographic study of contemporary women's practice and use of Western herbal medicine in the UK', unpublished PhD thesis, The Open University.

Nissen, N. (2010) 'Practitioners of Western herbal medicine and their practice in the UK: Beginning to sketch the profession', *Complementary Therapies in Clinical Practice*, 16(4): 181–6.

Noddings, N. (1988) 'An ethic of caring and its implications for instructional arrangements', *American Journal of Education*, 96(2): 215–30.

Noddings, N. (1990) 'Review symposium – A response', *Hypatia*, 5(1): 120–6.

Noddings, N. (1992) *The Challenge to Care in Schools*, New York: Teachers College Press.

Noddings, N. (1995a) 'Teaching themes of care', *Phi Delta Kappan*, 76(9): 675–83.

Noddings, N. (1995b) 'Caring', in V. Held (ed.) *Justice and Care: Essential readings in feminist ethic*, Boulder, CO: Westview Press.

Noddings, N. (2002) *Educating Moral People: A caring alternative to character education*, New York: Teachers College Press.

Noddings, N. (2003, first published in 1984) *Caring: A feminine approach to ethics and moral education* (2nd edn), Berkeley: University of California Press.

Noddings, N. (2005) 'Caring in Education', *Encyclopedia of Informal Education*. Online. Available HTTP: <www.infed.org/biblio/noddings_caring_in_education.htm> (accessed 15 October 2009).

Noddings, N. (2010a) 'Caring and empathy', *Abstracta Special Issue*, V: 6–12.

Noddings, N. (2010b) 'Moral education in an age of globalization', *Educational Philosophy and Theory*, 42(4): 390–6.

Noddings, N. (2010c) 'Moral education and caring', *Theory and Research in Education*, 8(2): 145–51.

NSPCC (2010) *Siblings in Care: Law and Practice*, Online. Available HTTP: <http://www.nspcc.org.uk/inform/research/questions/siblings_in_care_wda74187.html> (accessed 2 August 2011).

Nussbaum, M.C. (2006) *Frontiers of Justice: Disability, nationality, species membership*, Cambridge, MA: First Harvard University Press.

Nutbrown, C. (2006) *Threads of Thinking: Young children's learning and the role of early education* (3rd edn), London: Sage.

Nutt, L. (2006) *The Lives of Foster Carers: Private sacrifices, public restrictions*, Abingdon: Routledge.

Oakley, A. (1981) 'Interviewing women: A contradiction in terms', in H. Roberts (ed.) *Doing Feminist Research*, London: Routledge and Kegan Paul.

O'Brien, M. (2005) *Shared Caring: Bringing fathers into the frame*, Manchester: Equal Opportunities Commission.

O'Brien, M. (2009) 'Fathers, parental leave policies, and infant quality of life: International perspectives and policy impact', *Annals of the American Academy of Political and Social Science*, 624(1): 190–213.

O'Connor, B.B. (2000) 'Conceptions of the body in CAM', in M. Kelner and B. Wellman (eds) *Complementary and Alternative Medicine: Challenge and change*, London: Routledge, 39–60.

Ofsted (2009) *Early Years Online Self-evaluation Form (SEF) and Guidance – For Settings Delivering the Early Year Foundation Stage*. Online. Available HTTP: <http://www.ofsted.gov.uk/Ofsted-home/Forms-and-guidance/Browse-all-by/Other/General/Early-years-online-self-evaluation-form-SEF-and-guidance-For-settings-delivering-the-Early-Years-Foundation-Stage> (accessed 1 December 2009).

Oldfield, N. (1997) *The Adequacy of Foster Care Allowances*, Aldershot: Ashgate.

Oliver, M. (1996) *Understanding Disability: From theory to practice*, Houndmills: Palgrave.

Oliver, M. and Barnes, C. (2010) 'Disability studies, disabled people and the struggle for inclusion', *British Journal of Sociology of Education*, 31(5): 547–60.

Ong-Dean, C. (2009) *Distinguishing Disability: Parents, privilege, and special education*, London: University of Chicago Press.

Organisation for Economic Co-operation and Development (OECD) (2006) *Starting Strong II: Early Childhood Education and Care, Volume 2*, Paris: OECD Publishing.

Orlikowski, W.J. (2007) 'Sociomaterial practices: Exploring technology at work', *Organization Studies*, 28(9): 1435–48.

Osgood, J. (2006) 'Deconstructing professionalism in early childhood education: Resisting the regulatory gaze', *Contemporary Issues in Early Childhood*, 7(1): 5–14.

Owusu-Bempah, K. (2010) *The Wellbeing of Children in Care*, Basingstoke: Macmillan.

Papatheodorou, T. (2008) 'Some worldviews of early childhood in contemporary curricula', Inaugural Professorial Lecture presented at Anglia Ruskin University, Chelmsford, 20 October.

Parker, R. (1997) 'The production and purposes of maternal ambivalence', in W. Hollway and B. Featherstone (eds) *Mothering and Ambivalence*, London: Routledge.

Parker-Rees, R. (2007) 'Liking to be liked: Imitation, familiarity and pedagogy in the first years of life', *Early Years*, 27(1): 3–17.

Parkes, C.M. and Prigerson, H.G. (2010) *Bereavement: Studies of grief in adult life*, London: Penguin.

Parr, H. (2003) 'Medical geography: Care and caring', *Progress in Human Geography*, 27: 212–21.

Parreñas, R.S. (2001) *Servants of Globalization. Women, migration, and domestic work*, Stanford, CA: Stanford University Press

Parry, O. and Mauthner, N.S. (2004) 'Whose data are they anyway? Practical, legal and ethical issues in archiving qualitative research data', *Sociology*, 38(1): 139–52.

Parry, O. and Mauthner, N.S. (2005) 'Back to basics: Who re-uses qualitative data and why?', *Sociology*, 39(2): 337–42.

Parton, N. (2006) *Safeguarding Childhood. Early intervention and surveillance in a late modern society*, London: Palgrave Macmillan.

Paterson, C. and Britain, N. (2008) 'The patient's experience of holistic care: Insights from acupuncture research', *Chronic Illness*, 4: 264–77.

Payler, J. (2007) 'Opening and closing interactive spaces: Shaping four-year-old children's participation in two English settings', *Early Years*, 27(3): 237–54.

Penn, H. (2008) *Understanding Early Childhood: Issues and controversies* (2nd edn), Maidenhead: McGraw-Hill/Open University Press.

Pero, D. (2008) 'Political engagement of Latin Americans in the UK: Issues, strategies, and the public debate', *Focaal*, 51: 73–90.

Phillips, J. (2007) *Care*, Cambridge: Polity.

Philo, C. (1997) 'Across the water: Reviewing geographical studies of asylums and other mental health facilities', *Health & Place*, 3: 73–89.

Piersall, W. and Armstrong, H. (eds) (2011) *Mom Blogging for Dummies*, Hoboken, NJ: Wiley.

Pietroni, P. (1990) *The Greening of Medicine*, London: Victor Gollancz.

Piper, H. and Stronach, I. (2008) *Don't Touch! The educational story of a panic*, London: Routledge.

Popke, J. (2006) 'Geography and ethics: Everyday mediations through care and consumption', *Progress in Human Geography*, 30(4): 504–12.

Power, R. (2000) *A Question of Knowledge*, Harlow: Prentice Hall.

Pugh, A. (2005) 'Selling compromise: Toys, motherhood and the cultural deal', *Gender & Society*, 19: 729–49.

Pugh, A. (2009) *Longing and Belonging: Parents, children, and consumer culture*, Berkeley: University of California Press.

Pugh, G. (2010) 'The policy agenda for early childhood services', in G. Pugh and B. Duffy (eds) *Contemporary Issues in the Early Years* (5th edn), London: Sage.

Pullin Stark, P. (2007) 'An investigation into social cohesion in business meetings', unpublished PhD thesis, University of Birmingham.

Punch, S. (2005) 'The generationing of power: A comparison of child–parent and sibling relationships', *Sociological Studies of Children and Youth*, 10: 169–88.

Punch, S. (2008) '"You can do nasty things to your brothers and sisters without a reason": Siblings' backstage behaviour', *Children & Society*, 22: 333–44.

Qualifications and Curriculum Authority (QCA) (2000) *Curriculum Guidance for the Foundation Stage*, London: DfES Publications.

QCDA (2011) *National Curriculum*, Online. Available HTTP <http://curriculum.qcda.gov.uk/> (accessed 17 January 2011).

Raghuram, P., Madge, C. and Noxolo, P. (2009) 'Rethinking responsibility and care for a postcolonial world', *Geoforum*, 40: 5–13.

Ramji, H. (2006) 'British Indians "returning home": An exploration of transnational belonging', *Sociology*, 40(4): 645–62.

Ray, P.H. and Anderson, S.R. (2000) *The Cultural Creatives*, New York: Three Rivers Press.

Read, K. (2010) 'The implications of Every Child Matters and the Children Act for schools', *Pastoral Care in Education,* 23(1): 12–18.

Reay, D. (2000) 'A useful extension of Bourdieu's conceptual framework? Emotional capital as a way of understanding mothers' involvement in their children's education?', *Sociological Review*, 48(4): 568–85.

Reay, D. (2007) '"Unruly places": Inner-city comprehensives, middle-class imaginaries and working-class children', *Urban Studies*, 44: 1191–201.

Rees-Miller, J. (1995) *Linguistic features of disagreement in face-to-face encounters in university setting,* Stony Brook: State University of New York.

Rees-Miller, J. (2000) 'Power, severity, and context in disagreement', *Journal of Pragmatics,* 32(8): 1087–111.

Reynolds, T. (2001a) 'Black fathers and family lives in Britain', in H. Goulbourne and M. Chamberlain (eds) *Caribbean Families and the Trans-Atlantic World,* London: Macmillan.

Reynolds, T. (2001b) 'Black mothers, paid work and identity', *Journal of Ethnic and Racial Studies,* 24(6): 1046–64.

Reynolds, T. (2002a) 'Re-thinking a black feminist standpoint', *Journal of Ethnic and Racial Studies,* 26(3): 591–606.

Reynolds, T. (2002b) 'Analyzing the Black family', in A. Carling, S. Duncan and R. Edwards (eds) *Analyzing Families*, London: Routledge.

Reynolds, T. (2003) 'Black to the community: Black community parenting in Britain', *Journal of Community, Work and Family*, 6(1): 29–41.

Reynolds, T. (2005) *Caribbean Mothering: Identity and childrearing in the UK*, London: Tufnell Press.

Reynolds, T. (2006) 'Bonding social capital within the Caribbean family and community', Special Issue: Ethnicity and Social Capital, *Journal of Community, Work and Family*, 9(3): 273–90.

Reynolds, T. (2008) *Triangle Way Forward – A Brixton Parenting Project: Evaluation report*, London: Metropolitan Housing Trust.

Reynolds, T. (2009) 'Exploring the absent/present dilemma: Black fathers, family relationships and social capital in Britain', *Annals of the American Academy of Political and Social Science*, 624: 12–28.

Reynolds, T. and Zontini, E. (2006) *A Comparative Study of Care and Provision Across Caribbean and Italian Transnational Families*, Families & Social Capital ESRC Research Group Working Paper, No. 16, London: London South Bank University.

Reynolds, T. and Miah, N. (2007) *Black Asian and Minority Ethnic Employment Skills*, Lambeth: London Borough of Lambeth.

Reynolds, T. and Briggs, D. (2009) *Evaluation of RAW Leadership Programme*, London: Involve.

Ribbens, J. (1993) 'Facts or fictions? Aspects of the use of autobiographical writing in undergraduate sociology', *Sociology*, 27: 81–92.

Ribbens, J. (1998) 'Hearing my feeling voice: An autobiographical discussion of motherhood', in J. Ribbens and R. Edwards (eds) *Feminist Dilemmas in Qualitative Research: Public knowledge and private lives*, London: Sage.

Ribbens, J. and Edwards, R. (1995) 'Introducing qualitative research on women in families and households', *Women's Studies International Forum*, 18(3): 247–58.

Ribbens, J. and Edwards, R. (1998) *Feminist Dilemmas in Qualitative Research*, London: Sage.

Ribbens McCarthy, J. (2006) *Young People's Experiences of Loss and Bereavement: Towards an inter-disciplinary approach*, Buckingham: Open University Press.

Ribbens McCarthy, J. (2007) '"They all look as if they're coping, but I'm not": The relational power/lessness of "youth" in responding to experiences of bereavement', *Journal of Youth Studies*, 10: 285–304.

Ribbens McCarthy, J. (2012) 'The powerful relational language of "family": togetherness, belonging, and personhood', *Sociological Review*, 60(1): 68–90.

Ribbens McCarthy, J. and Edwards, R. (2000) 'Moral tales of the child and the adult: Narratives of contemporary family lives under changing circumstances', *Sociology*, 34(2): 785–804.

Ribbens McCarthy, J. and Edwards, R. (2011) *Key Concepts in Family Studies*, London: Sage.

Ribbens McCarthy, J., Edwards, R. and Gillies, V. (2003) *Making Families, Moral Tales of Parenting & Step Parenting*, Durham: Sociologypress.

Rinaldi, C. (2005) 'Documentation and assessment: What is the relationship?', in A. Clark, A.T. Kjørholt and Moss, P. (eds) *Beyond Listening*, Bristol: Policy Press.

Robinson, F. (2011) *The Ethics of Care: A feminist approach to human security*, Philadelphia, PA: Temple University Press.

Rogers, C. (2003) 'The mother/researcher in blurred boundaries of a reflexive research process', *Auto/Biography* XI (1&2): 47–54.

Rogers, C. (2005) 'A sociology of parenting children identified with 'special' educational needs: The private and public spaces parents inhabit', unpublished PhD thesis, University of Essex.

Rogers, C. (2007a) *Parenting and Inclusive Education: Discovering difference, experiencing difficulty*, Houndmills, Basingstoke: Palgrave Macmillan.

Rogers, C. (2007b) '"Disabling" a family? Emotional dilemmas experienced in becoming a parent of a learning disabled child', *British Journal of Special Education*, 34(3): 136–43.

Rogers, C. (2009) 'Hope as a mechanism in emotional survival: Documenting miscarriage', *Auto/Biography Year Book 2009*, Nottingham: Russell Press.

Rogers, C. (2011) 'Mothering and intellectual disability: Partnership rhetoric?', *British Journal of Sociology of Education*, 32(4): 563–81.

Rogers, C. (forthcoming) *Intellectual Disability and Social Theory: Philosophical and sociological debates on being human,* London: Routledge.

Ruddick, S. (1980) 'Maternal thinking', *Feminist Studies,* 6(2): 342–67.

Ruddick, S. (1983) 'Maternal thinking', in J. Treblicot (ed.) *Mothering: Essays in feminist theory,* Totowa, NJ: Rowman and Littlefield.

Ruddick, S. (1989) *Maternal Thinking: Toward a politics of peace,* Boston, MA: Beacon Press.

Ruddick, S. (1995) *Maternal Thinking: Towards a politics of peace* (2nd edn, with a new preface), Boston, MA: Beacon Press.

Ruddick, S. (1998) 'Care as labour and relationship', in M.S. Halfron and J.C. Harber (eds) *Norms and Values: Essays on the work of Virgina Held,* Lanham, MD: Rowman and Littlefield.

Runswick-Cole, K. (2007) '"The tribunal was the most stressful thing: More stressful than my son's diagnosis or behaviour": The experiences of families who go to the Special Educational Needs and Disability Tribunal (SENDisT)', *Disability and Society,* 22(3): 315–28.

Russell, P. (1997) 'Parents as partners: Some early impressions of the impact of the Code of Practice', in S. Wolfendale (ed.) *Working With Parents of SEN Children After the Code of Practice,* London: David Fulton.

Ryan, S. and Runswick-Cole, K. (2009) 'From advocate to activist? Mapping the experiences of mothers of children on the autism spectrum', *Journal of Applied Research in Intellectual Disabilities,* 22: 43–53.

Rybas, N. and Gajjala, R. (2007) 'Developing cyberethnographic research methods for understanding digitally mediated identities', *Forum: Qualitative Social Research,* 8(3): article 35.

Sacks, H., Schegloff, E. and Jefferson, G. (1974) 'A simplest systematics for the organisation of turn taking in conversation', in J. Shenken (ed.) *Language, Thought and Culture,* London: Academic Press.

Sanders, R. (2004) *Sibling Relationships: Theory and issues for practice,* Basingstoke: Palgrave.

Sayer, A. (2011) *Why Things Matter to People. Social sciences, values and ethical life,* Cambridge: Cambridge University Press.

Schaps, E. (2003) 'Creating a school community', *Educational Leadership,* 60(6): 31–3.

Schneirov, M. and Geczik, J.D. (1996) 'A diagnosis for our times: Alternative health's submerged networks and the transformation of identities', *Sociological Quarterly,* 37(4): 627–44.

Schneirov, M. and Geczik, J.D. (2003) *A Diagnosis of Our Times: Alternative health from lifeworld to politics,* Albany: State University of New York Press.

Schofield, G., Beek, M. and Sargent, K. with Thoburn, J. (2000) *Growing up in Foster Care,* London: BAAF.

Searle-Chatterjee, M. (1999) 'Occupation, biography and new social movements', *Sociological Review,* 47: 258–79.

Selleck, D. (2001) 'Being under 3 years of age: Enhancing quality experiences', in G. Pugh (ed.) *Contemporary Issues in the Early Years* (3rd edn), London: Paul Chapman/Coram Family.

Sevenhuijsen, S. (1998) *Citizenship & the Ethics of Care: Feminist considerations on justice, morality and politics,* London: Routledge.

Sevenhuijsen, S. (2000) 'Caring in the Third Way: The relation between obligation, responsibility and care in Third Way discourse', *Critical Social Policy,* 20(1): 5–37.

Sevenhuijsen, S. (2002) 'A Third Way? Moralities, ethics and families. An approach through the ethics of care', in A. Carling, S. Duncan and R. Edwards (eds) *Analysing Families: Morality and rationality in policy and practice,* London: Routledge.

Sevenhuijsen, S. (2003) 'The place of care: The relevance of the feminist ethic of care for social policy', *Feminist Theory,* 4(2): 179–97.

Shah, B. (2007) 'Being young, female and Laotian: Ethnicity as social capital at the intersection of gender, generation, race and age', *Ethnic and Racial Studies,* 30(1): 28–50.

Shakespeare, T. (2006) *Disability Rights and Wrongs,* Oxford: Routledge.

Sharp J.P., Routledge P., Philo C. and Paddison R. (2000) *Entanglements of Power: Geographies of domination/resistance,* London: Routledge.

Shields, R. (2003) *The Virtual,* New York: Routledge.

Shokeid, M. (1988) 'Anthropologists and their informants: Marginality reconsidered', *European Journal of Sociology,* 29(1): 31–47.

Silins, H. and Murray-Harvey, R. (2000) 'Students as a central concern: Schools, students and outcome measures', *Journal of Educational Administration,* 38(3): 230–46.

Silk, J. (2004) 'Caring at a distance: Gift theory, aid chains and social movements', *Social and Cultural Geography,* 5(2): 229–51.

Silverman, P.R. and Nickman, S.L. (1996) 'Concluding thoughts', in D. Klass, P.R. Silverman and S.L. Nickman (eds) *Continuing Bonds: New understandings of grief,* Washington, DC: Taylor & Francis.

Simon, A. and Ward, S. (2010) *Does Every Child Matter? Understanding New Labour's social reforms,* Abingdon, Oxon: Routledge.

Sinclair, I., Gibbs, I. and Wilson, K. (2000) *Supporting Foster Placements, Report One,* University of York, Social Work Research and Development Unit.

Siraj-Blatchford, I., Sylva, K., Muttock, S., Gilden, R. and Bell, D. (2002) *Researching Effective Pedagogy in the Early Years,* Research Report RR356, London: Department for Education and Skills.

Skinner, E., Kindermann, T. and Furrer, C. (2009) 'Motivational perspective on engagement and disaffection: Conceptualization and assessment of children's behavioral and emotional participation in academic activities in the classroom', *Educational and Psychological Measurement,* 69(3): 493–525.

Smart, C. (2007) *Personal Life,* Cambridge: Polity.

Smart, C. and Neale, B. (1999) *Family Fragments,* Cambridge: Polity.

Smith, A.B. (1993) 'Early Childhood Educare: Seeking a theoretical framework in Vygotsky's work', *International Journal of Early Years Education,* 1(1): 47–61.

Smith, D.M. (2000) *Moral Geographies: Ethics in a world of difference,* Edinburgh: Edinburgh University Press.

Smith, M. (ed.) (2004) 'Nel Noddings: The ethics of care and education', *Encyclopaedia of Informal Education,* Online. Available HTTP: <http://www.infed.org/thinkers/noddings.htm> (accessed 17 January 2011).

Smyth, J. (2006) 'When students have power: Student engagement, student voice, and the possibilities for school reform around dropping out of school', *International Journal of Leadership in Education,* 9(4): 285–98.

Sointu, E. (2011) 'Detraditionalization, gender and alternative and complementary medicine', *Sociology of Health and Illness,* 33(3): 356–71.

Sointu, E. and Woodhead, L. (2008) 'Spirituality, gender, and expressive selfhood', *Journal for the Scientific Study of Religion,* 47(2): 259–76.

Spencer-Oatey, H. (2000) 'Rapport management: A framework for analysis', in H. Spencer-Oatey (ed.) *Culturally Speaking. Managing rapport through talk across cultures,* London: Continuum.

Stake, R.E. (1995) *The Art of Case Study Research,* Thousand Oaks, CA: Sage.

Stewart, B. (2011a) 'Blogging the unspeakable within motherhood: Digital sociality and discourse', Under review.

Stewart, B. (2011b) [Personal Communication].

Stoppard, T. (1973) *Rosencrantz and Guildenstern are Dead*, New York: Grove City.

Sudbury, J. (1998) *Other Kinds of Dreams: Black women's organisations and the politics of transformation*, London: Routledge

Sveningsson, M. (2003) 'Ethics in internet ethnography', *International Journal of Global Information Management,* 11(3): 45–60.

Swann, J. and Leap, W.L. (2000) 'Language in interaction', in R. Mesthrie, J. Swann, A. Deumert and W.L. Leap (eds) *Introducing Sociolinguistics,* Edinburgh: Edinburgh University Press.

Takano, S. (2005) 'Re-examining linguistic power: Strategic uses of directives by professional Japanese women in positions of authority and leadership', *Journal of Pragmatics,* 37: 633–66.

Tannen, D. (2005) 'Interactional sociolinguistics as a resource for intercultural pragmatics', *Journal of Pragmatics,* 2(2): 205–8.

Taylor, J.S., Layne, L.L. and Wozniak, D.F. (2004) *Consuming Motherhood,* New Brunswick, NJ: Rutgers University Press.

Technorati (2010) *WHO: Bloggers, Brands and Consumers,* State of the Blogosphere 2010. Online. Available HTTP: <http://technorati.com/blogging/article/who-bloggers-brands-and-consumers-day/#ixzz1d3tQiYM0> (accessed 1 November 2011).

Theodosius, C. (2008) *Emotional Labour in Health Care: The unmanaged heart of nursing,* London: Routledge.

Thomas, C. (2007) *Sociologies of Disability and Illness: Contested ideas in disability studies and medical sociology,* Basingstoke: Palgrave Macmillan.

Thomson, R. and Holland, J. (2002) 'Young people, social change and the negotiation of moral authority', *Children & Society,* 16: 103–15.

Thomson, R., Kehily, M.J., Hadfield, L. and Sharpe, S. (2011) *Making Modern Mothers,* Bristol: Policy Press.

Tickle, L. (2008) 'A brother is not just for Christmas', *The Guardian.* Online. Available HTTP: <http://www.guardian.co.uk/education/2008/oct/14/children> (accessed 7 December 2011).

Tiongson, N. (1994) 'Education through the arts: The gift of tongues', in M.B. Dy Jr. (ed.) *Values in Philippine Culture and Education: Philippine philosophical studies 1,* Washington, DC: Council of Research in Values and Philosophy.

Tissot, C. (2011) 'Working together? Parent and local authority views on the process of obtaining appropriate educational provision for children with autism spectrum disorders', *Educational Research,* 53(1): 1–15.

Tong, R. and Williams, N. (eds) (2009) 'Feminist Ethics', *Stanford Encyclopedia of Philosophy.* Online. Available HTTP: <http://plato.stanford.edu/entries/feminism-ethics/> (accessed 17 January 2011).

Trevarthen, C. (2003) 'Infant psychology is an evolving culture', *Human Development,* 46: 233–46.

Trevarthen, C. (2004) *Learning about Ourselves, from Children: Why a growing human brain needs interesting companions,* University of Edinburgh: Perception-in-action. Online. Available HTTP: <http://www.perception-in-action.ed.ac.uk/PDFs/Colwyn2004.pdf> (accessed 16 January 2008).

Triseliotis, J. (1980) *New Developments in Fostering and Adoption,* London: Routledge and Kegan Paul.

Tronto, J. (1987) 'Beyond gender difference to a theory of care', in M.J. Larrabee (ed.) (1993) *An Ethic of Care: Feminist and interdisciplinary perspectives,* London: Routledge.

Tronto, J. (1989) 'Women and caring: What can feminists learn about morality from caring?' in A.M. Jaggar and S. Bordo (eds) *Gender/Body/Knowledge: Feminist reconstructions of being and knowing,* New Brunswick, NJ: Rutgers University Press.

Tronto, J. (1993) *Moral Boundaries: A political argument for an ethic of care,* London: Routledge.

Tronto, J. (1995a) 'Women and caring: What can feminists learn about morality from caring?' in V. Held (ed.) *Justice and Care: Essential readings in feminist ethics,* Boulder, CO: Westview Press.

Tronto, J. (1995b) 'Care as a basis for radical political judgments' (Symposium on Care and Justice), *Hypatia,* 10(2): 141–9.

Tronto, J. (2004) 'Vicious circles of privatised care', Presented at Rethinking Care Relations, Family Lives & Policies: An International Symposium, Leeds: CAVA, University of Leeds.

Tronto, J. and Fisher, B. (1990) 'Towards a feminist theory of caring', in K. Abel and M. Nelson (eds) *Circles of Care,* New York: SUNY Press.

Tucker, J.S. (2009) 'Foreword: Small world: Maternal blogging, virtual friendship, and the computer-mediated self', in M. Friedman and S.L. Calixte (eds) *Mothering and Blogging: The radical act of the MommyBlog,* Bradford, ON: Demeter Press.

United Nations (UN) (1989) *Convention on the Rights of the Child.* Online. Available HTTP: <http://www.ohchr.org/english/law/pdf/crc.pdf> (accessed 25 November 2010).

Utting, W. (1997) *People Like Us: The report of the review of the safeguards for children living away from home,* Department of Health: The Welsh Office.

Ve, H. (1989) 'The male gender roles and responsibility for children', in K. Boh, M. Bak, C. Clason, M. Pankratova, J. Qvortrup, B. Giovanni and K. Waerness (eds) *Changing Patterns of European Family Life: A comparative analysis of 14 European countries,* London: Routledge.

Vertovec, S. (2009) *Transnationalism,* Oxford: Routledge.

Victoria, M. (2009a) 'Power and politeness: A study of social interaction in business meetings with multicultural participation', *ESP across Cultures,* 40: 129–40.

Victoria, M. (2009b) 'Power and politeness: Social interaction in Philippine Higher Education classrooms', *Philippine Journal of Linguistics,* 40: 17–32.

Vincent, S. (2003) 'Preserving domesticity: Reading Tupperware in women's changing domestic, social and economic roles', *Canadian Review of Sociology and Anthropology,* 40(2): 171–96.

Vine, B. (2004) *Getting Things Done at Work: The discourse of power in workplace interaction,* Philadelphia, PA: John Benjamins Publishing.

Wacjman, J. (2010) 'Feminist theories of technology', *Cambridge Journal of Economics,* 34(1): 143–52.

Waerness, K. (1989) 'Caring', in K. Boh, M. Bak, C. Clason, M. Pankratova, J. Qvortrup, B. Giovanni and K. Waerness (ed.) *Changing Patterns of European Family Life: A comparative analysis of 14 European countries,* London: Routledge.

Walker, J., Manoogian, A., O'Dell, M., McGraw, L. and White, D. (2001) *Families in Later Life: Connections and transitions,* London: Pine Forge Press.

Walker, P. (2009) 'Incident Diary Reveals Ordeal of Mother who Killed Herself and Daughter', *The Guardian.* Online. Available HTTP: <http://www.guardian.co.uk/uk/2009/sep/24/fiona-pilkington-incident-diary> (accessed 7 December 2011).

Walkover, B.C. (1992) 'The family as an overwrought object of desire', in G.C. Rosenwald and R.L. Ochberg (eds) *Storied Lives: The cultural politics of self-understanding,* New Haven, CT: Yale University Press.

Wallman, S. (1984) *Eight London Households,* London: Tavistock.

Want, B. (2010) *Why Not Me? A story of love and loss*, London: Orion Publishers.

Waterhouse, N. (2000) *Lost in Care: Report of the tribunal of Inquiry into the Abuse of Children in Care in the formed county council areas of Gwynedd and Clwyd since 1974*, London: TSO.

Webb, L. (1974) *Purpose and Practice in Nursery Education*, Oxford: Basil Blackwell.

Weller, S. (2006). '"Sticking with your mates?" Children's friendship trajectories during the transition from primary to secondary school', *Children & Society online*, [cited 25 May 2007], available from http://www.blackwell-synergy.com/doi/abs/10.1111/j.1099-0860.2006.00056.x

Weller, S. (2007) 'Managing the move to secondary school: The significance of children's social capital', in H. Helve and J. Bynner (eds) *Youth and Social Capital,* London: Tufnell Press.

Weller, S. (2010) 'Time(s) to be creative! Sustaining young people's engagement in qualitative longitudinal research', in F. Shirani and S. Weller (eds) *Conducting Qualitative Longitudinal Research: Fieldwork experiences*, Timescapes Working Paper Series No. 2, Leeds: University of Leeds.

Weller, S. (in press) 'Evolving creativity in qualitative longitudinal research with children and teenagers', *International Journal of Social Research Methodology.*

Weller, S. (under review) 'Mapping emotions in different spaces of research and dissemination', *Emotion, Space and Society* (Special Issue edited by C. Caballero and S. Weller).

Wentzel, K., Battle, A., Russell, S. and Looney, L. (2010) 'Social supports from teachers and peers as predictors of academic and social motivation', *Contemporary Educational Psychology,* 35: 193–202.

Wheelock, J. (2002) '"Grandparents are the next best thing": Informal childcare for working parents in urban Britain', *Journal of Social Policy,* 31(3): 441–63.

Whitaker, A. (1984) *All in the End is Harvest: An anthology for those who grieve,* London: Darton, Longman and Todd.

White, P. (2006) 'Migrant populations approaching old age: Prospects in Europe', *Journal of Ethnic and Migration Studies*, 32(8): 1283–1300.

Whitehead, S. (2002) *Men and Masculinities*, Cambridge: Polity.

Wilding, R. (2006) '"Virtual" intimacies? Families communicating across transnational contexts', *Global Networks*, 6(2): 125–42.

Wilkins, M. (2009) 'Beyond cute: A mom, a blog, and a question of content', in M. Friedman and S.L. Calixte (eds) *Mothering and Blogging: The radical act of the MommyBlog*, Bradford, ON: Demeter Press.

Williams, F. (2004) *Rethinking Families,* London: Calouste Gulbenkian Foundation.

Williams, F. (2005) *Rethinking Families* (reprinted), London: Calouste Gulbenkian Foundation.

Williams, R. (2009) 'Fathering and ethnicity', *Community, Work and Family,* 12(1): 57–73.

Williams, R. and Hewison, A. (2009) *"We are Doing our Best": African and African Caribbean fathers' views and experiences of fatherhood, health and preventative primary care services*, Birmingham: Birmingham Primary Care Trust.

Wolf, D. (2004) 'Valuing informal elder care', in N. Folbre and M. Bittman (eds) *Family Time: The social organization of care*, London: Routledge.

Wolterstorff, N.P. (1987) *Lament For a Son*, Grand Rapids, MI: Wm B Eerdmans.

Woodthorpe, K. (2011) 'Using bereavement theory to understand memorialising behaviour', *Bereavement Care,* 30: 29–32.

Woodward, K. (2009) *Embodied Sporting Practices: Regulating and regulatory bodies,* Basingstoke: Palgrave Macmillan.

Woodward, V. (2008) 'Professional caring: A contradiction in terms?' *Journal of Advanced Nursing*, 26(5): 999–1004.

Wright, E.O., Gornick, J.C. and Meyers, M.K. (eds) (2009) *Gender Inequality: Transforming family divisions of labour,* London: Verso.

Yeates, N. (2009) *Globalising Care Economies and Migrant Workers: Explorations in global care chains,* Basingstoke: Palgrave.

Zelizer, V.A. (1985) *Pricing the Priceless Child: The changing social value of children,* New York: Basic Books.

Zontini, E. (2004) 'Immigrant women in Barcelona: Coping with the consequences of transnational lives', *Journal of Ethnic and Migration Studies,* 30(6): 1113–44.

Zontini, E. (2006) 'Italian families and social capital: Care provision in a transnational world', *Community, Work and Family,* 9(3): 325–45.

Zontini, E. (2010) *Transnational Families, Migration and Gender. Moroccan and Filipino women in Bologna and Barcelona,* Oxford: Berghahn.

Zontini, E. (under review) 'Growing old in a transnational social field: Mobility, identity and belonging'.

Index

References in **bold** indicate tables and those followed by a letter n indicate end of chapter notes.

abuse and neglect 43, 129
academic qualifications 34–5, 36
advertising and mommy blogging 93, 95, 102–3
affinities 185–6, 189, 190
African-Caribbean communities 82–91
African-Caribbean women 179
Afshar, Haleh 179, 180, 182
age and sibling relationships 161, 165, 167, 168
aggressive behaviour of children 43, 133, 136, 139, 140
ageing and care 171–82
Ahmad Nia, Shirin 107
alternative health care 72–81
anthropological neutrality 113–14, 115
Armstrong, Heather 92–3, 104n
attachment in foster caring 125–7
attachment theory 193
Attention Deficit Hyperactivity Disorder 45, 168
autistic spectrum disorders 45, 133
autobiographical experiences, use of in research 186–7
autonomy: and alternative health care 74, 79, 80; of elders 173, 178, 180, 182; of foster carers 128; relational 173, 179, 182, 185

Bahramitash, Roksana 106, 107
Baldassar, Loretta 174
Bamberger, Joanne 98, 99
Bangladeshis 177, 178
Barber, Tracy 38, 39
Beck, Ulrich 74, 80, 130, 178
Beck-Gernsheim, Elisabeth 74, 80, 130, 178

behavioural problems: aggression 43, 133, 136, 139, 140; disengagement blamed on 37; in foster children 124–5; and intellectual disabilities 139–41; psychological causes of 43, 45
behaviour management in infant schools 25
Behaviour Support Units (BSUs) 44–5, 46–52, 53n
Belenky, Mary 21
bereavement 184, 185–94; physical pain of 184, 190–2
bereavement care 183
bifocality 173
Big Society 142
Birth to Three Matters framework 19
Black and Minority Ethnic (BME) communities 82–91; mistrust of care services 87–8
blogging, mommy 92–104
Bloome, David 54, 55
body, care of after death 187–9
Bowlby, Sophia 4, 133, 162, 166; care over life course 157; caring by children 161, 167, 168
Brown, Penelope 54, 56–7, **58**, 60–1, 62, 65
bullying 161, 166–8
burden, care as 165, 175–6, 178

Caldwell, Bettye 26
Calixte, Shana 96, 98, 104n
Canada, mommy blogging 93, 97, 98, 100
capitalist consumption 92–104
care, definitions of 5
care/education conflict 20, 27, 37–8, 40, 56
care ethics see ethics of care

care profession: and gender 20; status of
     28, 172
care services, mistrust of 87–8, 180–1
'caring for' and 'caring about' 5, 108, 133,
     142, 172, 173
caring relationships 5, 30–2, 72–3, 79–80,
     179; exploitation in 31–2; father-child
     149–50; *see also* teacher-student
     relationships
cemeteries 183, 188
childcare: and early education 18–29;
     government policies in England 19–20;
     in Iran 109–10
childcare/work balance 100
children: disabled 132–43; foster 122–31;
     preservation of 23–4, 99, 146; 'putting
     first' 128–9, 148, 149; at risk 43, 44;
     see also students
Children Act (2004) 32–3, 43
children's services, reorganisation of 43
Child Support Agency 150
Chinese culture and bereavement 188
circle time 45, 47, 53n
citizenship 6, 70, 113
Citizenship Education 32
class and mommy blogging 98, 101, 104n
Climbié, Victoria 19, 29n, 43, 52n
Code of Conduct and Practice for
     Registered Teachers (2009) 46
commercialization of intimate life 93, 103
communities 69–115; African-Caribbean
     82–91; alternative health 72–81; and
     care of elders 179–80, 181–2; Iranian
     105–15; online 92–104
community centres 174, 177, 179–80, 182
community organisations, black-led 82–91
community responsibility, maternal 100–1
conflict avoidance 56
connected knowing 22, 26, 27, 28
Conners, Catherine 98, 102, 104n
Conradson, David 162, 163, 168
consumption, capitalist 92–104
contact centres, child 150, 151, 153n
conversation analysis 58–9, 65, 66n
court proceedings 150, 151
Criminal Record Bureau checks 44, 52
Culpitt, Ian 138
curriculum: alternative 35, 36; national 19,
     32, 45
Curriculum Guidance for the Foundation
     Stage (CGFS) 19

death, caring after 183–94
dependency and disability 133, 137

depression in women in Iran 107
deprivation 34, 43, 45, 83, 91n
developmental psychology 26, 28, 52
Dewey, John 22
disability 132–43
discourse analysis 54–65
discrimination: challenging 7; fears of
     racial 87, 90
disengagement in young people 30–41,
     43–4
division of labour, gendered 6, 84–6, 107,
     145, 147
divorce 144–53
Do Men Mother? (Doucet) 85, 99, 147
Donne, John 192
Doucet, Andrea 85, 89, 144, 147
Douglas, Ann 102–3
Down's syndrome 133

Early Childhood Education and Care
     (ECEC) 18–29
early years care, extended 137, 138
Early Years Foundation Stage curriculum
     (EYFS) 19, 20, 27
ECEC *see* Early Childhood Education and
     Care
ECM *see* Every Child Matters framework
educare 26–7
education 15–66; conflict with care 20, 27,
     37–8, 40, 56; early childhood 18–29;
     government policies and initiatives
     15–16, 19–20, 32–3, 42–4; secondary
     schools 32–40, 44–53; universities
     54–65; of women in Iran 106
Education Act (1944) 32
Education Reform Act (1988) 32
Edwards, Rosalind 10, 11, 129, 160, 161,
     162–9
elders, Italian migrant 171–82
Elfer, Peter 20, 24, 27
Ellis, Carolyn 186, 190
embodied relationality 183, 184, 186–94
emotional attachment in foster caring
     125–7
emotional care work 132–41
emotional intelligence 43–4
emotional literacy 44, 45
emotional responsibility, maternal 100
employment: parental 18, 20; of women in
     Iran 106–7, 108
empowerment and mommy blogging 101
England *see* United Kingdom
engrossment 30–1
environmental concerns 77, 79

equality 6, 7
Esfahani, Hadi Salehi 106, 107
ethical caring 5, 132, 134, 143n
ethics of care: in foster caring 128,
    129–30; and holism 72, 73–4, 79–81;
    relational 30–2, 33, 34, 37; of self 128,
    129; *see also* feminist ethics of care
ethnography, virtual 95–6
Evans, Ruth 161
Every Child Matters framework (ECM)
    19, 43–4, 45
exclusion from school 42–53
exploitative relationships 31–2
extreme care 133–4
EYFS *see* Early Years Foundation Stage
    curriculum

face 56–7, **58**, 59–61, 64, 65
families 119–53; and care of elders 172,
    173, 176, 178–9; and childcare support
    109–10; and consumption 93; disability
    and mothering 132–43; foster care
    122–31; post-divorce fathering 144–53;
    sibling relationships 160–70
Family Court 151, 153n
fathering: and black men 83–4, 88–9;
    father-child relationships 149–50;
    father-mother inequality 144–5, 147,
    149, 151, 153; optional nature of 145,
    149, 151; post-divorce 144–53
Featherstone, Brid 144, 145, 152
feminist ethics of care 4–7, 79–80, 86, 100,
    133, 184; aims of 146; and elders 172,
    173, 175, 182; and geographies of care
    162, 169; and post-divorce fathering
    145, 146–52; and relational self 193
Fernandez, Lee 26
Finland 25
Fisher, Berenice 3, 5–6, 112
formal care in education 15–16, 21, 28; *see*
    also professional care
form tutors 33, 40–1n
foster care 122–31
fostering growth 24–5
Foucault, Michel 73–4, 138
Francis, Doris 188
free school meals 34
Friedman, May 96, 104n
Furedi, Frank 33

Gardner, Katy 177, 178, 181
gender: bias within care profession 20; in
    father-child relationships 149–50; and
    race 82, 83–4

gendered differences: in community
    involvement 89–90, 180; division of
    labour 6, 84–6, 107, 145, 147; of elders
    174–9, 180; in parenting 144–5, 147,
    149, 151, 153; in sibling relationships
    161, 167
gender roles in Iran 107, 112–13
general care work 133, 134, 143n
General Teaching Council for England
    (GTCE) 46
geographies of care 161–2
Gerber, Magda 26, 27
Gibson, Linda 78
Gilligan, Carol 4, 6, 69, 79, 81, 182
globalisation 171–2, 176, 182
Goleman, Daniel 43–4
Gonyea, Judith 133
Goodfellow, Joy 24, 25, 26, 27, 28
Goss, Robert 193
government educational policies and
    initiatives 15–16, 19–20, 32–3, 42–4
green movements 79
grieving 188, 189, 192–4; *see also*
    bereavement
Guarnizo, Luis Eduardo 173
gun violence 88–9

Hancock, Sheila 189
hate *see* love/hate dualism
Hattar-Pollara, Marianne 107
health, holistic 77
health and safety 23, 180; *see also* safety
health care, alternative 72–81
health workers 181
Heidegger, Martin 31
Held, Virginia 69, 72, 79–80, 81
herbal medicine *see* western herbal
    medicine
Heshusius, Lous 25
hierarchical flows of care 161, 165, 166,
    167, 168, 169
Hill, Joanne 134
Hill Collins, Patricia 83, 86, 171, 173, 182
Hoagland, Sarah 31
Hochschild, Arlie Russell 103, 138, 171
holism 72, 73–4, 76, 77–81
home, working from 78
Hooyman, Nancy 133
Hunniford, Gloria 191–2
hygiene 23

identities: black masculine 83–91; of elder
    men 177; ethnic 179; gendered 83–4,
    90; moral 101, 148, 149, 151–2;

racialised 83–4, 86, 90; of siblings
163–9; of women as caregivers 86, 175,
176, 178, 182; *see also* self, sense of
inclusion policies, school 44, 50
independence: of elders 173, 182;
encouraging children's 25; expectation
of children's 132–3; *see also*
interdependency
individualisation 74, 178
individualism 73–4
inequality *see* gendered differences;
socio-economic disadvantage
informal care in education 16, 21–3, 26,
28, 38
inspection regimes, school 45
intellectual disability 132–43
interactional sociolinguistics 58–9, 65
interdependency 3, 162; and alternative
health care 73, 74; and disability 133,
137, 138, 142; of elders 182; of siblings
167, 168, 169
Iran 105–15
Italian migrant elders 171–82

Japanese culture: and bereavement 185,
188, 192, 193; women and power 55
Johnson, Jillian 98
justice and care 6–7, 141
Kağitçibaşi, Çiğdem 185

Kendall, Sally 36
Kinder, Kay 36
Klass, Dennis 185, 187, 188, 192, 193
knife crime 45, 88
knowing, women's ways of 21–2, 26, 27,
28
Kosonen, Marjut 161, 169

labour, gendered division of 6, 84–6, 107,
145, 147
language, power and care 54–65
Lawson, Victoria 162, 168
learning difficulties *see* intellectual
disability
learning styles of students 35, 36
Leffers, M. Regina 28
Lenz Taguchi, Hillevi 22
Levinson, Stephen 54, 56–7, **58**, 60–1, 62,
65
Lewis, C.S. 192
life course, caring across 157–94; caring
after death 183–94; migrant elders
171–82; sibling relationships 160–70
lifelong care 138–9

life politics 74, 77, 80
linguistic devices in caring relations 56–7,
59–65
linguistic politeness *see* politeness, theory
of
Lister, Ruth 70, 113
Lofland, Lyn 184
love, unconditional 130, 134, 135, 136
love/hate dualism 135, 136, 139, 142, 143n
love labouring 70, 120, 133, 135, 138
Lynch, Kathleen: carelessness in education
42, 44, 45; feminist ethics of care 4,
147; spheres of care 70, 120, 133–4,
143n, 152

McIntosh, Ian 168
McMillan, Margaret 18
Malaguzzi, Loris 27–8
'male pride' 87
marketing and mommy blogging 93, 95,
102–3
Mason, Jennifer 4, 185–6, 189, 190
maternal ambivalence 135; *see also* love/
hate dualism
maternal care 99–101; *see also* mothering
maternal thinking 22–6, 99–101, 103,
108–9, 112, 146
maternity leave 100
meals on wheels 180
Memel, Elizabeth 26
memorialisation 183, 184
men: black men and care work 82–91;
elder 176–8, 179, 180; as foster carers
123; *see also* fathering
mental health: of mothers of disabled
children 134; of students 43; of women
in Iran 107
mentoring young people 45, 88–9
methodologies *see* research methodologies
Meyer, Morgan 184
migrant elders 171–82
migration of care workers 171–2
mistrust of care services 87–8, 180–1
Mohseni Tabrizi, A. R. 107
mommy blogging 92–104
Money, Ruth 26
Moore, Henrietta 135
moral accountability 124–5
moral education 31, 32
moral identities: of fathers 148, 149,
151–2; of mothers 101
moral philosophy *see* ethics of care
moral responsibilities, maternal 101
moral theory, value of care for 5, 6, 7

Morand, David 63
Morgan, David 186
Morrison, Aimee 96–7, 98, 99, 101
mortality and bereavement 190
Morton, Frances 27
mothering: and consumption 93, 98;
    definition of 22; of disabled children
    132–43; maternal thinking 22–6,
    99–101, 103, 108–9, 112, 146;
    mother-child relationships 4, 5, 146;
    mother-father inequality 144–5, 147,
    149, 151, 153
motivational displacement 30, 31
mourning *see* bereavement
murder of disabled children 133–4

National Childcare Strategy 19
national curriculum 19, 32, 45
natural caring 5, 26, 132, 134, 143n
negligent care 129
neighbours and childcare support 109–10
neoliberalism 103
networks *see* communities
Nickman, Steven 193–4
Niikko, Anneli 23, 25
Noddings, Nel: care in education 25, 27, 31,
    35–6, 37–8, 39, 40; caring relationships
    30–2, 179; criticism of 31–2; feminist
    ethics of care 4–5; natural v ethical
    caring 5, 132, 134, 143n
nursery schools 18–19
Nutbrown, Cathy 27

obligation to care 134, 136, 139, 142; *see
    also* fathering: optional nature of; love/
    hate dualism
observation, child 20–8
Office for Standards in Education (Ofsted)
    19, 29n, 41n
Osgood, Jayne 20

pain of bereavement, physical 184, 190–2
palliative care 183
Papatheodorou, Theodora 20, 28
parenting: blamed for behavioural
    problems 43, 44, 45, 47–8; gendered
    differences 144–5, 147, 149, 151, 153;
    parent-child relationships and power
    161, 176, 179; values of 88; *see also*
    fathering; foster care; mothering
parenting classes 150, 151
parent-professional relationships 137–9,
    141
Parker, Rozsika 135

pedagogical theory 26, 28
Personal, Social and Health Education
    (PSHE) 32
Philippines 54–66
physical contact, policies against 51
physical pain of bereavement 184, 190–2
Pilkington, Fiona 134
Piper, Heather 44, 51
play, in education and care 20, 24, 25
playgroups 18–19
Plowden Report (1967) 19, 28n
policies and initiatives in education 15–16,
    19–20, 32–3, 42–4
politeness, theory of 56–7, **58**, 60–1, 62,
    65n
political theory, value of care for 6, 146
poverty, child 18, 19, 20; *see also*
    socio-economic disadvantage
power and care 54–65; for elders 176, 179,
    180, 182; in parent-child relationships
    161, 176, 179; in sibling relationships
    161, 164, 165–6, 169
'power with' and 'power over' 54, 56, 59,
    60, 65
practical care work 132, 133, 134, 136–9
practical thinking 22–3
prejudice *see* discrimination
presence 24, 25, 27, 100
preservation of the child 23–4, 99, 146
professional care: and disabled children
    137–9, 141; focus on in education 15,
    32–3, 40, 45–8, 49, 52–3; and foster
    care 122, 124, 125
protecting children *see* preservation of the
    child
psychology, developmental 26, 28, 52
psychotherapy 73, 74
Pugh, Gillian 20
Punch, Samantha 168
pupils *see* students

qualifications: for early years practitioners
    20, 29n; vocational and academic 34–5,
    36

race and gender 82, 83–4
racial discrimination, fears of 87, 90
regulation of care in education 33, 37, 40,
    45–8; *see also* professional care;
    statutory frameworks for care in
    education
relational autonomy 173, 179, 182, 185
relational care in education 15–16, 30–2,
    33, 34–40, 48–50

relational ethics of care 30–2, 33, 34, 37
relationality: concept of 185; embodied 183, 184, 186–94; and geographies of care 162
relational self: and alternative health care 69, 73–4; and bereavement 184, 190, 192, 193; and elders 182; and foster care 128
religious studies teaching 32
research ethics 3, 113–15
research methodologies: collective case studies 20–1, 29n; diary keeping 108; longitudinal studies 162–3, 169; questionnaires 108, 114; using autobiographical experiences 186–7; virtual ethnography 95–6
resentment of care-giving 175–6, 178
resistance: to giving care 178–9; to receiving care 181
responsibilities, maternal 99–101
Ribbens McCarthy, Jane 128, 129
rights, language of 7
Rinaldi, Carlina 25, 28
risk: children at 43, 44; of exclusion from school 42–53, 83; and teacher-student relationships 44, 46, 52–3
risk assessments 23
Ruddick, Sara 121; feminist ethics of care 4, 6, 146–7; maternal thinking 22–6, 99–101, 103, 108–9, 112, 146

sacrifice, care as 5, 80, 81, 178, 182
safety 23, 46, 52; *see also* health and safety
schools: infant 23, 25; nursery 18–19; secondary 32–40, 44–53; *see also* education
SEAL *see* Social and Emotional Aspects of Learning Programme
secondary schools 32–40, 44–53
self, relational *see* relational self
self, sense of 129, 164, 166; and alternative health care 73, 74, 79; of elders 175, 176, 178, 181, 182; *see also* identities
self-care: and alternative health care 72–4, 75–7, 79–80, 81; and elders 182; ethic of 128, 129; responsibility for 81, 168
self-discovery groups 72, 74, 81n
selflessness 5, 178; *see also* sacrifice, care as
Selleck, Dorothy 27, 28
separate knowing 21–2
Sevenhuijsen, Selma: caring as social activity 108, 112, 173; ethics of care 4, 6, 72, 106, 113; relational autonomy 173, 185

sexual citizenship 70, 113
Seyedan, Fariba 107
Sharp, Joanne 164, 166, 168–9
sibling relationships 160–70
Silverman, Phyllis 193–4
Singh-Mahal, Ajit 134
Smith, Anne 26–7
social activity, caring as 108, 112
Social and Emotional Aspects of Learning Programme (SEAL) 32–3, 44, 45, 47, 52
social development of children 25
social interaction theory 54; *see also* politeness, theory of
social justice 141
social media *see* mommy blogging
social model of disability 136
social services: lack of support from 124, 128; mistrust of 87–8, 180–1
socio-economic disadvantage 34, 43, 45, 83, 91n
sociolinguistics, interactional 58–9, 65
socio-political care work 132, 133
solidarity work 133, 134, 135, 141, 143n
special educational needs (SEN) 134, 143n
spiritual beliefs 188
standards agenda in education 45
state institutions, mistrust of 87–8, 180–1
status: of care profession 28, 172; of women in Iran 106–8
statutory frameworks for care in education 15–16, 19–20, 32–3, 42–4
'staying' by fathers 150–2
stereotyped images of black men 84, 89–90
Stewart, B. 97, 98, 99, 101
Stronach, Ian 44, 51
students: disengaged 30–41, 43–4; at risk of exclusion 42–53; *see also* teacher-student relationships
Sudbury, Julia 84
suicide 133–4, 141, 142
Sure Start programmes 19, 28–9n

teacher-student relationships: boundaries to 50–2; deficiency of care 34–8, 168; focus on professional care 44, 45–8, 52–3; power and care 55–6, 59–65; relational care 31, 33, 34–40, 48–50; and risk 44, 46, 52–3
teacher training 39, 40, 44
technology 95
thinking: maternal 22–6, 99–101, 103, 108–9, 112, 146; practical 22–3

Timescapes 162
transnationalism and caring 171–2, 178–9
Trevarthen, Colwyn 24, 25
Tronto, Joan 28, 38, 112, 160; feminist
    ethics of care 4, 5–6, 7, 100, 146, 173,
    184; research ethics 3, 113

unconditional love 130, 134, 135, 136
United Kingdom: education system 15–16,
    18–20, 32–3, 42–4; labour market
    demands 176; mommy blogging 93, 97,
    100
United Nations Convention on the Rights
    of the Child 19
United States of America: education
    system 31; mommy blogging 92–3,
    100
universities 54–65

Vertovec, Steven 173, 175
violence, gun 88–9
virtual ethnography 95–6
vocational courses 34–5, 36

Want, Barbara 191
Webb, Lesley 25
Western cultures and bereavement 185,
    188, 190
western herbal medicine (WHM) 72, 75,
    81n
'wise practice' 26, 28
Wolterstorff, Nicholas 189, 191
women: elder 174–6, 178–9, 180, 182;
    experiences of care 4, 6; identity as
    caregivers 86, 175, 176, 178, 182; roles
    of black women 83, 86; status of in Iran
    106–8; ways of knowing 21–2, 26, 27,
    28; *see also* mommy blogging;
    mothering
Women's Workshop on Qualitative Family
    and Household Research 9–12
Woodthorpe, Kate 184
working, alternative ways of 78–9

YMCA 150, 151, 153n

Zelizer, Viviana 127

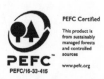

PEFC Certified

This product is
from sustainably
managed forests
and controlled
sources

www.pefc.org

PEFC/16-33-415

#0249 - 180416 - C0 - 234/156/13 - PB - 9781138781788